Cancer in Primary Care

Cancer in Primary Care

Edited by

Martin Gore PhD FRCP
Professor of Cancer Medicine
The Royal Marsden Hospital
London, UK

and

Douglas Russell MS BS BSc DRCOG MRCGP
Medical Director
Tower Hamlets PCT
London, UK

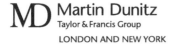
Martin Dunitz
Taylor & Francis Group
LONDON AND NEW YORK

First published in the United Kingdom in 2003
by Martin Dunitz, an imprint of Taylor and Francis Group plc, 11 New Fetter Lane, London EC4P 4EE

Tel.:   +44 (0) 20 7583 9855
Fax.:   +44 (0) 20 7842 2298
E-mail: info@dunitz.co.uk
Website: http://www.dunitz.co.uk

Although every effort has been made to ensure that drug doses and other information are presented accurately in this publication, the ultimate responsibility rests with the prescribing physician. Neither the publishers nor the authors can be held responsible for errors or for any consequences arising from the use of information contained herein. For detailed prescribing information or instructions on the use of any product or procedure discussed herein, please consult the prescribing information or instructional material issued by the manufacturer.

A CIP record for this book is available from the British Library.

ISBN 1 90186 526 6

Distributed in the USA by
Fulfilment Center
Taylor & Francis
10650 Tobben Drive
Independence, KY 41051, USA
Toll Free Tel.: +1 800 634 7064
E-mail: taylorandfrancis@thomsonlearning.com

Distributed in Canada by
Taylor & Francis
74 Rolark Drive
Scarborough, Ontario M1R 4G2, Canada
Toll Free Tel.: +1 877 226 2237
E-mail: tal_fran@istar.ca

Distributed in the rest of the world by
Thomson Publishing Services
Cheriton House
North Way
Andover, Hampshire SP10 5BE, UK
Tel.:   +44 (0)1264 332424
E-mail: salesorder.tandf@thomsonpublishingservices.co.uk

Composition by Scribe Design, Gillingham, UK
Printed and bound in Spain by Grafos SA

Contents

Contributors

Peter Blake MD MBBS BSc FRCR
Consultant Oncologist
Royal Marsden Hospital
London, UK

Irene Boeddinghaus MRCP
Clinical Research Fellow
The Royal Marsden Hospital NHS Trust
London, UK

Chris Boshoff MBChB MRCP PhD
Professor of Cancer Medicine
Wolfson Institute for Biomedical Research
University College London
London, UK

Michael Brada FRCP FRCR
The Royal Marsden Hospital
Sutton, Surrey, UK

Karen Broadley MB MS MRCP
Consultant, Palliative Medicine
The Royal Marsden Hospital
London, UK

Christopher Bunker MD FRCP
Consultant Dermatologist
Chelsea and Westminster Hospital and
Charing Cross Hospital
London, UK

David Cunningham MD FRCP
Consultant Medical Oncologist
The Royal Marsden Hospital NHS Trust
Sutton, UK

Gareth R Davies BSc MPH
Senior Health Analyst
National Public Health Service
Formerly Dyfed Powys Health Authority
Wales, UK

David Dearnaley MA MD FRCP FRCR
Reader in Prostate Cancer Studies & Honorary Consultant
Head of Urology Unit
The Royal Marsden NHS Trust
Sutton, Surrey, UK

Mitch Dowsett BSc PhD
Head of Department
Academic Department of Biochemistry
The Royal Marsden Hospital NHS Trust
London, UK

Ros Eeles MA PhD FRCP FRCR
Clinical Senior Lecturer & Honorary Consultant
Cancer Genetics & Clinical Oncology
Institute of Cancer Research & Royal Marsden NHS Trust
Sutton, Surrey, UK

Louise Fearfield MA MRCP
Consultant Dermatologist
Royal Berkshire Hospital
Reading, UK

Martin Gore PhD FRCP
Professor of Cancer Medicine
The Royal Marsden NHS Trust
London, UK

Kate Gregory MBBS MRCP MD
Consultant Medical Oncologist
Wessex Medical Oncologist
Royal South Hants Hospital
Southampton, UK

Clive Harmer FRCP FRCR
Consultant Clinical Oncologist
Department of Radiotherapy
The Royal Marsden Hospital NHS Trust
London, UK

Robert Huddart MBBS MRCP FRCR
Senior Lecturer and Honorary Consultant in
Radiotherapy and Oncology
The Institute of Cancer Research and The Royal Marsden
Hospital NHS Trust
Sutton, UK

Ian Jacobs MD MDCOG
Consultant Gynecological Oncologist
St Bartholemew's Hospital
London, UK

Stephen RD Jonhnston MA PhD FRCP
Senior Lecturer and Consultant Medical Oncologist
Department of Medicine (Breast Unit)
Royal Marsden Hospital
London, UK

Ian Judson MD FRCP
Professor of Cancer Pharmacology
Institute of Cancer Research
& Royal Marsden Hospital
Sutton, UK

Nick Maisey MRCP MD
Specialist Registrar in Medical Oncology
The Royal Marsden Hospital NHS Trust
London, UK

Jane Melia PhD MFPHM
Team Leader in Epidemiology
Institute of Cancer Research
Sutton, UK

Gillian Mitchell MBBS MRCP FRCR
Oncology Fellow
Peter MacCallum Cancer Centre
Melbourne, Australia

Sue Moss PhD MFPHM
Reader in Epidemiology and
Associate Director for the Cancer Screening Evaluation Unit
Institute of Cancer Research
Sutton, UK

Aurelia Norton MSc MRCP MRCPCH
Specialist Registrar
Department of Paediatrics
Royal Marsden Hospital
Sutton, Surrey, UK

Christopher Nutting BSc MBBS MRCP FRCR MD
Consultant and Senior Lecturer in Clinical Oncology
Royal Marsden Hospital
London, UK

Mary O'Brien MD MRCP
The Royal Marsden Hospital
Sutton, Surrey, UK

Nina Patel RGN RHV RSCN
Clinical Nurse Specialist, Paediatric Oncology
Royal Marsden Hospital
Sutton, Surrey, UK

Ray Powles MD BSc FRCP FRCPath
Royal Marsden Hospital
Sutton, Surrey, UK

Kathy Pritchard-Jones PhD FRCPCE FRCPCH
Consultant Paediatric Oncologist
Royal Marsden Hospital/Institute of Cancer Research
Sutton, Surrey, UK

Khalil Razvi
Subspecialty Fellow in Gynecological Oncology
Royal Marsden Hospital
London, UK

Gillian Ross PhD MRCP FRCR
Clinical Oncologist
Deputy Head, Breast Unit
The Royal Marsden Hospital NHS Trust
London, UK

Douglas Russell MS BS BSc DRCOG MRCGP
Medical Director
Tower Hamlets PCT
London, UK

Bhawna Sirohi MBBS DCH
Haemato-Oncologist
The Royal Marsden Hospital NHS Trust
Sutton, UK

Ian Smith MD FRCP FRCPE
Professor of Cancer Medicine
The Royal Marsden Hospital NHS Trust
London, UK

Val Speechley MA RGN RCNT Oncology Nursing Certificate
Deputy Director
The Cancer Resource Centre
London, UK

Kate Sumpter FRCP
Specialist Registrar in Medical Oncology
The Royal Marsden NHS Trust
London, UK

Merion Thomas MS FRCP FRCS
Consultant Surgical Oncologist
The Royal Marsden Hospital NHS Trust
London, UK

Glynis Tranter
Swansea NHS Trust
Wales, UK

Andrew Tutt PhD MRCP FRCR
Clinician Scientist Fellow
Breakthrough Breast Cancer Research Centre
Institute of Cancer Research
London, UK

Andy Webb BSc MBBS MRCP MD
Consultant Medical Oncologist
Sussex Cancer Centre
Royal Sussex County Hospital
Brighton, UK

Paula Wells PhD MRCP FRCR
Consultant in Oncology
Department of Radiotherapy
St Bartholomew's Hospital
London, UK

Foreword

Last week an old friend of mine died. She had been my patient for over a quarter of a century, and was almost exactly my own age. I had been her general practitioner through two of her pregnancies, dozens of consultations about her children when they were young, and her terminal cancer. She had presented to me with the initial symptoms. She had returned to me to discuss the sad news when the diagnosis was confirmed, she had sought my help for the side effects of the chemotherapy, and she had talked to me about how her death would affect her family. It genuinely was an honour to have been able to help her.

In that same week a shock headline in one of our less reputable daily papers had pointed out that cancer deaths were soaring. A quick reading of the story showed that the story could have equally well have been told as 'heart disease deaths are falling', but good news rarely sells newspapers. Nevertheless, this did bring home an important point. As primary and secondary prevention of one of our main killer disease becomes more effective, those patients who are protected from heart disease will live longer, and longer life inevitably predispose towards the ultimate development of cancer.

Of course, the very word 'cancer' is more a headline than a diagnosis. Different cancers are very different diseases, even though the public and the press cluster them all together in the same fearsome word. For many primary health care teams, the effective and caring management of cancer is one of the most satisfying aspects of their work. Because of the long term and very personal relationships we build with our patients, we are ideally placed to care for them either throughout the successful therapy for their cancer, or through the final stages of their lives.

Every member of the primary health care team will come to value this timely and important book. Whether you need to know about prevention or symptom control, genetics, psychology, teamwork, use of outside agencies or physiology, there is no doubt that our patients will benefit greatly from any practice team reading, sharing, and using this book.

This week, yet another old friend presented with cancer. This book will make a real difference.

Professor David Haslam
Chairman of Council
Royal College of General Practitioners

Preface

One in three people will develop some form of cancer and one in four people will die of cancer. At any one time, the average GP's practice of 5500 patients will have dozens of patients with some form of malignancy. The proposed new GP contract includes a quality target to maintain an accurate cancer disease registry and another to ensure all newly-diagnosed cancer patients have a comprehensive holistic review of their needs within at least six months of diagnosis. The physical and psychological management of patients with cancer is becoming more and more complicated and there are ever increasing expectations from patients and their relatives to 'get it right' from diagnosis to death. This adds to the burden on general practice, already struggling with access targets, NSF, NICE guidance and ever-increasing demands from many directions.

The two of us have each spent most of our respective careers in primary care and oncology and have felt for some time that there is no single reference point for general practitioners to access easily all the basic information necessary to care for patients with cancer and support their relatives adequately. We have therefore enlisted the services of a number of colleagues with specific and detailed experience of all the different aspects of cancer management including psychological support, cancer genetics, screening, palliative medicine, and the complications of cancer treatments. There is also a chapter that sets out a comprehensive list of places where patients can get more information and specific support. The bulk of the text is devoted to tumour-site specific chapters, which describe in concise terms all a GP might want to know about a particular cancer. Each section within these chapters is brief, so that information can be easily accessed. Many of our authors are internationally recognized experts in their field and they have kept to their brief of providing the kind of information that is required for the day-to-day management of a cancer patient. Most importantly of all, we hope that the text will help practitioners answer the questions patients and relatives inevitably ask a GP after a hospital appointment with their oncologist!

Oncology is not taught at medical school or to GP trainees in any detail. Very few GP trainee schemes have oncology modules or oncology experience as part of their rotation. This can leave a general practitioner feeling very exposed when faced with a patient who is suffering from a particular complication of therapy or who is anxious about treatment and prognosis. We hope that this text will be 'dipped into' by general practitioners, practice nurses and other healthcare professionals who are managing patients with cancer in the community, particularly when they are faced with specific problems or questions.

We have tried to make information easily accessible and practical. We would like to thank Johnathan Gregory who we originally approached with this idea and who was very helpful in the early days of the project. A special thanks goes to Andrew Prouse who is one of the Data Managers at the Royal Marsden Hospital – he has been enormously helpful in gathering information and putting the chapters together.

Martin Gore
Douglas Russell

SECTION 1

Organizing a cancer service

1 Cancer Services and Primary Care

Douglas Russell and Martin Gore

Cancer is a disease of major importance, because of its frequency, morbidity, mortality, and the emotional and psychological impact on patients and their families and carers. It also has very significant direct and indirect costs relating to its investigation, diagnosis, treatment, and follow-up.

The latest definitive figures for the UK show that there were 263,240 registrations of new cases of cancer in 1998 (129,450 in men and 133,790 in women). Provisional figures for 2001 for the UK show 154,460 people died from cancer [it is usual in cancer figures to exclude non-melanoma skin cancers (NMSC)]. In the USA in 1999 an estimated 1,221,800 people were diagnosed with cancer and 563,100 are expected to die from the disease.

Cancer is the second most important cause of death after cardiovascular disease in the developed world. In the UK, the evidence is that 40% of the population are affected by cancer at some time in their lives, and one in four of all deaths are from cancer. Cancer is mainly a disease of older people (*Figs 1.1–1.4*). Over 65% of new cases are diagnosed in those over 65 years old in the UK (50% in the USA), although certain cancers are particularly likely to affect particular age groups.

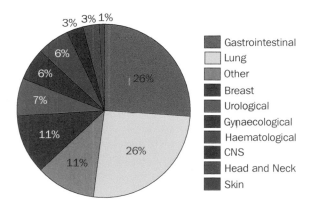

Figure 1.1. *Cancer deaths in those aged 0–14 years (Wales data).*

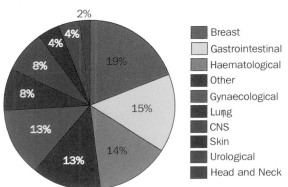

Figure 1.2. *Cancer deaths in those aged 15–44 years (Wales data).*

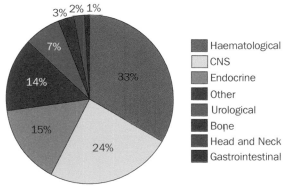

Figure 1.3. *Cancer deaths in those aged 45–69 years (Wales data).*

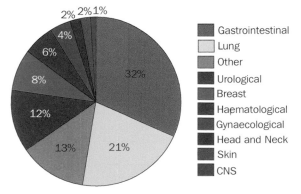

Figure 1.1. *Cancer deaths in those aged over 75 years (Wales data).*

The prevalence patterns of cancer types also changes over age cohorts (*Fig. 1.1*). In recent years an increasing cohort of childhood and adolescence cancer survivors has emerged because of improvements in treatment. In the UK, 60% of children with cancer are cured and it is estimated that 1 in1000 persons reaching young adulthood will be a cancer survivor.

Cancer is not a single disease, with over 200 different types of cancer. However, just four of them – lung, breast, large bowel (colorectal), and prostate account for half of all new cases in the UK.

Cancer Data

In considering progress in dealing with cancers it is usual to consider four measures: incidence, prevalence, mortality, and survival.

Incidence
Incidence is the number of new cases in the population each year, which is probably the best measure of trends in cancer risk. Cancer prevention aims to reduce the incidence. It is estimated that 50–60% of all cancers may be preventable (*see* Chapter 4). For a primary care organization of 100,000 patients, one might expect about 500 new cases of cancer per year (excluding NMSC).

Prevalence
Prevalence is the total number of patients currently alive within a population who have cancer. The populations that primary care teams care for vary in age–sex composition, so estimates of prevalence from standardized data need to be interpreted in the light of local circumstances. In England and Wales, of the patients diagnosed with cancer (excluding NMSC) in the 10 years between 1st January 1982 and 31st December 1992, in 1993 25% of men and 37% of women were alive (Office for National Statistics, 1999). These data suggest that in 1993 approximately 1.1% of the population at any one time lived with cancer. Since 1993, the proportion of elderly has increased, as have survival figures for many cancers, so the prevalence of patients living with cancer has almost certainly increased.

Mortality
Long-term reduction in mortality from cancer is a key indicator of progress against the disease. Cancer mortality rates in a given year depend on the number of cases diagnosed in the previous years, and on their survival. About a quarter of cancer patients die from other causes.

Survival
Survival is not only of crucial interest to the patient and family (it is likely to be one the first questions asked of the clinician after a diagnosis is made), but it is essential for monitoring the efficacy and equity of cancer treatment nationally.

Early Detection

A fundamental question for primary care is 'does early detection and intervention make a real difference to outcome?' It is essential that the public and clinicians in primary care understand the difference between screening and prevention (*see* Chapter 9). Screening is not the same as prevention. The aim of screening is to reduce the percentage of the at-risk screened population dying from the disease being screened for. Currently approved (UK) national screening interventions (for cancer) are:

- breast cancer for women aged 50–64 years invited every 3 years, and for those over 65 years on request of patient [or general practitioner (GP)];
- cervical cancer – all women aged 20–64 invited once every 5 years (every 3 years in Scotland); and
- bladder cancer screening for those considered to be at occupational risk.

Trials are currently under way to assess the appropriateness of population screening for colorectal cancer and ovarian cancer. It is explicitly advised *not* to offer population screening for prostate cancer using prostate-specific antigen (PSA) (National Screening Committee, 1998). A recent phenomenon has been the advent of commercially available PSA kits marketed direct to patients. Confounding factors in studies of screening that need to be considered include lead time bias, length time bias, and selection bias.

Lead time bias
Early detection results in diagnosing cancer at an asymptomatic stage of the disease, but the natural history remains unaltered by the early intervention. Patients apparently live longer, but screening has merely diagnosed them earlier.

Length time bias
Length time bias results in the diagnosis of less aggressive cancers. One group of patients may have rapidly progressive disease, while another has a more indolent type. Improved methods of screening may tend to diagnose a higher pro-

portion of slower growing (more indolent) cancers. Rapidly growing cancers with poorer prognosis may be missed by screening, and present as 'interval' cancers (i.e. during the interval between screening).

As life expectancy increases and methods of detection improve, increasing proportions of these slow-growing indolent cancers distort the apparent impact of cancer. This phenomenon has been described as 'pussycats and tigers'.

Selection bias

The difference in compliance rates with national screening programmes is known to vary. More disadvantaged communities are less likely to attend cancer screening. It is a major challenge for primary care teams to encourage compliance and reduce this cause of health inequality.

Populations at Risk

Early detection is particularly important for those at increased risk of cancer because of their genetic background, lifestyle, environment, occupation, or socioeconomic status. There is clear evidence that cancer patients with lower socioeconomic status have poorer survival outcomes (Coleman et al., 1999). Health care workers in primary care must address this issue if such health inequity and inequality is to be eliminated. The current reorganization of primary care in the UK to support greater multiagency working presents such an opportunity.

Nihilism versus enthusiasm

A balance needs to be struck between therapeutic nihilism and excessively zealous intervention that is not based on high-quality evidence. Such attitudes could apply to investigations, screening, treatment (particularly new treatments), counselling, or any other therapeutic area.

Good news

In the UK the incidence of lung cancer in men has been falling since the early 1980s, and is expected to continue to fall – reflecting changes in men's smoking habits. Conversely, in women lung cancer is expected to show a 5% rise between 1993 and 1996. In 1998, for the first time, USA data showed a favourable change of direction with a reduction in total incidence of cancer, and declining death rates from cancer. In addition 5-year survival rates continued to improve for most cancers (except lung).

In the USA the recently released health gain document *Healthier People 2010* (Surgeon General 2000) death rates from male lung, female breast, prostate, colon, and rectum cancers are reported as having decreased significantly during 1990–1996.

Other trends are:

- remarkable improvements in survival in many children's cancers (60% of children with cancer are cured and now go on to lead healthy adult lives; Cancer Research Campaign, 1998–1999);
- England and Wales prostate cancer mortality fell in 1996 and 1997, after a consistent rise throughout the 1980s and early 1990s (Office for National Statistics, 1999);
- the UK has also seen sharp falls in deaths from cervical cancer from 1991 to date; and
- there have been some startling increases in relative 5-year survival between patients diagnosed in 1971–1975 and those diagnosed in 1986–1990 (Coleman et al., 1999).

Prevention studies are under way for breast cancer with tamoxifen to see if the results of the first highly promising study in the USA can be reproduced.

Workload in Primary Care

A difficulty facing the primary care clinician in cancer care is the relative infrequency of cancer in a large patient workload. Maintaining a high index of suspicion requires familiarity with common warning signs and symptoms of the disease, and with the likely risk groups to be affected.

Early signs and symptoms of cancer are common presenting symptoms in general primary care practice. It has been estimated that as many as 5% of primary care medical consultations involve the ten common symptoms that could suggest cancer (Summerton, 1999); however, only a small number of these symptoms are due to cancer. The tables shown in cancer site-specific chapters (adapted from the NHS consultation document on ensuring early appropriate referral of suspected cancer patients) highlight key points and patient groups at risk.

The National Morbidity Survey of GP consultations in the UK (MSGP4) demonstrate an average consultation rate of 2.9 per 1000 patients registered, per annum (McCormick et al., 1995). Thus, a practice with a list of 10,000 would have 29,000 face-to-face consultations per annum. Of these, 1.2% were specifically about cancer (i.e. approximately one consultation per day).

Table 1.1. *Prevalence and incidence rates for cancers in a GP population (per 10,000)*

Cancer site	Prevalence	Incidence
Breast	30	10
Prostate	11	6
Large bowel (colorectal)	8	8
Trachea, bronchus, and lung	7	10
Non-melanoma skin	6	–
Bladder	4	3
Ovary	4	2
Cervix	3	1
Rectum	3	–
Uterus	2	1
Skin melanoma	2	–

Data adapted from NHS Cancer Care in England and Wales, December 2001.

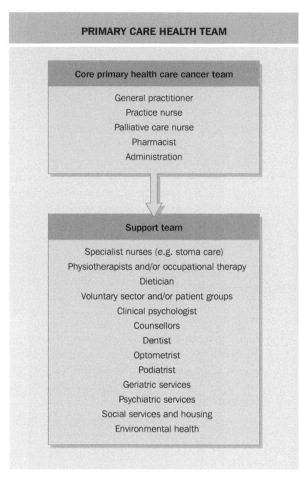

Figure 1.5. *Primary care health team.*

The data in MSGP4 only records rates for consultations specifically about cancer. This study took place in 1992, so it tallies with the estimate from population studies quoted earlier. Patients with cancer who attend for other reasons are not recorded as cancer consultations, and thus the true workload associated with such patients may be under-reported.

The same study (MSGP4) gave the results shown in Table 1.1 for prevalence rates of cancers in a GP population (defined as patients who consulted at least once in the study year for that condition, expressed as the rate per 10,000 patient years at risk (likely incidence and prevalence for cancers are shown in tables in each chapter). The appropriate incidence of new cases is also shown in Table 1.1.

The Role of Primary Care

Primary care has a tradition of being holistic, considering all patients in the context of physical, social, and psychological contexts. However, primary care is changing and although the GP or family physician remains a major player in primary care, it is more correct to consider primary care as a team of many professions and disciplines working together (Fig. 1.5 and Table 1.2).

Primary health care team
Many descriptions and definitions of primary care and primary care teams have been developed.

Primary care is often regarded as a 'gatekeeper' between self-care and specialized care. It is also a way of keeping care locally based, while making the most efficient and appropriate use of scarce resources to control high costs in cash-limited health care systems.

In the 1990s primary care became increasingly involved in purchasing or commissioning secondary care. An ethos developed that primary care should 'provide everything that it can provide efficiently and effectively, and purchase everything that it could not'. This new ethos challenged the role of traditional services that were hospital based, 'What do we need hospitals for anyway?'

A creative tension has developed between a traditional view of the primary health care team (PHCT) as a core group of generalists and of the PHCT as an ever-expanding group of subspecialist clinicians. Further, it is suggested that more secondary care specialists contribute in the form of outreach clinics.

Increasingly, GPs are acquiring additional skills and equipment to enable them to provide or undertake tasks previously the province of specialists in the hospital sector. Endoscopy, ultrasound, and near patient testing are becoming more usual in primary care settings.

GPs with a special interest are emerging in many disciplines, for example dermatology, diabetes, and gastroenterology (and possibly, in the future, oncology). Some GPs have already developed practice-based sigmoidoscopy in selected symptomatic patients for the early detection of colorectal cancer (Galloway, 2000), and others perform similar practice-based upper gastrointestinal endoscopy. Such schemes can reduce waiting times to days rather than weeks or months. A recent leading article discussed the possible contribution of primary care to a national initiative to improve the early detection of colorectal cancer (Jones and Kennedy, 1999).

Reconciling such approaches with the principles set out in the 1995 *Calman–Hine Report* will be a challenge for primary care. The solution may be for groups of primary care practices to work collaboratively, providing services for more than just their own practice patients. These GPs could work as part of the cancer team in a 'hub-and-spoke model' with the cancer unit and/or cancer centre.

Nursing and the professions allied to medicine have all greatly extended their role.

Drivers for change

Change in the provision of care for cancer patients is driven by political imperatives, public perceptions and needs, technological changes, and professional developments (Table 1.3). Shifts of care are:

- from hospital to community;
- to enhanced and extended primary care (practice nurses, social workers, psychologists, counsellors, physiotherapists, in-house pharmacists, specialist nurses, more outreach specialists in primary care);
- home-based care (increasing complexity of home support);
- from secondary to tertiary – requirement for 'critical mass' as in some of the rarer cancers.

Changes in primary care

As people are living longer, the proportion of the elderly is rising, and cancer sufferers are surviving longer, the prevalence of cancer patients may be expected to rise. Also, changing career patterns, with more part-time and flexible contract working, are changing primary care provision. Changes are also occurring in the way services are provided out of office hours, with more large cooperatives and treatment centres; these potentially cause problems in information transfer, continuity of care, and depersonalization of services.

Access to primary care is an issue, and it may not always be the route to hospital services. Accident and emergency units are increasingly used by some sections of the population. This has led to some redefining of primary care.

The debate continues as to whether fee for service is an efficient way to deliver primary health care. For example, in the USA it is estimated that 40,000,000 people do not have regular access to a usual primary health care provider (Surgeon General, 2000). The majority of these patients are younger males, particularly those from a more deprived background.

American insurance schemes vary tremendously in the extent of their health care provision, and limit access to certain hospitals, drugs, and even whether patients can have home care. A considerable number of health plans are related to employment, and thus unemployment followed by serious illness can be catastrophic for a family.

Changes in the role of doctors

Nurses have expanded their role and some have become nurse practitioners in their own right, working independently of doctors. The proliferation of nurse specialists has brought particular skills and benefits to cancer care. In the UK there are moves towards nurse prescribing after several successful pilot projects. Nurse-led triage at first point of contact is becoming commonplace, in the surgery, clinic, or via a telephone system ('NHS Direct' in the UK; 'Ask-a-Nurse' in the USA).

There has been a revolution in information via the internet for both patients and clinical staff. A patient who brings printouts from the net is a feature of many consultations, up to 20% and rising. It was estimated that by the end of the year 2000, 25% of all internet traffic will be health related.

Siting of Cancer Care

The proportion of patients treated by different sectors of the health-care system in the UK has changed little since 1948. The traditional proportions of the 'pyramid of care' do not apply to cancer patients, as virtually 100% will go to secondary or tertiary care sectors. Increasingly, these sectors have been re-evaluated and there is a recognition that patients must be

Table 1.2. *Practical contributions to cancer care by the primary health care team*

Administrative

- Increasing involvement in the commissioning of cancer services
- Systematic collection and coding of cancer data (site of tumour and histology)
- Increasing use of new technology to facilitate information transfer as efficiently as possible
- Maintenance of the accuracy of the Health Service administrative register – accurate addresses and post codes (zip codes), without which population-based call and recall screening cannot function properly
- The potential for using pooled budgets to address inequities in the introduction of new drugs should be examined

Patients at risk

- Family history
- Occupational risk
- Lifestyle risk (e.g. smoking, alcohol consumption)
- Appropriate evidence-based interventions for patients at risk
- Continuing education about the contribution of genetics to identifying patients at increased risk; selection and referral of suitable patients to expert cancer genetic services

Diagnosis/Referrals

- Keep up-to-date comprehensive information detailing specialist teams in the area for each common cancer site
- Point(s) of contact within the local area centre should be known so that information on teams servicing the rarer cancers can be accessed easily
- Making available specific telephone consultation times for results to be given or to discuss recent appointments
- Have clear systems and protocols for referral of patients to appropriate cancer units and cancer centres
- Systematic audit of the above systems
- Refer patients to teams that participate in clinical trials
- Act as a patient advocate when referring cancer patients
- Acting as a link and coordinator of services

Prevention/screening

- Adopt cancer prevention as a high priority within health promotion, with prime emphasis on evidence-based smoking cessation strategies, but also promote healthy diet and exercise regimes
- Encourage maximum patient participation in national cancer screening campaigns; identify non-attenders and address their concerns and fears

Information

- Provide access to internet information sites for patients and carers
- Interpret and explain information for patients and their families and carers

Medical care

- Encourage holistic patient-centred care
- Work as an integrated primary care team that provides access to and coordinates all the personnel and agencies that provide cancer care
- Ensure psychological and social factors are addressed in cancer care, for both the patients and their families

- Be responsible for continuing general medical care of cancer patients in parallel with their cancer treatment
- Ensure that information is shared appropriately
- Collaborate with shared and continuing care for cancer patients (e.g. the provision of continuing tamoxifen prescriptions, depot hormone insertions in prostate cancer)
- Collaborate with community and hospital drug information pharmacists on drug information when faced with unfamiliar new treatments
- Ensure provision of treatment to minimize symptoms during therapy

Support

- Assist in the organization, coordination and prioritization of transport for patients undergoing treatment
- Offer to put patients in contact with support groups
- Help patients to access advice regarding employment and financial matters
- Offer to counsel and give information to family members to remove this burden from the patients and their immediate families
- Specific support needs to be considered for children and adolescents if their mother, father, or sibling is the patient
- Certification and insurance reports

Palliative care

- Provide palliative care including referral to hospices and specialist palliative care teams
- Links to and coordination of services with voluntary agencies, such as in the UK Macmillan cancer relief, and Marie Curie nurses
- Put patients in contact with appropriate support groups, in respect of information, social support, employment counselling, insurance counselling, transport arrangements, and sources of financial assistance and benefits
- Organize appropriate terminal care in conjunction with the wishes of the patient and their family and/or carers
- Arrange bereavement counselling
- Accurate and complete death certification

Education

- Continuous professional development plans must include cancer care. Areas that require particular attention include prevention, screening, genetics, and new treatments
- Each member of the primary care team should regularly update the others on new developments in their particular area of expertise

referred to specialists and be seen as a matter of urgency.

While there is evidence from the literature that delays of up to 3–6 months from referral to hospital appointment had no effect on outcome, there is no doubt from the patient perspective that speed is of the essence. From April 2000 the NHS has introduced targets for patients with urgent referral for possible cancer to be seen within 2 weeks of referral. Clearly, any delay at the practice office in dictating, typing, signing, and sending such a letter must be kept to an absolute minimum. The use of electronic templates, with data drawn directly from the electronic patient record, may be of assistance.

Chapter 2 describes how cancer services have been and are being reorganized. The rationale for the changes were the unacceptable variations in the outcomes for some cancers between regions in the UK, and between countries in the Western world.

In 1995 a report in the UK set out a framework for commissioning high-quality cancer care and also defined general principles for care, and the central role of primary care (Calman–Hine report, 1995). Many healthcare systems have now set targets to reduce cancer morbidity and mortality.

Distance from specialist centres and the difficulties in travel to and from these centres are a major consideration

Table 1.3. *Drivers for change*

Political imperatives

- Cost containment
- Quality improvement
- Accountability (corporate and clinical governance)
- Life-long learning and professional revalidation
- Cancer plan

Public

- Increased knowledge
- Information revolution
- Increased preparedness to challenge 'experts'
- Bad publicity for medicine
- Increased consumerism, 'I want it, I want it all, and I want it NOW'

Technology

- Information technology and communications (e.g. internet literature searches, mobile communications, e-mail)
- Minimally invasive surgery
- Interventional radiology
- Telemedicine – e.g. transmission of X-rays, ultrasound scans, magnetic resonance imaging and/or computed tomography images, pathology results, clinical data, and remote video conferencing at multiple sites
- New scanning techniques – magnetic resonance, positron emission, spiral computed axial tomography
- Day case units
- New drugs
- Genetics

Professions

- Decreasing public trust in professions
- Increasing litigation
- Evidence-based medicine
- Clinical and corporate governance

for patients and their carers. Clinicians should guard against the temptation to second guess the patient in this matter. Most patients will travel further and endure greater inconvenience for high-quality cancer care than they will for more mundane conditions that are not life-threatening. The most appropriate site for treatment may vary at different episodes during the patient cancer experience depending on local expertise and the individual's condition at the time. For example, long distance travel by ambulance may be inappropriate when a patient is suffering from the side effects of treatment. Time is precious to cancer patients and their families and days spent travelling to and from treatment centres can represent significant proportions of remaining life. Distance is particularly relevant when considering the options for where palliative care should take place, in contrast to those cases for which induction of remission is the aim.

To assist PHCTs in assessing cases for referral, the Department of Health has produced a consultative document that sets out criteria by which to assess patients by cancer type, and suggests sample referral forms (Department of Health, 1999). These are reproduced in this book as appendices to the appropriate cancer site chapters.

The Cancer Journey

The cancer journey for any given patient can be divided into five, and for some, six stages.

1. Health promotion and screening
2. Suspected malignany and referral
3. Diagnosis
4. Treatment
5. Follow-up
6. Palliative care

A key role for primary care is to organize and facilitate the patient through the cancer journey. To assist in this it is advisable to appoint a 'key worker' as the main point of contact for each cancer patient. At different points of the cancer journey that key worker may change, according to circumstances.

Cancer charities and the World Health Organization (WHO) declared six principles in the *Charter of Paris 2000*:

- All people affected or potentially affected by cancer should have equal access to information concerning the disease origin, prevention, and current standards for detection, diagnosis, and treatment.
- Open and collaborative communication between people with cancer and health care professionals and scientists is essential.
- A commitment to total patient well being includes not only clinical care but also information and psychosocial support.

- People with cancer throughout the world have the opportunity to become informed, organized, and influential.
- The professional medical community, recognizing the power and benefit of an informed and active public, will help facilitate popular commitment to both the scientific process and the practice of evidence-based medicine.
- The medical research, industry, and policy communities will regard informed patient advocates as key strategic partners in all aspects of the fight against cancer, including the standards of care and survival.

The patient perspective

Analysis of patient and relatives complaints paints a sobering picture. A survey of hospice patients estimated that up to 30% of those receiving palliative care were at some stage subject to delay, prevarication, or missed treatment opportunities that resulted in an otherwise treatable condition becoming inoperable or beyond the possibility of inducing a remission.

Evidence from cancer charities indicates that up to 90% of contacts from patients or their families are to obtain some or more information about their condition and prospects. It appears that most clinicians – including those in primary care – could do better at imparting information. Primary care has a clear role in 'interpreting' and reinforcing the more specialized information that patients receive from the team that cares for them at their cancer centre or unit. All parties are agreed that cancer services should be 'patient-centred', but the failings of current practice are highlighted by the many studies in this area:

- The majority of patients in one study (National Cancer Alliance, 1996) felt that adequate and appropriate information was *not* available. Leaflets, while important, were no substitute for enough time in discussion. It is not enough to ask 'any questions?', because patients 'do not know what they do not know'.
- The 'attitude' or approach of health professionals and their communication skills is a frequent cause of distress and complaint (*see* Chapter 27 for a discussion).
- The large number of team members involved in the 'Cancer Journey' potentially compromises continuity of care. Effective teamwork and

continuity of care is enormously reassuring to patients. Nearly 90% of patients involved in the study reported that continuity of care was of *maximum importance* (National Cancer Alliance, 1996). This has significant implications for primary care teams, which are becoming larger, and for the increasing use of out-of-hours deputizing and cooperative services. The more people are involved the greater the number of communication channels, as calculated from the formula $(n^2-n)/2$, where n = the number of team members. Thus a team of 10 will have $(100-10)/2$ = 45 communication channels between team members. The difficulty is compounded when all the secondary care team members are added. The patient could have contact with 30–40 different members of this secondary team, which includes surgeon, medical oncologist, haematologist, radiation oncologist, and all their junior staff, radiologist and radiographer, pathologist and technicians, pharmacists, oncology nurses, chemotherapy nurses, specialist nurses (breast care, stoma care, etc.), palliative care nurses, appliance technician, dietician, physiotherapist, occupational therapist, clinical psychologist, social services, councillors, religious pastoral care, secretaries, clinic clerical staff, transport staff, and support groups and charities.

- Many patients highlighted difficulties with the GP. Many felt their initial presentations were dismissed or ignored, resulting in needless delay in diagnosis. If patients feels that their GP did not take them seriously or delayed referral, the patients become very reluctant to involve their GP in future care, and want to access the specialist unit on *all* matters directly. Good communication between hospital and GP is also vital – the GP must know what has happened during the last appointment and/or admission.
- Privacy during consultations needs to be both physical and aural – this was rated as the most important factor by some patients.
- There is a balance to be struck between speed and 'time to think'. Speed is highly valued in the context of referral. Conversely, time for patients to think and reflect when treatment options are being considered is also important, and doctors should be happy to facilitate second opinions.

Patients' expectations

A major concern for patients is whether their primary care clinician knows where to send a patient for a particular cancer care service. All too often they fear the referral is determined more by personal acquaintance and convenience than by knowledge of the best available facilities, skills, and treatment protocols:

- Patients want to know that they are being seen by a cancer team that achieves results commensurate with the best available.
- Patients want factual information.

- Many patients would like the opportunity to talk to other patients and/or carers who have experience in the treatment they are about to undergo.
- Many also wish to access support groups.

Where a cure is not possible, quality of life can be improved by optimal anticancer treatment, including chemotherapy, radiotherapy, and effective palliative care and support. Maintaining a good overall state of mental health is essential if quality of life is to be preserved. This includes physical, psychological, and social functioning and it should be a medical priority (*see* Chapter 27).

References

Calman K, Hine D. *A Policy Framework For Commissioning Cancer Services – report by the expert advisory group on cancer to the chief medical officers of England and Wales.* London: 1995.

Coleman M, Babb P, Damiecki, *et al. Cancer Survival Trends England and Wales 1971–1995.* London: Office for National Statistics Series SMPS No 61, 1999.

Cancer Research Campaign Scientific Yearbook. London: Cancer Research UK, 1998–1999, pp 43–44.

Department of Health. *Referral Guidelines for Suspected Cancer – Consultation Document.* London: Department of Health, 1999 (also available at http://www.doh.gov.uk/cancer, comments proforma at http://www.doh.gov.uk/cancer/proforma.htm)

Galloway J. *J Primary Care Soc Gastroenterol.* 2000; **8**:.

Heyrman J, Spreeuwenbergh C, eds. *Vocational Training in General Practice.* Leuwen; Katholieke Universiteit Leuven, 1987.

Jones R, Kennedy T. The early detection of colorectal cancer in primary care. *Br J Gen Pract.* 1999; **49**: 956–8.

McCormick A, Fleming D, Charlton J. *Morbidity Statistics from General Practice.* Fourth National Study 1991–1992 Series MB5 No 3. London: Office Population Census and Surveys, 1995.

National Screening Committee. *First Report of the National Screening Committee.* London: Department of Health, April 1998.

Office for National Statistics. *Health Statistics Quarterly 04 Winter 1999.* London: Office for National Statistics England and Wales, 1999.

Olesen F, Dickinson J, Hjortdahl P. General practice: time for a new definition. *BMJ.* 2000; **320**: 354–7.

Summerton N. *Diagnosing Cancer in General Practice.* Oxford: Radcliffe Medical Press, 1999.

Surgeon General. *Healthier People 2010.* Understanding and Improving Health. Washington, DC: US Department of Health and Human Services, 2000.

The National Cancer Alliance. *Patient-Centred Cancer Services? What Patients Say.* The National Cancer Alliance, 1996.

Stott N. *The Nature of General Medical Practice.* Report from General Practice No. 27. London: Royal College of General Practitioners, 1996.

World Health Organization. Charter of Paris 2000. Geneva: World Health Organization, 2000.

2 Organization of Cancer Services

Douglas Russell

Cancer is a major public health problem throughout the world. There are striking variations of incidence and prevalence in different countries, and even by region within countries. Cancer deaths vary by sex, race, ethnicity, and country. Some of these differences may result from genetics, lifestyle factors (such as smoking, diet, and alcohol consumption), and environment (sunlight, pollution, carcinogens, ionizing radiation, infection), but at the population level there also seems to be a clear association between socioeconomic status and survival figures.

Analysis of outcomes within the UK highlights differences for cancer patients that might be attributable to variations in clinical practice and in the organization of services. This prompted the publication of a report, named after the England and Wales Chief Medical Officers of the time (Calman and Hine, 1995).

The report set out advice and recommendations on:

- how purchasers and/or commissioners of cancer services should expect such services to be organized;
- general principles governing the provision of cancer care (*Table 2.1*);
- the relationship of cancer services with primary care (*Table 2.2*).

In commissioning and/or purchasing cancer care it is necessary to move away from contracts in which cancer services are not clearly identifiable by tumour site. The process must be capable of discriminating between the different diseases and the detailed needs of particular groups of patients (Scottish Cancer Co-ordinating and Advisory Committee, 1996).

The proposed new GP contract has, in the 'Quality and Outcomes' section, two indicators specific to cancer. The first requires the practice to produce a register of all cancer patients (excluding nonmelanoma skin cancer) from April 2003. The second involves a demonstration of the coordination of patient care between the Practice and secondary care and that, within 6 months of diagnosis, each patient has had a review of their support needs.

Sectors of Cancer Care

Health care in the UK and similar systems has traditionally been regarded as a 'pyramid of care', with the relative proportions of health care episodes seen in each successive layer of the system being in an approximate ratio of 10:1. Cancer care is an exception to this rule in that virtually all patients with cancer should be seen by secondary care at least, and

Table 2.1. *General principles governing the provision of cancer care*

1. All patients should have access to a uniformly high quality of care in the community or hospital wherever they may live to ensure the maximum possible cure rates and best quality of life. Care should be provided as close to the patient's home as is compatible with high-quality, safe, and effective treatment.
2. Public and professional education to help early recognition of the symptoms of cancer and the availability of national screening programmes are vital parts of any comprehensive programme of cancer care.
3. Patients, families, and carers should be given clear information and assistance, in a form they can understand, about the treatment options and outcomes available to them at all stages of treatment from diagnosis onwards.
4. The development of cancer services should be patient centred and should take account of patients', families', and carers' views and preferences as well as those of professionals involved in cancer care. Individuals' perceptions of their needs may differ from those of the professionals. Good communication between professionals and patients is especially important.
5. The primary care team is a central and continuing element in cancer care for both the patient and his or her family, from primary prevention, pre-symptomatic screening, initial diagnosis, through care and follow-up, and (in some cases) death and bereavement. Effective communication between sectors is imperative in achieving the best possible care.
6. In recognition of the impact that screening, diagnosis, and treatment of cancer can have on patients, their families, and their carers, the psychosocial aspects of cancer care should be considered at all stages.
7. Cancer registration and careful monitoring of treatment and outcomes are essential.

Table 2.2. The relationship of cancer services with primary care

1. The close relationship between primary care and secondary care services within the cancer unit and cancer centre is emphasized in the recommendations. The development of primary health care teams will enhance patient care.
2. The relationship should be one of partnership in continuing care rather than one involving the permanent or temporary transfer of responsibility for the patient.
3. To judge the quality of care provided by their local cancer services, general practitioners (GPs) require information about what constitutes 'best care', both organizationally and for individual cancers.
4. Local guidelines for the identification and management of symptoms that indicate a high risk of malignancy need to be established for each cancer, with reference to nationally agreed and rigorously evaluated standards.
5. The cancer services need to establish local referral patterns in co-operation with primary care. These should be flexible, recognizing the extent to which many GPs wish to be involved with the diagnostic process.
6. Secondary and tertiary care services must recognize that, simultaneously with their medical management of the patient, the primary care team is providing psychological and emotional support, acting as a link and advocate with secondary and tertiary sectors, providing and translating information, and dealing with parallel non-cancer illness.
7. The importance of communication, appropriate in time and content, between primary care and the specialist services cannot be over-estimated. Any changes in patient management should be made known to all involved in the patient's care. As with referral, local procedures for this need to be established.
8. Discharge information should reach relevant members of the primary health care team on the day of discharge; it should include details of diagnosis, a management plan, including drugs, other agencies involved, and information given to the patients and their families.
9. Primary health care teams must ensure that clinical changes are notified to the next patient contact.

perhaps by tertiary care. Calman and Hine (1995) went on to describe the three different levels of care, and the features typical of each.

Level 1: primary care

Primary care is considered in the Calman–Hine report to be the focus of care. However, in the 7 years since this report was published primary care has changed, and still is changing (see below).

Level 2: designated cancer unit

The designated cancer unit is normally in a district general hospital that is of a size adequate to support clinical teams with sufficient expertise and facilities to manage the more common cancers.

Level 3: designated cancer centre

The designated cancer centre should provide expertise in the management of *all* cancers, including the more common cancers within their local geographical area, and those referred from cancer units. Such centres should have specialist diagnostic and therapeutic techniques including radiotherapy. Experience of implementing these designations has, in some cases, proved difficult.

Multidisciplinary Teams

A number of expert reports have emphasized the importance of working in multidisciplinary teams to ensure the best possible outcomes for cancer patients (Calman and Hine, 1995; Scottish Cancer Co-ordinating and Advisory Committee, 1996). A specialist multidisciplinary cancer team is defined as;

❝A group of specialists, working together under appropriate leadership to achieve an accurate speedy diagnosis, and decide, implement and monitor effective treatment and care as determined by locally and nationally agreed evidence-based guidelines and protocols. The team must communicate effectively with patients, professionals and within itself and audit its outcomes. Individual members must keep up-to-date in their own fields. ❞

Further definitions of terms used in this statement are:

- *Group:* The team comprises core and associate members. The membership will vary depending upon the tumour site.
- *Specialist:* Specialization of core team members is defined in terms of training, experience, research, and time commitment. The associate team specialization should include a formal commitment by the named individual to the team, but the individual is not necessarily involved in the care of all patients.
- *Working together:* The core team must meet regularly, be given appropriate resources, and respect the principles of effective team working. Members of the associate team attend the regular meetings as and when appropriate.

- *Leadership:* An appropriate senior clinical specialist is designated to lead the team. He or she will provide evidence for his or her specialist interest, as described above. He or she will be responsible for the team and for an annual review of its membership, processes, patient satisfaction, and clinical outcome. This person does not necessarily have to be a doctor.
- *Effectively:* The team will ensure that all those involved in the care of the patient, including the primary health care team (PHCT), are fully informed of the treatment plan that has been agreed with the patient.
- *Up-to-date:* There are many ways that staff can maintain their knowledge over time. Apart from the professional obligation to adopt a culture of life-long learning, there are available professional continuing education, formal course and training, and distance learning programmes. Conferences, symposia and peer group activity also contribute to up-sating knowledge.
- *Guidelines:* Guidelines describe the key principles that determine the clinical management of particular cancers.
- *Protocols:* Protocols provide the details of particular treatments that follow the clinical management decisions outlined in the guidelines.
- *Audit:* The team will set aside separate time for audit, the results of which will be published.

Specific recommendations about the composition of specialist multidisciplinary teams for cancer care are beyond the scope of this book, but can be found in the Clinical Outcomes Group expert reports published by the NHS Executive. Cancer-specific guidelines available on the Internet also contain specific recommendations about the composition of such teams.

Targets

The NHS in the UK has attempted to demonstrate progress in health care by setting targets. The first of these initiatives was the *Protocol for Investment in Health Gain (Wales, 1990)*, which pioneered the concept of patient-centred services that added 'years to life and life to years'.

Over time the targets have been modified, and other countries have adopted similar approaches. In Wales the current targets are:

1a. Reduce the European Standardized Mortality Rate for lung cancer in men under age 75 years by at least 53% by the year 2010.
1b. Reduce the European Standardized Mortality Rate for lung cancer in women under age 75 years by at least 21% by the year 2010.
2. Reduce the European Standardized Mortality rate for breast cancer in women aged 50–74 years by at least 30% by the year 2002.
3. Reduce the European Standardized Registration Rate for invasive cervical cancer in women by at least 50% by the year 2002.

In England the 1992 *Health of the Nation* strategy identified cancer as one of five key areas in which progress was required. Cancers of lung, breast, cervix, and skin were identified specifically. Numerical targets were set for reduction in the incidence and/or mortality of these cancers within a period of 10–15 years.

The most recent strategic document for England, *The NHS Cancer Plan 2000*, has superceded previous plans – its aims are:

- To ensure that people with cancer get the right professional support and care, as well as the best treatments;
- To tackle the inequalities in health that mean unskilled workers are twice as likely to die from cancer as professionals;
- To build for the future through investment in the cancer workforce, research and preparation for the genetics revolution, so that the NHS never falls behind in cancer care again.

The Surgeon General in the USA has published a document, *Healthy People 2010*, that contains in Section 3 on 'Cancer' a large number of targets relating to reductions of death rates for lung, breast, cervical, colorectal, oropharyngeal, prostate, and melanoma cancer deaths, as well as targets for cancer prevention measures, and includes a target for cancer survival – from a baseline of 59% of persons with invasive cancer of any type living 5 years after diagnosis to 70% by 2010, a target of 19% improvement.

The Department of Health has commissioned a series of studies into the organization and provision of cancer services according to tumour type. The recommendations are evidence-based as far as is possible and published under the generic title of 'Guidance on Commissioning Cancer Services: improving outcomes'. The documents that cover breast, lung, colorectal, and gynaecological cancers have been published and the process is under way for urological and upper gastrointestinal cancers. These publications provide an important resource to all those involved in cancer care.

Cancer Collaboratives and Cancer Networks

The EUROCARE study showed that cancer patients in England and Wales had poorer survival rates than patients in other European countries in the study. This study in part prompted the Calman–Hine report, which referred to a network of care. The Calman–Hine report was not intended to be a blueprint but to allow commissioners to make well-informed and wise decisions with regard to the provision of local cancer services. It recognized that health services cannot do everything for everybody and there had to be some prioritization within available resources. More recently, the concept of a cancer network has become a reality and is no longer viewed as optional. Historically, the first cancer network was set up in Scotland, and there are now 34 cancer networks throughout England, and similar organizations exist in Wales, Scotland and Northern Ireland. These cancer networks are approximately aligned to the newly formed strategic health authorities in England, although they do not exactly match

geographically. Typically, a network consists of a cancer centre and its surrounding cancer units, which tend to be based in district general hospitals. Each network relates to a number of primary care organizations and their constituent practices. The networks are governed by boards and the delivery of care is overseen by tumour-site-specific groups, which consist of clinicians, nurses and managers. Primary care organizations have direct representation on the cancer network boards through nominated lead clinicians.

Multidisciplinary discussion of individual patients' management, peer review, audit and education are fundamental functions within the individual tumour site specific groups. Cancer networks are also used as the framework for local research networks, which link to the National Cancer Research Network. Palliative care teams are of course closely related to their cancer network.

In 1999 cancer services collaboratives were set up by the government in nine areas in England. These projects were driven by project leaders concentrating on a patient-centred approach. They key part of these projects was patient journey (pathway) mapping, which identified bottlenecks in the system that lead to delays in diagnosis and treatment. These collaboratives have played a major part in some of the changes that are now being made to reduce delays in cancer care. There are now tumour-site-specific collaboratives in breast, lung, cervix, ovary and prostate (Kerr *et al.*, 2002).

Further Reading

Expert Advisory Group on Cancer. A Policy Framework for Commissioning Cancer Services – A report to the chief medical officers of England and Wales (Calmon–Hine Report). London: 1995.

Kerr D, Bevan H, Gowland B, *et al.* Redesigning cancer care. *BMJ* 2002; **324**: 164–6.

Scottish Cancer Co-ordinating and Advisory Committee. *Commissioning Cancer Services in Scotland*. Edinburgh: Scottish Office Department for Health, 1996.

3 Organization of Palliative Care Services

Douglas Russell and Glynis Tranter

Palliative care is sometimes incorrectly understood as terminal care. The two are not the same – terminal care is a subset within palliative care. Palliative care has been defined as 'the active total care of patients and their families by a multi-professional team when the patient's disease is no longer responsive to curative treatment'. Palliation can begin at the point of diagnosis, continue throughout the rest of the 'patient journey' and, for the family and carers, extend beyond death into bereavement care. It can accompany continued curative treatment.

Principles of Palliative Care Provision

1. It is the right of every person with life-threatening illness to receive appropriate palliative care wherever they are.
2. It is the responsibility of every health care professional to practise the palliative care approach and to call in specialist palliative care colleagues as the need arises, as an integral component of good clinical practice, whatever the illness or its stage.

The responsibility for ensuring that these defined rights of patients and their families can be met, and that health care professionals may be enabled to fulfil their responsibilities, lies with the commissioners and providers of the service. The philosophy of the palliative care service is to provide a palliative rather than curative approach, an acceptance of death and a focus on the psychological and social needs of the patients and their carers (Griffin, 1991). Palliative care adds life to years, curative care adds years to life.

The Palliative Care Approach

- A focus on quality of life
- Pain and symptom control
- A holistic approach to care planning
- Care encompassing the patient their family and their carers

- Respect for patient autonomy and choice
- Open and sensitive communication with patients, carers and professionals
- High standards of medical and nursing care

Palliative Care Teams

Palliative care skill is a core skill of all health care professionals dealing with patients who have life-threatening disease. This applies whether in primary, secondary or tertiary care settings and in a clinic, a ward or the community.

The National Hospice Council have divided palliative care into three areas:

1. The palliative care that should be part of all patients management.
2. The palliative intent that accompanies anti-cancer treatments given by surgeons, radiotherapists and medical oncologists.
3. The care that is offered by specially trained multiprofessional teams.

The primary care team members that have already been referred to in Chapter 1 integrate at all of these three levels. Much palliative care takes place in primary care, but there are specialist palliative care teams, often associated with cancer units and centres, and also existing in the voluntary sector.

Specialist palliative care is delivered by a multiprofessional team, who should possess recognized palliative medicine training. They should work collaboratively to address the areas set out below. A specialist palliative care team might include:

- consultant in palliative care medicine;
- nurse specialist in palliative care;
- other nurses (e.g. stoma, breast, Macmillan, Marie Curie);
- psychological medicine–nursing input;
- pharmacist;

- social worker;
- physiotherapist and occupational therapist;
- dietician;
- spiritual counsellor; and
- care assistant.

There should be no artificial barriers between the different sectors. The care model used should be the one that is most appropriate for the patient, with the patient fully involved in the care planning process. Palliative care depends on integrated teamwork, with the patient as the central focus.

Patient Requirements

Each patient will have certain fixed determinant of their requirements:

1. Clinical status
   - the type of cancer;
   - the stage and prognosis of the disease;
   - impact of current treatment;
   - future treatment options.
2. Sociodemographic variables
   - age;
   - marital status and presence of a social partner;
   - ethnicity (language and culture);
   - education;
   - socioeconomic status; and
   - environment.

Attention will be given by the palliative care team to relief and rehabilitation in six domains, which are modifiable to improve the patient's experience:

1. Physical (or physiological) symptoms:
   - pain, fatigue, nausea, dyspnoea, anorexia, pruritus.
2. Psychological and cognitive:
   - anxiety, depression, agitation, confusion, motivation.
3. Social relationships:
   - family, carers, friends;
   - available support systems;
   - knowledge and use of community support systems.
4. Economic demands:
   - income, savings, insurance, benefits, housing, transport;

- flexibility of employment;
- suitability of home for medical equipment and aids.
5. Hopes and expectations:
   - milestones, understanding of prognosis, communication between care team and patient;
   - perception of quality of life;
   - perceptions of illness.
6. Spiritual beliefs and value system:
   - religion, sense of purpose and meaning, spirituality.

Palliative Care Interventions

Interventions include:

- family and friend interventions (communication, delivering care, meeting needs, taking responsibility for tasks, reducing burdens);
- social interventions (spiritual activity, pastoral care, support groups);
- medical provider interventions (communication and regular contact with patient, advance care planning, 'living will' approaches);
- health care system interventions (symptom relief, pain service, hospice, hospital at home); and
- social interventions (health care system coverage, employer welfare programmes, insurance coverage, voluntary sector care provision).

These domains are addressed in relevant chapters in this book.

It is recommended that the palliative care team should have an identified, named key worker for each patient, and that this person (and how and when to contact him or her) is known to everyone involved.

Organizing Palliative Care

Changes in the way primary care is delivered over 24 hours, the introduction of deputizing and cooperative arrangements for GPs and the increasing use of call centres for out-of hours care makes it imperative that good communication systems exist and that hand-over arrangements are foolproof.

Patient-held records are a sensible way of ensuring that all team members are aware of relevant facts. This also helps to ensure that the patient is fully involved in the care planning process. Certain patient groups are at much higher risk of receiving fragmented care – those with low income, urban-dwelling minorities, patients living alone with no social support and those in remote rural settings.

Primary care teams organize the prescription or supply of appropriate drugs and delivery systems. They must also ensure that the family and carers are able to cope with them (e.g. syringe drivers for subcutaneous delivery of analgesics). Research shows that poorly controlled pain dramatically increases the physical and psychological burdens of carers.

Preparing for the Inevitable

The issue of advance care planning and 'living wills' is controversial but may be discussed with some patients. Patients can also find it helpful to discuss enduring powers of attorney with family members earlier rather than later. Primary care team members may need to assume the role of patient advocate with third-party insurers and benefits agencies.

The primary care team should assume the responsibility of finding out whether relatives and those close to the patient are aware of any poor prognosis. With the patient's consent the team should offer to speak to appropriate relatives and carers.

The patient's cultural beliefs about death and his or her attitudes towards burial, cremation and even possibly *post mortem* examination should be known to team members.

Organizing Nursing Care

There is often confusion about the roles of the nurses involved in palliative care provision – the Marie Curie nurses, Macmillan nurses and district nurses. The nurse's role has tended to be seen as primarily a traditional bedside caring role, but this has been extended to incorporate assessment of family needs, coordination of care provided by all agencies, and counselling and teaching of patients and relatives.

The involvement of nurses in the holistic care of dying patients has been extensive. Caring for the dying patients and the family extends all the fundamental skills that a nurse should have.

There is need to provide support for cancer patients irrespective of whether they live in an urban or rural setting or in a sparsely or densely populated area. This could be addressed by supporting joint appointments between cancer units and community services, with individual staff working across the current divide.

Specialist palliative care nurses

Specialist nurses in the UK are mainly originally funded by the Cancer Relief Macmillan Fund and are known as Macmillan Nurses. Their role is to provide advice about symptom control and pain relief and emotional support to the patient and the family and to act as a resource and liaison point with the specialist palliative care services. Macmillan nurses do not take over responsibility from the district nurses for practical nursing. As district nurses take an increasing role in planning care for their patients, delegating practical tasks to nursing assistants, the interface between the district nurses and the Macmillan nurse has in some areas become unclear. The role of the district nurse is well established; however, there are potential conflicts over the responsibility for care.

The role of the Marie Curie nurses differs in that they provide a nursing service that includes hands-on practical nursing and complements the community nursing service.

The Cameron Report (1996) recommended that to benefit patients, who are currently cared for in a wide range of settings, a mixed option of care should have both practical and resource benefits. To support this, models such as networks of specialist nurses who can support generalist nurses in the field should be developed. A robust network system would enhance communication between members of the multidisciplinary health care team at all levels.

Clinical nurse specialists

The clinical nurse specialist role has been refined and developed in recent years and a number of specialist posts in cancer services have developed. These includes breast care, cytotoxic chemotherapy, stoma care, palliative care and paediatric oncology.

Specialist nurses are able to effect health gain both as coordinators of multidisciplinary teams and as practitioners in their own right and they should be available in all health care settings. Examples of health gain from the adequate provision of specialist nursing care include:

- *alleviation of psychological distress associated with breast cancer by early detection and help with identified problems;*
- *improved symptom control for the terminally ill with early involvement of specialists in palliative care nursing;*
- *improved functional ability for patients with cancer of the colon through the psychoeducational interventions of stoma nurses;*

- improved continuity of care for patients undergoing chemotherapy through the development of the role of the chemotherapy nurses; and
- improved quality of life for patients through the application of techniques for the reduction of lymphoedema developed by lymphoedema nurses.

Extending the role of nurses

There is a general shortage of doctors in the UK and during 1983–1993, the number of general practitioner trainees in England and Wales dropped from 1769 to 1653. Extending the role of the specialist nurse is therefore crucial in providing adequate cancer care. There are changes in health care, however, that are currently causing polarization between the need for specialization of skills and equipment at one end and community-based generic services at the other. Parallel to this is the perception of patients, families and carers that only a specialist nurse will give the right advice.

The extended role of the nurse within the primary health care setting is important for facilitating multidisciplinary team working. Evaluation of nurse prescribing projects has proved that nurse prescribing is successful, and safe and effective working practices have been established. The scheme has been shown to be popular with nurses, GPs and patients. Patients do not complain about being treated by a nurse prescriber and GPs do not report that it is necessary to query a nurse's prescription. Over half of the GPs in one report said that nurse prescribing had saved them time and that they were having to sign fewer nurse-generated prescriptions. Team working within the primary health care team had also been enhanced (Legge, 1997).

Similarly, a study undertaken to evaluate the nurse-led telephone consultations produced substantial changes in the management of 'on-call' for GPs (Latimer *et al.*, 1998).

There was a reduction in the overall workload of for GPs by 50% and callers had quicker access to health information and advice. There was no associated increase in the number of adverse events and this model of out-of-hours primary care is safe and effective. The study highlighted the fact that the telephone consultation is becoming an increasingly accepted approach to patient care and improves public access to clinical information and advice. The nurse-led telephone consultation not only replaced telephone advice given by a doctor but resulted in reductions in both home visits and surgery attendances out of hours.

Caring for the carers

The multidisciplinary team should provide support for health care staff involved in palliative care. This includes training, education, audit and research related to palliative care. The broad aim of the team is to facilitate improvements in the services rather than to de-skill staff involved in palliative care.

Carers need to be involved in decisions on patient management. For instance, it should not be forgotten that, for most patients dying at home, the major burden of care falls on the family. In the UK the family is supported by community nurses within the Primary Health Care Team (PHCT). The PHCT have often known the patient long before the terminal illness and will continue to care for the family afterwards. The PHCT may also care for people in residential nursing homes. Family and carers experience changes in their functioning during the process of adjustment to impending loss. They are often registered with the same GP practice as the patient and require the services of the same PHCT. The continuing care of the patient must also encompass the continuing professional care of the close family or carers (Finlay, 1999), particularly when difficult decisions are taken.

References and Further Reading

Cameron, I. *Cancer Services in Wales: a Report by the Cancer Services Co-ordinating Group.* Cardiff: Welsh Office, NHS Wales; 1996.

Finlay I. Families as secondary patients. *Palliat Care Today* 1999.

Griffin, C. *Dying with Dignity.* London: Office of Health Economics; 1991.

Lattimer V, George S, Thompson F, et al. Safety and effectiveness of nurse telephone consultation in out of hours primary care: randomised controlled trial. *BMJ* 1998; **317**: 1054–9.

Legge A. Nurse prescribing is a success. *BMJ* 1997; **314**: 461.

Palliative Care 2000: Commissioning through Partnership. London: National Council for Hospice and Specialist Palliative Care Services; 1999.

Managing Patients with Cancer

4 Cancer Symptoms and Their Management

Karen Broadley

Symptom control in cancer is essential, both when an individual is being managed actively or when palliation is more appropriate as no further anti-cancer treatment is possible. Symptoms may occur as a result of:

- the disease itself (e.g. pain because of bone metastases);
- the treatment received (e.g. mucositis or nausea caused by chemotherapy);
- a problem associated with cancer (e.g. chronic obstructive pulmonary disease in lung cancer); and
- a completely unrelated condition such as arthritis.

Management of the symptoms can be achieved by active management of the cancer, but this may take time to be effective and will not be possible for most situations. Symptom control measures should be instituted immediately.

Pain

The World Health Organization ladder

Pain is the most common and the most feared symptom for a cancer patient. Up to 50% of people present with pain at the time of diagnosis and this increases to 75% of patients with more advanced disease. With the introduction of the World Health Organization (WHO) guidelines it is now known that cancer pain can be relieved in 80–90% of patients. The remaining 10–20% have more difficult pain and need more complex treatments.

The WHO ladder (*Fig. 4.1*) requires that medication be given regularly. If pain persists, then stronger analgesia is required on the next step of the ladder. At each step, use of non-opioids and adjuvant drugs is considered. Step 1 medication includes paracetamol or aspirin, with paracetamol up to 1g every 6 hours (q6h; four times a day) being the drug of choice in the UK. Non-steroidal anti-inflammatory drugs can

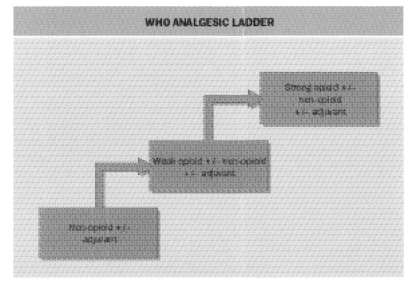

Figure 4.1. WHO analgesic ladder.

Table 4.1. *Alternative opioids*

Drug	Preparation	Indication	Comment
Diamorphine	Injection	Parenteral opioid required	More soluble than morphine
Fentanyl	Transdermal patch	Alternative to morphine, useful for poor compliance, or where alternative route of delivery required	Not suitable for rapidly changing analgesic requirements
Methadone	Liquid, tablets and injection	Alternative to morphine, possibly a specific role in neuropathic pain	Long half-life, beware of toxic metabolite accumulation
Oxycodone	Liquid, tablets and suppositories	Alternative to morphine, fear of morphine	Used widely for chronic pain in the USA
Hydromorphone	Tablets and injection	Alternative to morphine	Widely used in North America, injection available on named patient basis
Dextromoramide	Tablets and suppositories	Incident pain (e.g. prior to dressing changes)	Short duration of action, not useful for chronic pain mainly for breakthrough
Pethidine	Tablets and injection	Not indicated for chronic pain	Short duration of action, tablets poorly absorbed, accumulation of toxic metabolites with regular use

be included at this step. For step 2 the weak opioids are the drugs of choice, such as dihydrocodeine or dextropropoxyphene in combination with paracetamol (co-proxamol). Although the latter is an effective combination, care must be taken in general with combination products as each of the drugs in the medication may not be being taken at its optimum dose. Tramadol can also be a useful step 2 drug.

At step 3, the drug of choice remains morphine. For severe pain, immediate-release morphine liquid or tablets can be given every 4 hours with the same dose being used for breakthrough pain. A common starting dose is 10mg of morphine. Nausea may occur in up to 50% of individuals and commonly lasts for a few days. An antiemetic such as haloperidol 1.5mg at night should be made available and should be prescribed regularly if nausea occurred with weaker opioids. Constipation is always a side effect of opioid drugs and a laxative should be prescribed with morphine.

Alternative opioids

Other opioids are available for oral, rectal, subcutaneous, and transdermal delivery. While morphine is the gold standard, indications for using alternative opioids may arise for persistent, unacceptable side effects with the morphine, or for specific reasons that a different route of delivery may be appropriate. For example, a transdermal patch may improve compliance in an elderly patient or

be appropriate for someone who is having difficulty swallowing. In some situations, the alternative opioid is used because of a fear of morphine. The most commonly used alternative opioids appropriate for chronic pain control are given in *Table 4.1.*

Adjuvant drugs

Some pains are not fully responsive to morphine and adjuvant drugs are needed. The most difficult to manage is neuropathic pain. This is pain in an area of abnormal sensation, which may be experienced as burning, lancinating, stabbing, or aching pain. Adjuvant drugs such as the tricyclic antidepressants or anticonvulsants are generally prescribed first. Amitriptyline and dosulepin (dothiepin) may be useful, commencing on a low dose at night, which can be increased slowly over a period of days. Although the onset of action may not be for 10 days, it is generally faster than an effect seen in depression. Tricyclic antidepressants may be of particular benefit when the individual has difficulty in sleeping at night or when the patient experiences depressive symptoms. Their usefulness is limited because the side effects of a dry mouth and sedation are poorly tolerated.

Anticonvulsants, such as sodium valproate carbamazepine and gabapentin, have also been used effectively. While anecdotally they have been used for stabbing pain, the other types of neuropathic pain also respond. Again, the starting dose is

Table 4.2. *Commonly used adjuvant analgesic drugs for neuropathic pain*

Drug category	Examples	Typical doses
Tricyclic antidepressant	Amitriptyline, dosulepin (dothiepin)	Low starting dose (initially 10mg in the elderly, 25mg in general; effective dose varies from 50 to 150mg at night
Anticonvulsant	Sodium valproate, carbamazepine, gabapentine	Initially 100mg q12h to be increased slowly (gabapentin q8h)
Oral local anaesthetic	Mexiletine, flecainide	Flecainide 50–100mg q12h, mexiletine 150mg q12h to q8h
Corticosteroid	Dexamethasone, prednisolone	Up to 16mg of dexamethasone a day
Calcium antagonist	Nifedepine, diltiazem	Variable
Miscellaneous	Baclofen, clonzepan	Variable

low, with an increase being made every few days. An analgesic response is thought to occur within 10 days. Side effects of the anticonvulsants include nausea and vomiting, tremor, and dizziness.

Table 4.2 gives other drugs used in neuropathic pain.

Nausea and Vomiting

Nausea and vomiting are common symptoms that cause distress in around 50% of patients with advanced cancer. Although they commonly present together, they may occur separately. The causes are multiple, and are given in *Table 4.3*. If the cause is correctable, then this should be treated directly.

If not known, the most likely cause should be considered with an appropriate antiemetic prescribed on a regular basis. For continuous nausea or vomiting, the use of subcutaneous infusion is suggested (*see Table 4.4*).

Table 4.3. *Causes of nausea and vomiting*

Metabolic:
  hypercalcaemia
  uraemia
Raised intracranial pressure – cerebral metastases
Drug-induced
Chemotherapy
Radiotherapy
Gastrointestinal cause:
  constipation
  gastric distension and stasis
  bowel obstruction
Pain
Anxiety

Constipation

Difficulty in the passage of faeces is a common event in the severely ill. Medication used, particularly analgesics and the new antiemetics, cause constipation, which is then aggravated by a poor diet and general ill health. Specific causes, such as hypercalcaemia, should be ruled out, and treatment with regular laxatives commenced. Softeners, such as docusate, should be combined with a stimulant, such as danthron or senna, and taken regularly. Bulk-forming laxatives should be avoided. Enemas and suppositories may be needed to treat a severe case of constipation. The best treatment is preventative and laxatives should always be prescribed when strong analgesics are given.

Cachexia

Cachexia is a combination of weight-loss anorexia, weakness, and fatigue, which may be present in different degrees. The clinical picture is one of progressive wasting, together with deteriorating function. The incidence is particularly high in patients with lung cancer and in those with cancer of the gastrointestinal tract. Although this syndrome results from changes in carbohydrate, protein, and liver metabolism, other factors such as decreased appetite, nausea and vomiting, and (in particular) bowel obstruction contribute. A corticosteroid such as dexamethasone 6–8mg a day or a progestagen, such as medroxyprogesterone acetate 160mg a day, could be tried, but should be discontinued if not effective.

Table 4.4. Commonly used antiemetic drugs, their route of administration and uses

Drug	Usual dosages and route of administration	Typical dose in 24 hour subcutaneous infusion	Specific uses, apart from general antiemetic
Cyclizine	50mg q8h, oral, subcutaneous, intravenous	150mg over 24 hours	Bowel obstruction, vertigo
Haloperidol	1.5–3mg q24h or q12h, oral, subcutaneous, intravenous	3–10mg over 24 hours	Opioid-induced nausea, bowel obstruction, uraemia
Domperidone	10–20mg oral, 30–60mg per rectum, q8h or q6h	Not available	Gastric stasis
Metoclopramide	10mg q8h, oral, subcutaneous, intravenous	30mg over 24 hours 30–60mg over 24 hours	Gastric stasis, chemotherapy induced nausea
Prochlorperazine	5–10mg q8h, oral; 3–6mg q12h, buccal; 5mg q8h, 25mg stat per rectum	Not Suitable	Vertigo
Levopromazine	6.25–12.5mg q24h or q12h, oral or subcutaneous	25–150mg over 24 hours	Bowel obstruction and where sedation is required
Hyoscine hydrobromide	200–400mcg q8h, subcutaneous; 1 mg transdermal (lasts 3 days)	800–1200μg over 24 hours	Bowel obstruction where cramping is also a problem
Ondansetron	4–8mg q12h, oral or intravenous	Has been used as a continuous infusion, 8mg	Chemotherapy-induced nausea, bowel obstruction, and uraemia induced nausea
Granisetron	1mg q12h, oral; 3mg intravenous	Not known	Chemotherapy-induced nausea
Dexamethasone	4–16mg a day, oral, intravenous, or subcutaneous	4–16mg (tends to precipitate when mixed with other drugs at high doses)	Raised intracranial pressure, liver metastases

Anorexia

Anorexia is a common symptom and one that causes most distress to carers. Refusal to eat food that has been carefully prepared may create anxiety and tension. It is essential to elucidate specific causes that can be treated or managed appropriately. General advice about food preparation, giving only small and frequent meals, and often simply allowing individuals to voice their fears may be all that is needed, together with reassurance.

Fatigue

Cancer causes fatigue through a number of mechanisms, including tumour necrosis factor release, electrolyte disturbances, hypercalcaemia, and poor nutrition. Psychological factors such as anxiety and depression can exacerbate fatigue, as can co-morbid factors such as pain, poor sleep patterns, and infection. Many patients have concurrent diseases which can also cause

fatigue (e.g., cardiac failure). Travelling to hospital or the GP's surgery is very tiring if the patient is in anyway incapacitated.

All forms of cancer therapy have the potential to cause fatigue and in the case of chemotherapy and radiotherapy this can last for some weeks or months after the cessation of treatments. Treatment of cancer-related fatigue includes altering the patients activity to fit their ability. It should be explained that rest is not detrimental and can be very helpful, as it may allow for periods of well-being and greater activity.

Corticosteroids and progestogens may reduce fatigue, although the former needs to be used with caution. Other measures that may improve a patient's energy level include good nutritional and psychological support and the correction of anaemia and electrolyte imbalances.

Dysphagia

Difficulty in swallowing is a common problem with head and neck cancer or in oesophageal cancer. If pain is a causative

Table 4.5. Causes of breathlessness

Caused by disease	Specific treatment
Upper airway obstruction	Humidified air to reduce sticky secretions; consider tracheostomy if the cause is disease progression
Nasal obstruction	Surgery, stenting, or laser treatment
Superior vena cava obstruction	Radiotherapy or superior vena cava stenting
Lung metastases	Symptomatic treatment
Lymphangitis carcinomatosis	Trial of high-dose corticosteroids (12–16mg dexamethasone a day)
Pleural effusion	Aspirate and consider pleurodesis if recurrent
Associated with the disease	
Pulmonary emboli	Anticoagulation as long as bleeding is not a problem
Bronchopneumonia	Antibiotics and bronchodilators
Chronic obstructive airways disease	Bronchodilators

factor, management of this (including treatment of painful infections such as candida in the oesophagus) may allow increase in food intake. Where dysphagia results from an obstructive lesion or from damage to structures involved in swallowing, further management may be needed. An agreement should be made between the staff, the patient, and the carers as to what the feeding goal is. Advice should be given on liquidizing normal food, together with the prescription of food supplements as recommended by a dietician. Temporary feeding via a nasogastric tube may cover a period in which active management of the dysphagia using surgery or radiotherapy is undertaken. Feeding gastrostomy tubes are often placed endoscopically or under imaging when major head and neck surgery is to take place. These methods of feeding are rarely appropriate in a more terminal cancer patient.

Lymphoedema

Lymphoedema can occur in the limbs, trunk, genitals, or facial areas and is caused by damage to the lymphatics through progression of cancer, radiotherapy, or surgery. A concomitant hypoproteinaemia and venous obstruction can also aggravate the condition. Management of lymphoedema includes massage, skin care, support hosiery, and movement to keep the joints supple. It is essential to protect the skin and avoid damage. A lymphoedematous limb is particularly prone to infection, which can sometimes present insidiously. Slight redness and an increase in pain may be the only presenting signs. Where infection has occurred, antibiotics should be commenced rapidly with the intravenous route preferred in many instances. After two infections then prophylactic antibiotics are suggested.

Other complications of lymphoedema include discomfort and sometimes severe pain, together with altered function of a limb and an unacceptable appearance to the patient.

Management should include regular analgesia, and in some situations a trial of diuretics or corticosteroids could reduce the limb or facial swelling.

Breathlessness

Breathlessness is a common symptom in late cancer and is poorly treated. The range of the problem is from mild breathlessness after heavy exertion, to breathlessness that interferes with daily activity, such as dressing, to the most problematic and distressing, breathlessness at rest. Where a cause is known and treatment is possible and appropriate (e.g., drainage of a pleural effusion), this should considered (*Table 4.5*). However, often a specific cause cannot be found, but the most likely causes are chronic lung disease together with generalized weakness and debility. Anxiety is often a concomitant feature that makes the symptom worse.

For mild-to-moderate breathlessness advice on general coping methods can be given by an occupational therapist or physiotherapist. Relaxation therapies can be empowering. Pharmacological treatment includes reducing anxiety with short-acting benzodiazepines (lorazepam 0.5–1mg orally or sublingually q6h–q8h), or midazolam subcutaneously when more rapid treatment is required. Morphine given in small doses regularly may relieve breathlessness; 2.5–5mg q4h is a suggested starting dose. If the patient is already on morphine for pain, then increasing the regular morphine may help.

Fistulae

Fistulae are common between the oropharynx and the skin in head and neck cancer, and in abdominal or pelvic cancer between the bladder and bowel or between the bowel and vagina. A fistula may occur as a result of cancer treatment (surgery or radiotherapy), but more commonly it is a result of progressive cancer together with the side effects of previous therapies.

Management depends on the clinical situation. When the condition is not complicated by progressive cancer, the treatment is generally active with surgical excision of the fistula and bypass while healing occurs. When the cause is progressive cancer, surgery is rarely an option and care is focused on supporting the patient and reducing unpleasant symptoms.

Continual leakage of fluid onto the skin can cause excoriation, so barrier creams are essential. In head and neck cancer absorbent dressings can be applied and, if sialorrhoea (ptylism) is a complication, the use of hyoscine by the buccal or transdermal route may help. Fistulae between the bowel and vagina are problematic as the discharge is continuous and dressings are difficult to hold in place. An offensive odour may lead to isolation.

Changes in stool consistency may help reduce the output from a faecal fistula. Where there is constipation, keeping the stool soft may allow for more active bowel movements and less pressure on the weakened area. Where the stool is liquid, increasing the consistency with codeine phosphate 30–60mg q6h or loperamide 2mg q6h can be of benefit. If liquid loss continues on this medication, a trial of octreotide (somatostatin analogue) sc 300–600μg in 24 hours may improve the situation.

Wounds and Bed Sores

Patients with advanced cancer are at increased risk of developing pressure sores because of impaired vascular and lymphatic systems together with poor nutritional status. Skin over bony prominences is particularly affected, with the skin initially being reddened and sore and finally breaking down. Superficial lesions can be very painful.

The best management is to avoid the development of a skin break by regular passive or active movements and by pressure-relieving mattresses or cushions. These are readily available in the community. Once a bed sore occurs in a patient of this group, it rarely heals in spite of good nursing care.

Once a bed sore has developed, the mainstay is of relief of discomfort with regular analgesia and protective dressings.

The advice of specialist wound care nurses should be sought. Infection is a common occurrence and can increase pain severity. Systemic antibiotics may be appropriate in this situation. Colonization with anaerobes can lead to an offensive smell, which can be reduced by application of metronidazole gel.

Superficial bleeding can be reduced with alginate dressings and, if more severe, oral antifibrinolytic drugs such as tranexamic acid 1g q6h can be taken.

Mouth Care

The main mouth problem for a cancer patient is dryness (xerostomia) caused by a decrease in saliva, damaged oropharynx, and mouth breathing. Infection with candida is common and this, together with xerostomia, can cause taste changes. The reduction in saliva can be caused by drugs (e.g. opioids and anticholinergics) or arise from treatment of the disease with surgery or radiotherapy that results in damaged or absent salivary glands.

Improvement in symptoms with saliva substitutes (methylcellulose) or stimulants such as sugar-free chewing gum can improve a dry mouth. Good oral hygiene is essential and mouth infections should be sought and treated when they occur.

Fractures

Bone metastases are common in some malignancies and may be asymptomatic or cause pain. With a 30–50% destruction of the cortex of a long bone the risk of fracture is high and prophylactic pinning should be considered.

Where a fracture has occurred, treatment constitutes immobilization of the bone and administration of adequate analgesia. A decision as to whether surgical management is appropriate depends on the individual's clinical condition. A fracture of the humerus can be managed with a sling or by binding the arm to the chest. However, active management with pinning allows greater comfort on movement, as fractures caused by cancer rarely heal.

A fracture of the femur is generally managed surgically unless a patient is extremely unwell. Pain can be relieved for a short time by the use of a femoral nerve block, but an epidural gives better and continued pain control where surgery is not appropriate. After surgery, speed of rehabilitation is dictated by the health of the patient; unrealistic goals should not be set.

Pruritus

Pruritus (the urge to scratch) is caused by many things and aggravated by dry skin.

Cancer itself, as in Hodgkin's lymphoma, can cause itch, as can cholestatic jaundice and renal failure. A reaction to a drug such as morphine or infection with scabies is also a cause. Treatment of the condition, withdrawal of the offending drug, and treatment of infestation may lead to rapid relief (except scabies for which itch can last a long time after an effective remedy has been applied).

In all cases, practical advice such as moisturizing the skin with aqueous cream and avoidance of hot baths and soap should be given.

The general use of an antihistamine may be useful, but topical agents should be avoided. Other drugs reported to be of some benefit include histamine blockers such as cimetidine, corticosteroids, and the non-steroidal anti-inflammatory drugs. Ondansetron has been shown to be effective in the itch of renal failure and cholestatic jaundice.

Physical Methods of Improving Care

Improvements in the home situation may be the key factor to enable an ill patient to be managed at home. Use of specialist beds, hoists, commodes, and mattresses can ease the burden for the carers of a sick person. Equipment can be installed rapidly when required, but this needs input from each member of the multidisciplinary team, particularly the district nurse, physiotherapist, and occupational therapist.

End of Life

In the last days of life, good symptom control and psychological support for the patient, the family, and the carers becomes an imperative. A number of practical issues that may need to be addressed are given in the box.

Practical issues at the end of life

Incontinence
Sheaths or catheterization should be considered.

Restlessness
Causes such as pain, urinary retention and constipation need to be excluded. Therapies include the use of midazolam or levomepromazine if no cause is found.

Agitated delirium
Haloperidol, levomepromazine, or midazolam can be used.

'Death rattle'
To dry secretions hyoscine or glycopyrronium can be used.

Terminal haemorrhage
Patients should be sedated to relieve anxiety. Options include midazolam and diamorphine.

References and Further Reading

Twycross R. Symptom *Management in Advanced Cancer*. Abingdon: Radcliffe Medical Press, 1997.

Twycross R, Wilcock A, Thorp S. *Palliative Care Formulary*. Abingdon: Radcliffe Medical Press, 1998.

Doyle D, Hanks GWC, MacDonald N, eds. *Oxford Textbook of Palliative Medicine*. Oxford: Oxford Medical Publications, 1998.

Kayle P. *Decision Making in Palliative Care*. Northampton: EPL Publications, Meditec UK, 1999.

5 Psychological Aspects of Cancer in Primary Care

Douglas Russell

Cancer as a disease carries an incalculable burden of psychological morbidity for patients and their families and carers. One of the major contributions primary care can make is to address and minimize this morbidity.

Patients complain about lack of clarity from clinicians and difficulties in communication (National Cancer Alliance, 1996). Communication skills of doctors in particular were seen as particularly important, especially at the point of diagnosis, or when 'breaking bad news'. Patients want doctors to be sensitive, gentle, and honest. Doctors should avoid the use of euphemisms for cancer such as 'lump', 'growth', 'tumour', 'neoplasm', 'malignancy', '-oma', unless it is clearly established that the patient understands the terms. Patients want doctors not to be afraid of using the word 'cancer' even though pedantically the word carcinoma is only strictly correct for malignant neoplasms arising from epithelial tissue. It is not reasonable to expect patients to understand the precise variations in meaning and implication unless specifically explained.

Breaking Bad News

Patients are naturally extremely anxious at the point of diagnosis. They may have unrealistic beliefs and expectations. There may be myths and beliefs that need to be explored and discussed.

- Allow sufficient time
- Ensure that the discussion takes place with both physical privacy and aural privacy (i.e. out of hearing of others, and away from extraneous distracting noise)
- Encourage the patient to be accompanied by a relative or friend.
- Give a 'warning shot' to prepare the ground for bad news
- Be prepared to leave the patient (and family member or friend) alone for a while and come back and discuss matters again after an interval
- Be prepared to allow a second opinion; however,

be realistic about the balance between the need for a speedy decision and allowing a patient time to think
- Reinforce the discussion with written material. Published evidence shows that many patients find tape recordings of the interview helpful. The research showed that those with more hopeful messages listened to the tape up to eight times and those with less encouraging messages listened at least once or twice
- Be prepared for natural psychological and emotional reactions from patients and their families. Shock, disbelief, denial, anger and guilt are all recognized components of grief reactions. Such grief can be for a future that now no longer appears as expected. Anger can be directed inwards – guilt, self-blame – or externally – to doctors and health professionals. This can be particularly likely when patients believe that there has been delay in referral or diagnosis, which they perceive has adversely affected their chances of effective treatment
- Break bad news incrementally. Progress stepwise, allowing questions and clarification at each stage
- It can be a kindness to offer to speak to relatives, in-laws, parents and children on behalf of the patient. Such an offer to the patient may be appreciated
- Be prepared to give detailed information, particularly about treatment, timing, likely side-effects and measures to deal with them, and expected outcomes (although patient's responses to information vary – see below)
- Primary care clinicians should be cautious about giving definite survival likelihood figures. General statements based on the most recent cancer registry data can be used as a guide, but remember that survival depends on a number of factors – some general, such as socioeconomic status and coexisting disease, and some specific, such as tumour type and stage and hormone receptor

status. Cancer unit and cancer centre specialists are in a much stronger position to give details of current experience of best achievable results on the basis of clinical trials

- Avoid glib or patronizing statements, such as 'enjoy your remaining time'
- Do not remove all hope, as in 'there is nothing to be done'. The transition from curative to purely palliative care requires careful and tactful management
- Offer information sources and contacts (see Chapter 30)
- Do not just talk to the patient, but listen as well
- 'Check in' with the patient – feelings, reactions, further support information requirements, time to think and so on
- Be prepared to 'pick up the pieces' – if not yourself, then by offering support and contact with others, specialist nurses, counsellors, patient support groups, follow up appointments

Quantity of Information

Patients vary in how much information they want. One study in lung cancer (Meredith *et al.*, 1996) patients showed that:

- 95% wanted to know if their disease was cancer;
- 79% wanted as much information as possible;
- 15% did not want any information;
- 6% only wanted to know if the news was 'good';
- 91% wanted to know the chances of a cure;
- 86% wanted to know about all possible treatments; and
- 94% wanted to know about side-effects of treatment.

As far as who should give the diagnosis this same study showed that:

- 60% wanted it to be the hospital doctor;
- 14% wanted it to be the GP;
- 2% wanted it to be a nurse; and
- 24% expressed no preference.

Patient Attitudes

A qualitative study showed that patients varied in their attitudes, with older male patients wanting the least informa-

tion (Leydon *et al.*, 2000). The study was performed at a major UK cancer centre and describes three over-arching attitudes to cancer and strategies for coping with it that limited the patient's wish for further information.

Faith

Faith in the doctor's expertise and knowledge precluded the need for further information (apparently demonstrating continued value in the 'paternalist' model of patient doctor relationship).

Hope

Hope was considered essential for coping and could be maintained by avoiding potentially negative information (perhaps a form of denial).

Charity

Charity to fellow patients – including the recognition that scarce resources (including information and explanation) had to be shared, which meant that limited information was accepted as inevitable.

Intrapersonal denial and psychotherapeutic interventions was the subject of another study in which the outcome was decrease in denial in the intervention group while the control group had an increase in denial (Connor, 1992). Such differing messages from the evidence base emphasizes the importance of having a mutually negotiated and agreed model for the individual patient–clinician relationship. It is important to remember that even though the patient may not want immediate information, the same may not be true for relatives.

Ethical Models of Patient–Clinician Relationships

There is much emphasis in modern medicine on the autonomy of the individual patient – the so-called patient-centred approach. This constitutes the liberal ethical model of doctor–patient relationship. In the past the two dominant ethical principles affecting the doctor–patient relationship were *primum non nocere* – first do no harm (or non-maleficience) – and do the patient some good (beneficience). These two combine to form the paternalist approach, which can conflict with the patient-centred approach and which clinicians should now guard against adopting. Surveys of cancer patients show that they want information – much more than they are usually given. Patients also feel that doctors are sometimes callous or unfeeling in their dealings with patients. There is research evidence that doctors overestimate their effectiveness in patient communication, and also overestimate expected survival.

Some patient requests conflict with what a physician is allowed to do by law, or by professional codes. Euthanasia is such an example. Increasingly physicians are expected to take into account the financial and other finite resources available for health care. The principle of distributive justice, or equity, applies. This can be extremely difficult for specialists to bear when new treatments become available that are extremely expensive. Increasingly primary care have to become involved with deciding between conflicting priorities.

In negotiating with patients and their families and carers, obtaining consent is not just a matter of obtaining a signature on a consent form. Informed consent involves taking into consideration the views and mores of the patient and reaching a negotiated consent that is the shared model of the doctor–patient relationship.

Specific Psychological Problems

Many patients will wish to discuss alternative and complementary therapies. Although some such therapies remain highly controversial, it is important to value and respect the patient's autonomy in making choices. The clinician's job is to help to make those choices as well informed as possible.

Depression and anxiety are common in patients with cancer. More than a third of dying patients may be depressed, and more than half of patients with advanced cancer feel sad, anxious and irritable. Suicide rates are higher for the terminally ill than the general population. Antidepressants, cognitive and behavioural psychological interventions, anxiolytics and counselling should all be considered as part of the cancer care therapeutic armamentarium.

The usual instruments or questions and rating scales for use in the general population may not be appropriate for use in the cancer patient (e.g. reference to weight loss or appetite may be inappropriate). There are well validated instruments that are suitable (Cohen *et al.*, 1995; Portenoy *et al.*, 1994; Bruera *et al.*, 1991; EORTC, 1993).

Women who have been treated for gynaecological cancer are prone to problems with social adjustment and depression, and most are anxious about recurrence. There is consistent evidence for cancer patients in general that a variety of cognitive and behavioural techniques can be beneficial. Techniques such as relaxation training and education with information accompanied by counselling can reduce side-effects of therapy and alleviate psychological and functional disturbances.

A meta-analysis of 116 studies, based on data from 5236 patients with cancer, showed statistically significant benefits for intervention in all seven outcomes assessed (Devine and Westlake, 1995):

- anxiety;
- depression;
- mood;
- nausea;
- vomiting;
- pain; and
- knowledge.

Some research has demonstrated that some clinicians have difficulty in coping themselves with the psychological stress of communicating with cancer patients. This can exhibit itself by 'blanking' questions, avoidance, not listening or hurried conclusion of consultations. Clinicians require training in communication techniques with cancer patients, and they probably need those skills updated on a regular basis.

The UK National Health Service Executive has published Guidance on Commissioning Cancer Services, which has collected a large number of critically appraised published evidence on psychosocial interventions in cancer patients.

Readers interested in a more comprehensive list of references are directed to the Cochrane database of systematic reviews, and the set of Improving Outcomes in Cancer publications.

Sexual Problems

- Clinicians should not shy away from discussing sexuality with patients. It is natural for many patients to lose interest in sex during cancer treatment
- It is important to instigate symptom control and action to address anxiety and depression early in the patient's illness
- Patients with gynaecological cancer have particular problems, and advice from a palliative care nurse specialist attached to the cancer centre may help.
- Cancer charities have very helpful, patient-friendly leaflets and information websites that can be helpful
- Hormonal treatment can produce a premature menopause for women

- Treatment for cancer of the prostate can produce difficulties with ejaculation and erection, and even continence. Hormones used after primary treatment can cause flushing and impotence
- Radiotherapy and chemotherapy can have detrimental effects on sexuality and sex drive. Patients may well find this difficult to raise as a topic, but good cancer care should make it comfortable for then to do so

Cancer in Children

- Special skills are needed when dealing with children who have cancer, children of cancer patients, and also with adolescents
- Parents have particular difficulty in coping with a diagnosis of cancer for their child, and offering a second (or even third) opinion may help them while they adjust. Anger is very common at this stage, as is guilt. Parents will often blame themselves for delay caused by their not recognizing when the cancer began
- Telling children about cancer in terms they understand is difficult. Children are not miniature adults, and have different concepts about the world at different ages
- Separation and loneliness are particularly frightening to children under the age of 5 years. They should be reassured that parents will be back even when they leave for a short while

- Children will ask questions about death. Refusal to discuss questions may aggravate a child's distress
- Siblings will be affected by the diagnosis, and confusion and fear are common. Honesty and openness are the best policy. All children need to know that cancer is not contagious
- Authorities agree that continuation with schooling is vital. Increasing numbers of children survive cancer and they will need to be able to relate to their peer group and compete in an adult world
- Adolescents have particular issues. They perceive parental overprotection as undermining their emerging independence. Frustration with limitations imposed by the disease and the treatment regime may exacerbate a natural tendency to rebel against authority figures. This can include parents as well as members of the clinical team
- Patient support groups and charities have a lot of very useful information to help families through these very challenging situations

Useful websites

http://www.nhsdirect.nhs.uk
http://crc.org.uk/
http://cancerbacup.org.uk/
http://cancer.gov/cancerinformation
http://cancer.gov/cancerinfo/types/childhoodcancers

References and Further Reading

Bruera E, Kuehn N, Miller M J, Selmser P, Macmillan K. The Edmonton symptom assessment system (ESAS): a simple method for the assessment of palliative care patients. *J Palliat Care.* 1991; **7**: 6–9.

Cohen SR, Mount BMM, Strobel MG, Bui F. The McGill quality of life questionnaire: a measure of quality of life appropriate for people with advanced disease: a preliminary study of validity and acceptability. *Palliat Med. 1995:* **9**: 205–19.

Connor SR. Denial in terminal illness: to intervene or not to intervene? *Hospice J.* 1992; **8**: 1–15.

Devine E, Westlake S. The effects of psychoeducational care provided to adults with cancer: meta-analysis of 116 studies. *Oncol Nurs Forum.* 1995; **22**: 1369–81.

Leydon GM, Boulton M, Moynihan C, *et al.* Cancer patients information needs and information seeking behaviour: in depth interview study. *BMJ.* 2000; **320**: 909–13.

Meredith P, Symonds P, Webster L, *et al.* Information needs of cancer patients in West Scotland: cross sectional survey of patients' views. *BMJ.* 1996; **313**: 724–6.

Portenoy RK, Thaler HT, Kornblith AB, *et al.* The Memorial symptom assessment scale: an instrument for the evaluation of symptom prevalence, characteristics and distress. *Eur J Cancer.* 1994; **30**: 1326–36.

The European Organisation for Research and Treatment in Cancer (EORTC). Quality of Life Questionnaire (QLQ-C30): a quality of life instrument for use in international clinical trials in oncology. *J Natl Cancer inst.* 1993; **85** 365–76.

The National Cancer Alliance. *Patient-Centred Cancer Services. What Patients Say.* 1996.

Managing Side-Effects of Cancer Therapy

Kate Gregory and Andrew Tutt

Introduction

Unfortunately, many cancer treatments are associated with detrimental effects on patients. Chemotherapy can cause severe nausea and vomiting and hair loss, and may have implications for future fertility. Radiotherapy effects are more localized and depend on the site being treated, but long-term effects include second malignancies and infertility. Surgical treatments, too, can be mutilating and leave patients and their relatives having to struggle with feeding tubes and stomas. In this chapter we describe the main side-effects associated with cancer therapies and suggest strategies to manage them.

Chemotherapy

General side-effects

Many patients have a dread of receiving chemotherapy. They often know or have read about people who have suffered severe side-effects with treatment. Generally speaking, side-effects are preventable and many supportive measures can make treatment more tolerable. Side-effects of chemotherapy common to most agents are summarized in *Table 6.1*. More specific toxicities are outlined in *Table 6.2*.

Acute side-effects

Many of the acute side-effects of chemotherapy are common to the majority of agents. One of the side-effects that patients find particularly difficult to cope with is lethargy. This is a particularly difficult problem as there is no magic wand to be waved. It is obviously important to rule out infection, anaemia, or progressive disease (e.g. liver metastases) as a cause. Once this has been done, all that can be done is to reassure the patient that extreme lethargy and tiredness is a common side-effect of treatment.

Nausea and vomiting

Emesis is greatly feared by patients commencing chemotherapy. However, with the advent of the 5-hydroxytryptamine

Table 6.1. *General side-effects of chemotherapy*

Acute
Nausea and vomiting
Mucositis
Myelosuppression (neutropenic sepsis, need for transfusion)
Alopecia
Lethargy
Palmar–plantar syndrome
Peripheral neuropathy
Weight gain

Delayed
Cardiomyopathy (anthracyclines)
Infertility
Second malignancies

Table 6.2. *Toxicities of specific chemotherapy agents*

Acute	Effect
Cisplatin	Emesis, peripheral neuropathy, renal impairment
Taxanes	Alopecia, peripheral neuropathy
Vinca alkaloids	Peripheral neuropathy, jaw pain, constipation
Anthracyclines	Alopecia, cardiomyopathy (either idiosyncratic or dose-related)
Cyclophosphamide	Haemorrhagic cystitis
Mitomycin C	Haemolytic uraemic syndrome
Bleomycin	Lung fibrosis, hypersensitivity reactions
5-Fluorouracil	Palmar–plantar syndrome
Ifosfamide	Encephalopathy

Table 6.3. *Emetogenecity of chemotherapy agents in current use from the most emetogenic to the least*

Cisplatin

Mustine

Dacarbazine

Carboplatin

Dactinomycin

Cyclophosphamide

Daunorubicin

Cyclophosphamide (oral)

Epirubicin

Etoposide

Mitozantrone

5-Fluorouracil

Paclitaxel

Docetaxel

Mitomycin C

Methotrexate

Bleomycin

Melphalan

Vinblastine

Vincristine

Vinorelbine

($5HT_3$) antagonists, control of emesis should be possible for the vast majority of patients. Certain drugs, particularly cisplatin, are highly emetogenic (*Table 6.3*) and it is vital that patients receive adequate anti-emetic prophylaxis, since once emesis is established it can be difficult to control. A combination of intravenous dexamethasone (8 mg) and granisetron (1–3 mg) before chemotherapy and of oral metoclopramide (20 mg three times daily) and dexamethasone (2 mg three times daily) for 3 days after treatment is usually adequate to prevent nausea and vomiting. For patients who have significant problems despite this combination, consideration should be given to prescribing additional agents such as cyclizine (50 mg three times daily), lorazepam (1–2 mg twice a day), or methotrimeprazine (6.25–25 mg twice a day). If patients have persistent vomiting at home then they should be re-admitted to hospital to allow for the instigation of intravenous anti-emetics. Anticipatory nausea and vomiting can become a problem as a course of chemotherapy proceeds. Lorazepam (1–2 mg) taken the night before and on the morning of chemotherapy can be extremely effective in treating this problem.

Mucositis

Mucositis can be associated with any chemotherapy regime because of immunosuppression and the cytotoxic effect on a rapid turnover of oral mucosa. It is also more specifically associated with certain drugs such as methotrexate. To some extent it can be prevented by regular mouth care and the use of mouth washes, such as nystatin (1 ml four times daily) and chlorhexidine. For patients with established mucositis, sucralfate (5–10 ml four times daily) can speed the healing of ulcers. Paracetamol gargles or even oromorph can be used to control the pain. Oral candidiasis is a common problem and is best treated with fluconazole (50 mg once daily for 7 days).

Alopecia

The prospect of losing their hair is of great concern to many patients. Not all chemotherapy combinations cause alopecia; the main groups of drugs that cause hair loss are the anthracyclines (used in many combinations to treat breast cancer, lymphoma, small cell lung cancer, and myeloma) and the taxanes (used in ovarian and metastatic breast carcinoma). Commonly used drugs for the adjuvant treatment of bowel cancer and the treatment of non-small cell lung cancer do not tend to cause hair loss. In some institutions, methods of scalp cooling are offered to try and prevent hair loss. However, success is not guaranteed and it is usually advisable for patients to be counselled for hair loss and to have a wig organized at the beginning of their treatment. During chemotherapy it is not advisable for patients to have their hair chemically treated (permed or dyed) as this can further weaken the hair and lead to accelerated loss.

Bone marrow suppression

Neutropenia is one of the most potentially serious side-effects of chemotherapy. For most agents the nadir is at 7–10 days. Patients should be provided with information from their oncology centre as to the signs and symptoms to watch for and the action to take should these arise. Many hospitals encourage patients on chemotherapy to contact the unit directly. All patients on chemotherapy who present to their general practitioner (GP) with non-specific symptoms should have an urgent full blood count performed. Patients who are neutropenic and septic require urgent admission to a specialist unit for treatment with intravenous broad-spectrum antibiotics. Different units have different policies as to the management of non-septic neutropenic patients; in some centres patients are given prophylactic antibiotics (e.g.

ciprofloxacin or augmentin) to cover the period of neutropenia, in others patients are admitted for neutropenia, and in some units patients are given granulocyte colony stimulating factor (GCSF) to promote recovery of the neutrophil count. GCSF is administered subcutaneously; patients may complain of joint aches and pains, in which case paracetamol is usually the most effective treatment.

It is not advisable for patients to receive live vaccines during chemotherapy and for up to 6 months afterwards.

Anaemia is common in patients on chemotherapy and can have a marked impact on the quality of life. At present anaemia is managed with blood transfusion, but studies are ongoing into the potential role of erythropoietin in these patients. However, cost constraints are likely to make widespread use of this agent unrealistic.

Marked thrombocytopenia, such as is likely to cause significant bleeding problems, is unusual with standard-dose chemotherapy. Most units perform a platelet transfusion only when the platelet count is $<10 \times 10^9$, unless there is active bleeding or infection. In patients with chronically low platelets (e.g. after bone marrow transplantation), tranexemic acid can be used to prevent bleeding problems.

Palmar–plantar syndrome

Palmar–plantar syndrome (reddening/soreness and pain of palms and soles) is particularly associated with 5-fluorouracil (5-FU) treatment and may be so severe that patients can experience difficulty in walking. Pyridoxine at a dose of 50 mg three times daily can alleviate the condition somewhat, but in the more severe cases it is necessary to stop 5-FU if it is a continuous infusion, or a dose reduction may be necessary if the 5-FU is being administered intermittently.

Peripheral neuropathy

Peripheral neuropathy can be associated with the platinum drugs (particularly cisplatin), the taxanes (docetaxol and paclitaxel) and the vinca alkaloids (vincristine, vinblastine, and vinorelbine). Patients typically complain initially of pins and needles or tingling in the hands and feet, but the vinca alkaloids can also be associated with jaw pain and paralytic ileus. There is no specific treatment for the neuropathy and patients may require dose reductions or even a change of drugs if their symptoms are severe or progressive. The neuropathy should improve on halting treatment, but complete resolution does not always occur.

Delayed side-effects of treatment

Fortunately, the majority of the side-effects of chemotherapy, while unpleasant, are reversible and short-lived.

However, a few potentially very serious long-term side effects of treatment can have a very profound impact on a patient's quality of life.

Infertility

Infertility is a potential complication of any combination of chemotherapy, although it is more likely to occur in patients who receive high-dose chemotherapy. For male patients, sperm banking should be discussed if future fertility is likely to be an issue. This can be organized urgently if the need to commence treatment is pressing. For female patients the situation is more complicated; if a patient is in a stable relationship and treatment is not urgent, then embryos can be preserved. New experimental techniques in egg retrieval and ovarian biopsy may provide options in the future, but at the present time these are not widely available and their success is uncertain.

For most patients who have been treated for cancer it is generally advisable to wait for 2 years after completion of treatment before contemplating trying for children. This is partly because the effects of chemotherapy on the developing ovum and sperm are unknown, but also to ensure the cancer has been successfully treated.

Anthracycline-induced cardiomyopathy

Anthracyclines can cause a dilated cardiomyopathy, either as an idiosyncratic reaction or as a dose-dependent phenomenon. Patients who receive concurrent radiotherapy to the cardiac region are more prone to this. Liposomal anthracyclines may be less cardiotoxic and are undergoing trial at the present time. Patients who develop this complication are best treated under the guidance of a cardiologist with angiotensin-converting enzyme (ACE) inhibitors and diuretics, but the outlook is poor.

Second malignancies

Second malignancies are a rare complication of previous chemotherapy and radiotherapy. Patients treated with alkylating agents may be particularly prone to developing secondary myelodysplastic syndrome and leukaemias.

Hickman lines

Although not strictly speaking a side-effect of chemotherapy, patients are increasingly being sent home with central access lines in situ. These are inserted for a number of reasons, including the administration of continuous-infusion 5-FU, to facilitate the administration of chemotherapy in patients with poor venous access and in patients on long programmes of chemotherapy (e.g. in the treatment of leukaemia). Skin-tunnelled catheters are most commonly used in this setting, as this removes the exit site from the entry point in the vein and thus reduces the risk of infection. Nevertheless, the main complication of these lines remains infection and the line should always be considered as a potential source of sepsis in these patients; with any infection a prompt referral back to the oncology centre for treatment and removal is essential. The other main problem associated with these lines is thrombosis. Suspicion is raised by pain in the arm and shoulder, swelling and erythema, and distended superficial veins. The presence of a clot is best demonstrated by ultrasound or a linogram. The majority of centres use low-dose anticoagulation (e.g. warfarin 1 mg once daily) to try to prevent this complication.

Radiotherapy

General side-effects

In contrast to chemotherapy, radiotherapy is delivered to a specific region of the body. Side-effects are usually limited to this region and vary according to the site, total dose, and size of each individual treatment-dose delivered. The total doses referred to in this chapter are generally given in fractions of 2 Gy. Palliative treatments require side-effects to be minimal. They deliver a few relatively large radiotherapy fractions that result in a low total dose and minimal inconvenience to the patient. Curative (radical) treatments must deliver much higher doses to be successful and are given in many small fractions to improve the therapeutic ratio. Except in the treatment of lymphoma, seminoma, and some childhood tumours, this therapeutic ratio is narrow and a balance must be struck between an increasing prospect of radiotherapy cure with increased dose and an acceptable risk of long-term side-effects.

Patients are often concerned at the prospect of treatments that involve radiation and assume they will suffer the full spectrum of side-effects associated with total body irradiation (TBI). This is not the case. Most acute side-effects can be ameliorated with good supportive care. A risk of serious long-term complications of >5% is generally considered unacceptable by most oncologists. Improvements in radiotherapy delivery that allow three-dimensional shaping of radiation fields to the tumour volume and the use of smaller, more frequent radiation doses may significantly improve the therapeutic ratio in radical treatments.

Table 6.4. *Acute and intermediate side effects of radiotherapy at specific sites*

Site	Acute	Intermediate
Skin	Erythema Dry desquamation Moist desquamation Hair loss	Mild oedema
Oral cavity	Dry mouth Mucositis	
Upper aerodigestive tract	Mucositis Dysphagia	
Mediastinum and thorax	Transient obstruction caused by tumour oedema	Pneumonitis – dry cough and dyspnoea
Abdomen	Nausea Small bowel enteritis	
Pelvis	Small bowel enteritis Cystitis Proctitis	
Lower pelvis and perineum	Proctalgia Vaginal mucositis Perineal desquamation	
Central nervous system	Raised intracranial pressure caused by tumour oedema Nausea	Somnolence syndrome

Specific side-effects

From a patient's perspective it is most useful to categorize side-effects dependent upon the area irradiated and the natural history of symptoms.

Side-effects usually occur in three distinct phases:
- acute – occurring during or within 6 weeks of treatment;
- intermediate – 6 weeks to 6 months after treatment; or
- late – more than 6 months after treatment.

The acute and intermediate side-effects of radiotherapy at several common sites are summarized in *Table 6.4*. Some acute side-effects may occur despite the lower doses delivered for palliation. Significant late side-effects from palliative treatments are very rare because of the low radiation dose and the patient's often limited life expectancy.

Acute side-effects

Skin

Erythema and desquamation

Modern radiotherapy spares the epidermis from receiving the full tumour dose. Radical or adjuvant radiotherapy doses are generally in the range of 35–65 Gy and cause acute erythema within both the beam entry and exit sites. This occurs within 3 weeks and may progress to areas of dry and then patchy moist desquamation. It is worst in areas of maximum skin dose, within skin creases, and in areas exposed to friction (e.g. the inframammary fold, natal cleft, and perineum). Skin does not repair until after the completion of radiotherapy and no evidence supports the routine use of antibiotics, talcs, and creams. Early management is aimed at symptom alleviation. Contrary to popular belief, it is perfectly acceptable to wash the treated areas with a mild soap, but the areas should be dried without rubbing. Aqueous cream may prevent skin dryness, and cotton or Lycra underwear reduces friction. Hydrocortisone 1% cream can reduce itching and therefore exacerbation of the reaction through scratching, but it should not be used on areas of moist desquamation. Some creams contain metal ions and should not be used as they increase skin dose. Commonly used skin-care guidelines are given in *Table 6.5*. Significant skin reaction is rare with palliative treatments.

Table 6.5. *General skin care guidelines*

Creams	All patients who have radical treatment to their breast, mastectomy site, buttocks, axilla, groin, face, head, neck, or genital areas are given moisturizing cream or aqueous cream to be applied at least twice daily to their treatment area from the start of treatment. The frequency may be increased as the skin becomes drier.
Hygiene	The treatment area can be washed carefully. The skin within the treatment area should be patted, not rubbed, dry. If the patient has treatment marks that need to be preserved, this must be explained. Patients may still wash with their usual soap and water, unless this stings, in which case they should use a milder soap. Hair can be washed gently using the usual shampoo, even if the hair is in the treatment field. For patients who have treatment marks on the scalp, hair washing must be discussed on an individual basis. An electric razor is best if patients wish to continue shaving an area within the treatment field.
Clothing	Clothing that covers the treatment field should not cause friction (e.g. bras and belts).
Specific guidelines for radiation-damaged skin	
Pruritus	For patients with intractable pruritus 1% hydrocortisone can be used twice daily. It should be used sparingly after the moisturizer.
Erythema	Continue to apply the moisturizing cream generously and as frequently as the patient wishes until the skin returns to its normal state.
Moist desquamation	For slightly exuding moist desquamation continue to use moisturizing cream and cover with a non-adherent dressing. Other dressings to consider are Jelonet together with a non-adherent dressing, or Granuflex.
Heavily exudating wounds	Dress with a hydrophilic dressing (e.g. Allevyn) and change only when 'strike-through' occurs. No creams should be used with this dressing. (NB: Patients who continue to receive treatment have dressings removed during the treatment to prevent an increase in skin dose.)

Hair loss

Hair loss occurs at skin doses of 5–10 Gy or more, and therefore occurs with both curative and palliative treatments. Loss occurs within the area of beam entry or exit and begins 2 weeks after the start of therapy. At palliative doses or the curative doses for lymphoma or seminoma, hair regrowth begins 8–9 weeks after treatment. At skin doses of >50 Gy, which occur in some curative treatments, loss is likely to be permanent and cannot be prevented.

Upper aerodigestive tract

Mucositis

Mucositis is the dominant acute toxicity associated with the treatment of cancers of the head, neck, and mediastinum. The oral mucosa has the most rapid cell turnover and mucositis therefore occurs after 10–14 days. Oesophageal mucositis begins a little later. Symptoms become maximal in the final week of treatment and the following week, and then rapidly resolve over the next 2–3 weeks. It is crucial to maintain good mouth care and good fluid and nutritional intake. Edentulous patients should clean dentures daily, but wear them as little as possible. The mouth should be cleaned with sponge sticks. Dentate patients should continue to brush their teeth twice daily with a mild fluoride toothpaste. Pain control should be aggressive. Topical aspirin gargles, aspirin in a mucilage vehicle, and mucaine may be used, but systemic opioid analgesia is often required. Candidal infection should be excluded and treated if necessary with nystatin (1 ml four times daily) or fluconazole (50 mg once daily) until the mucosa has healed after radiotherapy. Saline is a useful regular gargle, but mouthwashes that contain alcohol must be avoided. The drinking of spirits and smoking also worsens mucositis. Patients must be weighed weekly and assessed by a dietician. Temporary enteral feeding should be started in those patients who do not maintain their weight.

Xerostomia

The irradiation of some volume of the major salivary glands is almost unavoidable in the treatment of both head and neck cancer and in Mantle field irradiation for Hodgkin's disease. This leads to a noticeable dryness of the mouth within the first week of therapy. It is usually possible to avoid bilateral total parotid irradiation, and therefore subsequent compensation by other glands occurs. Reduced salivary flow makes good mouth care essential and the services of a dental hygienist are useful.

Pneumonitis

Pneumonitis is not strictly an acute event as it occurs between 6 weeks and 6 months after therapy in those who have had >10% of their lung volume irradiated. It may occur in both radical and palliative lung cancer treatments and in the treatment of extensive intrathoracic lymphoma. It is a rare (<3%) complication of modern breast and chest-wall radiotherapy for breast cancer. Pneumonitis is the major dose-limiting toxicity for TBI in the context of bone marrow transplantation.

Patients present with dry cough, dyspnoea, and occasionally fever. There is usually an infiltrate, strictly limited to the irradiated volume, on chest radiographs. The severity of symptoms depends on baseline lung function, but it is usually mild. The mainstay of treatment is a reducing course of corticosteroids. Symptoms are transient and resolve over a few weeks. In those treated with TBI, pneumonitis may contribute to transplant mortality.

Transient tumour oedema in a large intraluminal lung or oesophageal tumour may cause obstruction and worsen the symptoms. This can be prevented or treated with a short course of dexamethasone.

Abdominal irradiation

Abdominal irradiation is rarely performed in a radical context, except for the treatment of infra-diaphragmatic lymphoma or testicular seminoma. Partial abdominal irradiation occurs with the palliative treatment of spinal metastases, bulky para-aortic lymph node metastases, and tumours of the pancreas and kidney.

Acute enteritis

The small bowel is the major acute dose-limiting structure. Single palliative treatments of <8 Gy and small-volume fractionated treatments usually produce few symptoms because of the daily mobility of the small bowel. Reduced bowel mobility (caused by the presence of adhesions) or treatment with larger volumes lead to an acute enteritis. Maintenance of good fluid and electrolyte intake, reduction of green vegetable intake, and the judicious use of codeine phosphate or loperamide is required. Symptoms reduce over 2–3 weeks following therapy. Severe symptoms may require a treatment break, but this must be weighed against any detrimental effects on tumour control.

Nausea and vomiting

Abdominal irradiation can induce moderate nausea and vomiting. This can be prevented effectively with use of metoclopramide, domperidone, or cyclizine. In severe cases, $5HT_3$ antagonists provide superior control to other agents.

Pelvic irradiation

Low-dose palliative treatments for pelvic bone metastases usually produce very few side-effects. Radical radiotherapy for bladder, prostate, rectal, or cervical cancers is associated with acute toxicity because of the irradiation of at least partial volumes of adjacent organs.

Radiation enteritis
Radiation enteritis may occur particularly in those who have had previous abdominal or pelvic surgery, as discussed above.

Radiation cystitis
Frequency, dysuria, and occasionally stranguria may occur 4–6 weeks into radical treatment courses that involve the bladder, bladder base, and prostate. Symptoms are identical to those of bacterial infection, which is commonly associated, and so a weekly midstream urine sample is taken. Treatment is symptomatic.

Radiation proctitis
Radiation proctitis most commonly occurs in the radical treatment of prostate cancer, and more rarely following intra-cavitary radiotherapy for cervical cancer. Patients may complain of anal pain, tenesmus, and passage of mucous per rectum. Symptoms begin 4–6 weeks after starting therapy and resolve over 2–6 weeks after therapy. Topical anaesthetic creams and suppositories such as cinchocaine with prednisolone are helpful. Preparations containing metal ions or bismuth should be avoided.

Acute perineal and vaginal reactions
Where possible the penis and scrotum are taped out of the radiation field and are shielded. Vaginal mucositis may lead to vaginal adhesions and is treated prophylactically with a daily vaginal douche. Where pelvic fields extend inferiorly, skin reactions are often worst in the natal cleft, perianal region, and the vulva. Twice-daily shower cleansing and application of Drapolene are helpful. Anal soreness may be helped with a topical local anaesthetic cream such as cinchocaine with prednisolone. Soft cotton or Lycra underwear absorbs sweat and reduces friction.

Haematological toxicity
Haematological toxicity is not usually significant as most radiotherapy fields include small marrow volumes only. Large-volume treatments, such as those used for supra- or infra-diaphragmatic Hodgkin's disease or large spinal or pelvic fields treated during or shortly after chemotherapy, may cause marrow suppression. The full blood count is checked and patients are rested from treatment using criteria similar to those used for chemotherapy-induced marrow suppression.

Central nervous system irradiation
Nausea and vomiting
Nausea and vomiting is rare in the absence of increased intracranial pressure, which must always be excluded. Acute tumour oedema may occur early in the treatment and should be treated aggressively with dexamethasone 16 mg daily in divided doses. Osmotic diuresis is rarely required. Large fractions of palliative radiotherapy (>4 Gy) may induce nausea, which is managed with anti-emetics as described above.

Exacerbation of spinal cord compression
Exacerbation of spinal cord compression may arise from tumour oedema early in the treatment, and should be prevented by prophylaxis with dexamethasone. Worsening symptoms prompt reconsideration of neurosurgical spinal decompression.

Somnolence syndrome
Somnolence syndrome is not strictly an acute complication as it tends to occur 4–6 weeks after cerebral radiotherapy. Patients complain of somnolence and lethargy, caused by transient white matter demyelination and oedema. The symptoms usually last for 1–2 months and may be helped by a reducing course of dexamethasone.

Late or delayed complications of radiotherapy
The scope of this chapter precludes a detailed discussion of this subject and we concentrate on the least rare complications, their prevention, and management.

The maximization of the therapeutic ratio between tumour control and late complications is central to modern radiotherapy. This relies on the combination of high-energy, skin-sparing irradiation, sophisticated three-dimensional treatment planning that minimizes normal tissue irradiation with the use of small daily treatment doses. As a result many patients' fears of the severe radiotherapy complications suffered by older relatives are now thankfully unfounded.

Skin
A degree of subcutaneous fibrosis and subsequent cutaneous telangiectasia and atrophy occur after skin doses of >60–65 Gy. This may occur following the treatment of skin tumours, in the area overlying the tumour bed following breast radiotherapy, and in skin overlying the macroscopic tumours in the head and neck.

Skin necrosis is very rare. Trauma or surgical incision within heavily irradiated skin may lead to a necrotic ulcer. Other predisposing factors are advanced age, diabetes, and irradiation of the skin over the back and lower limb. Management of a necrotic ulcer is conservative and involves eradication of underlying infection, and improvement in both diabetic control and tissue oxygenation. Surgical debridement must be avoided unless excision margins extend into unirradiated skin.

Upper aerodigestive tract

Oral cavity

The most common late complication is xerostomia. Meticulous treatment planning to minimize parotid irradiation is essential, but dryness is sometimes unavoidable. Artificial saliva may provide relief, but some doctors favour pilocarpine. A handy small bottle of mineral water is a simple alternative. Good mouth care and regular attendance at a dental hygienist prevent the onset of caries.

Osteoradionecrosis of the mandible occurs to various degrees in 2–10% of patients with tumours of the oral cavity treated with radical radiotherapy. It is imperative that any necessary dental extraction is carried out before treatment. Dental extraction following radiotherapy should be undertaken only after consultation with the head and neck oncology team, as the risk of necrosis rises dramatically. Small areas of necrosis settle with conservative measures.

Oesophageal stenosis

Return of dysphagia may result from tumour occurrence, but fibrotic stenosis may occur after radical treatment of oesophageal or centrally sited lung tumours. Dilatation or stenting provides relief.

Lung

The dominant late complication is pulmonary fibrosis within the treatment field, which may occur after both radical and palliative treatments. Careful patient selection before treatment and good radiotherapy planning should prevent significant new respiratory symptoms.

Occasionally haemoptysis may occur several years after successful radical therapy because of bleeding from a telangiectatic intraluminal vessel. Haemoptysis earlier than this usually indicates recurrence.

Abdominal and pelvic complications

Small bowel

The low total radiation doses used in large-field treatments of seminoma and abdominal lymphoma are not associated with significant long-term complications. If abdominal adhesions tether the small bowel within the small high-dose volume used to treat pelvic tumours, regions of permanent small bowel damage may result. This often requires no more than a reduction in dietary bulk, but in 1–2% of patients surgical correction of an area of stenosis may be required. Meticulous radiotherapy planning reduces this risk.

Bladder

Radical radiotherapy to the whole bladder causes a reduction in overall bladder capacity, which is commonly noted by patients after an extensive transurethral bladder resection in particular. Superficial mucosal telangiectasia may cause intermittent haematuria, which should always prompt exclusion of an underlying recurrence.

Prostatic radical radiotherapy may be complicated by urethral stricture in 3–4% of patients. As the risk is greatest in patients who have had previous transurethral prostatic resection, such radiotherapy should be avoided in patients known to have prostate cancer.

Rectum

High-dose radiotherapy >65–70 Gy to the anterior rectal wall may (rarely) occur following radical prostate radiotherapy or intracavitary therapy for cervical cancer. This can lead to intermittent rectal bleeding and mucous discharge. In rare severe cases (<1%) rectal injury may require surgical intervention. Usually, conservative management is sufficient and symptoms gradually settle over months or a few years.

Sexual function

Radical radiotherapy to the vagina in cervical and vaginal carcinomas leads to vaginal dryness and can cause stenosis, adhesions, and consequent impairment of sexual function. Regular use of a vaginal douche during therapy and regular use of a vaginal dilator after the acute mucositis settles can avoid stenosis and adhesions. If regular sexual intercourse resumes after therapy dilators are unnecessary. The use of vaginal lubricant is usually required.

Male erectile dysfunction occurs as a result of radical prostate radiotherapy in approximately 30% of men, but the exact risk is difficult to assess for any particular age group. Overall, these figures compare favourably with radical prostatectomy. Interstitial radiotherapy techniques currently under evaluation seem to reduce further the risk of impotence. The use of silenafil or sublingual apomorphine may be appropriate (endorsed SLS).

Female fertility

Radiotherapy doses used for adjuvant and radical radiotherapy to the pelvis cause infertility and early menopause. Pelvic radiotherapy in women is most commonly given for gynaecological malignancy, which may preclude subsequent pregnancy in any event.

For cases in which ovarian irradiation is minimal (<1.5 Gy), as in the context of para-aortic nodal irradiation for lymphoma, ovarian function is usually preserved. If nodal irradiation extends into the pelvis, but the ovarian dose can be reduced to <5 Gy by ovarian transposition and shielding, ovarian function may be preserved in some younger women. Embryo storage may be appropriate for some woman.

Male infertility

Radiation doses >2–3 Gy to the testis produce permanent azoospermia. The testes are usually protected from the scattered radiation of abdominal or pelvic fields by their enclosure in lead gonad shields. Nevertheless, patients are offered sperm banking where there is any concern about the testicular dose.

Couples are usually advised to avoid conception for 1 year after therapy when the gonadal dose is thought to be significant. The evidence to support this practice is scarce.

Discussion of the effects of cranial irradiation on fertility is beyond the scope of this chapter.

Neurological complications

Radiation brachial plexus injury

Thankfully, radiation brachial plexus injury, a complication of supraclavicular and axillary radiotherapy, is now exceedingly rare (<1%). Modern radiotherapy practice minimizes the risk of overlap of treatment fields and emphasizes the need for small doses per fraction. Patients are no longer treated with a full axillary dissection and radiotherapy. The concomitant use of chemotherapy and radiotherapy is also avoided in those who receive axillary radiotherapy.

Radiation transverse myelopathy

Radiation transverse myelopathy is also extremely rare (<1%), as the total radiation dose to any point in the spinal cord can be predicted accurately and limited.

Risk of second malignancy

There is a very small increased incidence of tumours following large-volume radiotherapy at any site. This risk is significantly less than 1% and must be set against a requirement for the best therapy to eradicate the patient's present tumour. There is greater concern for an increased risk of breast cancer in women irradiated in their teens and early twenties for Hodgkin's disease using 'Mantle field' radiotherapy techniques. These women may require follow-up in a breast clinic. They are also particularly at risk for smoking-induced lung cancer and should be advised accordingly.

Further Reading

Laufer MR. Reproductive issues for cancer patients/survivors (editorial). *J Clin Oncol.* 1999; **17**: 2631–2.

Livesey EA, Brock CGD. Gonadal dysfunction after treatment of intracranial tumour. *Arch Dis Child.* 1998; **63**: 495–500.

Muscari EL, Aikin JL, Good BC. Premature menopause after cancer treatment. *Cancer Pract.* 1999; **7**: 114–21.

Radford JA, Shalet SM, Lieberman BA. Fertility after treatment for cancer. *BMJ.* 1999; **319**: 935–6.

Sussman N. Reactions of patients to the diagnosis and treatment of cancer. *Anticancer Drugs.* 1995; **6 (Suppl 1)**: 4–8.

Principles of
Cancer Care

7 Cancer Prevention

Douglas Russell and Gareth Davies

It is easy to be tempted into a nihilistic view of the potential return of efforts directed at cancer prevention, but epidemiological studies suggest links between cancers and possible avoidable causes. Many cancer prevention strategies require macro-interventions at population or governmental level and, although there is increasing evidence that interventions at the personal level can make a difference, in relatively few cases is there a scientifically proven cause and effect link. Nevertheless, two out of three cancer deaths may be preventable.

The public is exposed to information overload in the media and many of the messages are contradictory and confusing. There is also massive interest in 'alternative' medicine. In the scientific press our state of knowledge is in flux, since published trials can produce conflicting results. Clinical staff need to develop their critical appraisal skills in order to give patients the best advice, and primary care organizations should ensure that clinicians and patients have access to reliable sources of unbiased, expertly evaluated information. Increasingly, such access is available via the NHS net.

Aetiology

20 years ago, Doll and Peto (1981) estimated the proportion of cancer deaths attributable to various (potentially avoidable) causes (*Table 7.1*). This was an early attempt at quantifying the environmental contribution of factors such as diet, tobacco, alcohol, occupation and radiation to cancer causation.

Cancer has a complex causation but at least four basic factors are involved:

- inherited genetic abnormalities;
- viruses;
- ionizing radiation; and
- chemicals.

In addition, some cancers are hormone-sensitive or hormone-dependent and alterations or defects in normal immune mechanisms may promote certain cancers.

The fact that not all people who have an inherited autosomal-dominant genetic mutations predisposing to cancer develop the disease (incomplete penetrance) was explained by the 'two-hit' hypothesis, using retinoblastoma as the model. This early explanation of a rare cancer has evolved into the 'multi-hit' theory of cancer causation, in which multiple steps are required in a cascade of events leading to the malignant transformation of a cell. There appear to be a number of distinct processes associated with carcinogenesis. In one model, the following series of events can be envisaged:

1. Exposure to the relevant agent
2. Metabolism of the agent
3. Interaction between the agent and a cell constituent – most importantly, DNA ('initiation')
4. Repair of DNA damage, death of the cell or persistence and replication of a clone of abnormal 'damaged' cells
5. Growth of the abnormal clone into a focus of pre-neoplastic cells ('promotion')
6. Growth of the tumour and its spread to other parts of the body ('progression')

For cancers associated with radiation (both ionizing and ultraviolet) and viruses the mechanism may be different.

Table 7.1. *Proportion of cancer deaths attributable to various causes*

Causative factor	Estimated proportion of cancer deaths attributable to factor (%)
Smoking	30
Diet	35
Alcohol	3
Sexual behaviour	7
Occupation	4
Industrial products	<1
Medical procedures	1
Geophysical factors (including ultraviolet light)	3
Infections	Uncertain

Genetics

The main genetic associations of clinical relevance in primary care concern with breast cancer, ovarian cancer and colon cancer (particularly familial adenomatous polyposis (FAP) of the colon), and hereditary non-polyposis colorectal cancer (HNPCC).

In the past few years there have been great advances in our understanding of the biology and chemistry underlying sporadic cancers and the inheritance of familial cancers. This new knowledge, and continuing advances in genetics flowing from the human genome project, is likely to cause a significant shift of emphasis in primary care with regard to cancer. A list of 2000 patients in primary care will have 40–50 people with at least one first-degree relative affected by breast, ovarian, endometrial or colorectal cancer at any one time, and inevitably a proportion of these cases will have a hereditary component.

Genetic counselling servcies are being introduced but primary care will increasingly have a gatekeeper role in identifying those people at increased risk and arranging their referral, while containing inappropriate demand for genetic services. It follows that detailed family history taking is an increasingly important task in primary care for managing the appropriate use of the cancer genetic services.

Prevention

Cancer prevention includes primary and secondary prevention:

- primary prevention involves measures to stop the disease process before it starts (e.g. avoiding environmental ot dietary elements linked to an increased cancer risk);
- secondary prevention involves detecting the disease in a precancerous or treatable stage early in its course when cure is achievable.

Primary care health teams (PCHTs) should include cancer prevention within their own health promotion programme. Primary care organizations (primary care groups or trusts and local health groups) should have cancer prevention as a major part of their health action plans and health improvement programmes. It is likely that the role of primary care will shift from a diagnosis, referral, treatment and support function to a cancer predicting and cancer prevention service. This fits well with the anticipatory care model at the heart of family practice. PCHTs already hold chronic disease registers for asthma, diabetes and coronary heart disease. A practice cancer register is a logical next step, together with a register of those with a significant family history of cancer. Agreement and standardization on clinical terming and coding conventions will become necessary.

Many important cancer prevention actions act at a higher population level than the PCHT. These include:

- taxation of tobacco and alcohol;
- advertising restrictions or bans on tobacco advertising;
- restricting sponsorship by tobacco and alcohol companies;
- environmental health, and health and safety legislation; and
- radiation regulation.

Primary care organizations will need to form alliances with other local agencies to affect determinants of health in relation to cancer but within the context of prevention strategies for other diseases.

Smoking cessation

One out of every two smokers will die from smoking-related disease, most of them in middle age; cancer and cardiovascular disease are the two most common causes of smoking-related deaths. Cigarette smoking causes 80–90% of all lung cancer. It is also implicated in the causation of cancers of the bladder, uterine cervix, stomach, oesophagus, oropharynx, kidney and pancreas and in leukaemia. Overall, smoking in the UK is estimated to be strongly associated with 33% of all cancer deaths.

The single most important and effective health improvement measure that primary care can undertake is to assist existing smokers to stop and in reducing the adoption of smoking by young people. It is estimated that 23% of 11-year-olds in England have tried smoking. This rises to 63% of girls and 59% of boys by the age of 15 years. Nicotine is highly addictive and addiction to nicotine is usually established in adolescence, with only 10% of new smokers starting after age 18.

All patients should have their smoking status recorded and regularly updated. Note should be made of passive smoking in non-smokers. A record of 'non-smoker' may disguise the fact that the person has stopped the day before after 20 years of smoking and may start again a week later. 'Never smokers' after the age of 25 are unlikely to start smoking.

In the UK, male smokers are declining in numbers but the number of young female smokers is continuing to rise. This is likely to result in changes in causes of death (e.g. it is expected that lung cancer will overtake breast cancer as the leading cause of death from cancer in women in the UK early this century). Rises in female deaths from lung cancer are already being reported in the USA.

Brief advice from a doctor (approximately 3 minutes) has been shown to lead to 2% of patients stopping smoking at 1 year. Increasing the duration of the advice (10 minutes) can double the effect to 4%. Individual and group counselling and behaviour modification can help smokers to stop. Proactive telephone counselling can also help but it is not as effective as face-to-face interventions. Adding nicotine replacement therapy (NRT) can nearly double the effectiveness of advice fom health professionals to 8%. Inhalers and sprays appear better than patches, which in turn appear better than gum.

Self-help materials used alone do not appear to be effective in helping patients to stop smoking. There is insufficient evidence of effectiveness to recommend acupuncture, hypnosis, antidepressants, anxiolytics, aversive therapy (including silver acetate) or nicotine antagonists in smoking cessation.

Workplace-based initiatives have good success rates, with long-term average cessation rates of 13%. Anti-smoking media campaigns produce small changes in the proportion of smokers but do so in large populations. Every 1% increase in the real (inflation-adjusted) price of cigarettes leads to a fall in consumption of 0.5%. Unfortunately this does not appear to hold true for the most deprived social groups, where consumption remains constant.

Since June 2001 all types of NRT have been available on NHS prescription in England. Patient group directives is a recently introduced mechanism that enables other health professionals engaged in smoking cessation support to make NRT available to patients without them having to see a doctor for a prescription.

Bupropion has been shown to be helpful in selected highly motivated people. It is an antidepressant but is not used for this purpose in the UK. It may be more effective if used in combination with NRT. Patient motivation should be assessed before it is prescribed and it should be started while the patient is still smoking. The patient should set a 'quit date' within the first 2 weeks of treatment. After 3 days the dose will need to be increased. An assessment of progress and compliance should be made midway through the 8-week course of treatment. Even if a patient fails to quit on the first attempt, it may be worth considering a repeat attempt at a later date after reassessment of patient's motivation. As with any drug, bupropion should only be used in accordance with the manufacturer's data sheet.

Both bupropion and NRT have been found to be effective only in conjunction with structured support and advice, both of which can help to prevent weight gain that otherwise might occur on smoking cessation.

Pregnant women who smoke should be identified and offered individual prenatal counselling on smoking cessation as part of routine antenatal care. Pregnant women are more likely to give up if given personally tailored advice from health professionals. Prenatal counselling of about 10 minutes, including individual advice, from a health professional with self-help material can double cessation rates from 8% to 15%.

Alcohol

Alcohol is mainly associated with an increased risk of cancers of the oral cavity, pharynx, larynx, oesophagus and liver. Alcohol intake is measured in units, each assumed to contain 8–10 g of alcohol. One unit of ethanol is one half pint of beer, one glass of wine or one single pub measure of spirits (one-sixth of a gill). Some beers, particularly 'export' lagers, are stronger. 'Beer' is meant to be no more than 4% alcohol by volume. Many wines are stronger than 11% alcohol by volume. A 'glass' of wine is one-sixth of a 700 ml bottle. Spirits vary in strength as does the size of a 'measure'. Spirit single measures are one-twenty-sixth of a standard 700 ml bottle of no more than 37% alcohol by volume.

Patients should be advised to limit their intake to 14 units per week for women and 28 units per week for men. There is some evidence that a small regular intake of alcohol may have benefits in the prevention of cardiovascular disease. Consumption is best spread out evenly over time rather than in binges.

Brief interventions have been shown to be effective in persuading patients to moderate their intake. Case records in primary care should be regularly updated to show the level of alcohol intake. Most patients when asked will underestimate their intake. Use of the four-point 'CAGE' questions has been shown to be effective in identifying patients at increased risk of alcohol-related disease or social problems:

- Has your alcohol consumption been **Criticised**?
- Have comments about your drinking made you **Angry**?
- Have you felt **Guilty** about your drinking?
- Have you ever needed an **Eye-opener** in the morning?

Patients with a positive response to two questions are at increased risk of alcohol-related ill health. Three or four positive responses indicates a very high probability of alcohol-related health problems.

Diet and exercise

The American Institute for Cancer Research published a review of a global perspective on the evidence for and against elements of diet and cancer in 1997. It suggested that the correct diet, an ideal body weight (body mass index of 20–25) and physical activity (brisk exercise lasting at least 30 minutes three times weekly) could reduce cancer risk by 30–40%. A diet rich in fruit and vegetables may confer protection against many types of cancer. The normal advice is to eat five portions of fruit and/or vegetables daily which amounts to approximately 440 g (or 16 ounces).

Diets thought to increase the risk of cancer are those that include a high fat content; smoked, cured or pickled foods; excessive salt; and mouldy foods (where carcinogenic toxins may develop). Calories from fat should make up no more than 30% of the total intake. High-fat diets are particularly linked with cancer of the prostate and with colorectal cancer.

Many of the claims made for the protective effects against cancer of diet and exercise remain controversial. A recent large study of dietary fibre supplementation failed to show an expected reduction in the risk of developing colon cancer, and it is clear that more research is needed before categorical statements can be made. There is a large study in progress involving 400 000 people in nine European countries (EPIC) who are being followed prospectively to establish links between diet and cancers.

However, it still seems sensible to continue to support healthy eating and exercise as a general lifestyle health promotion because this will have a beneficial impact on other diseases such as cardiac disease and diabetes, in addition to a possible impact on the incidence of cancer.

Food supplements

Food supplements are not a substitute for a healthy diet but might be necessary in certain clinical situations of impaired eating or convalescence. Excessive supplementation may indeed be harmful (e.g. selenium). One study in lung cancer patients who smoked showed that increasing beta-carotene (vitamin A) intake worsened prognosis. However, low dietary levels of vitamin A and beta-carotene are associated with increased levels of lung cancer. No convincing evidence exists for specific protective effects against lung cancer for antioxidant micronutrients (vitamins A, C and E and selenium). Patients should be cautioned against fad diets and

supplements promoted at high cost that promise cancer prevention or cure.

Sunlight exposure

Exposure of the skin to ultraviolet radiation in sunlight is associated with an increased risk of skin cancers. People with fair skin with freckles and moles, particularly if they have fair hair and blue or grey eyes, are most vulnerable. People who have dark hair and eyes who tan easily without burning are at less risk. People with pigmented skin are least at risk of skin cancer. The message from experts is clear:

- avoid recreational sun exposure;
- there is no such thing as a safe tan;
- whenever possible stay in the shade;
- when sun exposure is unavoidable, give priority to clothing; and
- sunscreens are to be used as an adjunct on body areas that cannot be protected by clothes or a hat.

This advice, although clear, may be an oversimplification. Fair-skinned people with intermittent skin exposure appear to be at more risk than those who work outdoors all day. The intensity of sunlight and ultraviolet radiation varies with the degree of filtering by the atmosphere, and latitude, altitude and time of day are also important since they all affect the amount of ultraviolet light reaching the skin. It should be remembered that reflection of sunlight from water or snow can increase ultraviolet exposure.

Many specialists remain wary of the long-term use of sunbeds. Patients must weigh up the risks and benefits of tanning, and if they choose to use sunbeds they should pay careful attention to the manufacturer's safety instructions.

The use of sunscreens is also considered controversial by some, in that they may confer a false sense of security in susceptible people. Sunscreens can give the false impression that if they are applied it is safe to sunbathe. Sunscreens should last 2 years if stored below 25° C. It is probably wise, however, to replace a susncreen each year.

Infections

HIV infection is associated with malignancy (see Chapter 28).

The immature uterine cervix may be particularly sensitive to human papilloma virus types 16 and 18, which are postulated as being linked to increased risk of cancer of the uterine cervix. Age of first sexual experience is declining: 50% of 16-year-old girls are sexually active in the UK, and significant numbers of 14-year-olds will have had more than one sexual partner. Primary care team promotion of safe sex messages and encouragement of the use of condoms could have cancer prevention effects as well as the effects on the reduction of sexually transmitted diseases and teenage pregnancies.

There is evidence that homosexual males practising anal intercourse are more at risk of anorectal cancer.

Schistosoma haematobium infection is associated with bladder cancer in parts of Africa and the Middle East. There is now a vaccine available against schistosomiasis.

Hepatitis B and C are associated with hepatic cancer. Hepatitis B can be immunized against but not all patients will seroconvert. It is worth giving a booster immunization after the initial course but if seroconversion still fails then further immunization is not advised.

Screening

Screening for cancer is discussed in Chapter 9.

Body awareness

Patients are encouraged to take responsibility for themselves and their own health. Public education to encourage body awareness seeks the advantage of early recognition, presentation, referral and treatment. The hope is that more cancers will be detected at an earlier stage, with consequently smaller tumours, less likelihood of extension to surrounding tissues, less likelihood of metastasis and better chances of improved outcomes. PCHTs are well placed to promote body awareness in the course of new patient registration checks, routine medical examinations, in well man clinics and well woman clinics, and health promotion clinics.

Chemoprevention

Female hormones may reduce the risk of ovarian cancer but conversely may slightly increase the risk of breast cancer.

Tamoxifen and other agents continue to be under investigation as a chemoprevention agent in breast cancer. Recent results are conflicting and a large trial (IBIS) is in progress to try and resolve the question. Tamoxifen is associated with a small increase in the incidence of endometrial cancer.

Non-steroidal anti-inflammatory drugs are reported to be associated with a reduced risk of colon cancer.

Ionizing radiation

Ionizing radiation can cause cancers, and there is concern that patients should not have too many X-ray examinations, particularly repeated contrast media studies. Radio-isotopes are a source of radiation that can vary significantly in effect depending on the type of radiation – alpha, beta or gamma.

Alpha-particle radiation externally does not penetrate very far through skin but can have very much greater effects if ingested, injected or inhaled. Radon gas is an environmental radiation source that is more common in areas built on granite, and some houses may need modification. Repeated investigations have failed to demonstrate causal links between nuclear power stations and clusters of leukaemia; however, potential risks exist and scrupulous safety standards are required.

Survivors of cancer who have been successfully treated by radiotherapy may be at increased risk of other cancers later in life. The risk is increased if chemotherapy and radiotherapy are used together.

Radiologists, radiographers, dental staff, laboratory and science workers, wherever there is radiation exposure, need special safety measures to protect them.

The most recent report of the National Radiation Protection Board suggests there may be some small elevation of relative risk due to high-intensity electromagnetic fields, but the absolute risk is still very small.

Occupational risk

Certain industries carry occupational exposure risks that may put workers at increased risk of cancers. Bladder cancer is associated with certain industrial exposures such as rubber, cable manufacture and certain dyes. Occupational exposure to benzene is associated with leukaemia. Exposure to other hydrocarbons may increase the risk of lung cancer. Workers underground may have increased exposure to radon.

It is the responsibility of employers and employees in these situations to ensure that all health and safety procedures are soundly established and scrupulously observed.

Cancer-Site-Specific Prevention Messages

Lung

- Do not start smoking
- Stop existing smokers from smoking
- Avoid passive smoke exposure
- Avoid asbestos
- Avoid radon
- A diet high in fruit and vegetables may reduce risk
- A diet high in fat and alcohol possibly increases risk
- Physical activity and vitamins C and E possibly reduce risk, although evidence is weak

Breast

- Encourage full participation in national screening campaign. Outcomes are substantially improved by early detection. Mammography is the most effective method for detecting these early malignancies
- Being overweight is a breast cancer risk factor for post-menopausal women
- Genetic risk assessment for earlier mammography and regular assessment may be appropriate (see Chapter 8)
- A diet high in fruit and vegetables may reduce risk
- Age of first pregnancy affects risk, as does age at menopause
- Tamoxifen may assist in prevention

Oropharynx

- Do not smoke
- Restrict alcohol consumption to moderate intake
- Smoking and alcohol combined as risk factors explains 90% of oropharyngeal cancers
- Closer integration of dentistry into primary care teams is desirable to enable early identification of mouth cancers
- Advise against the chewing of beetle nuts

Oesophagus

- Do not smoke
- Restrict alcohol consumption to moderate intake
- Long-standing gastro-oesophageal reflux and duodenal ulceration is associated with Barrett's oesophagitis, with risk of adenocarcinoma of oesophagus

Stomach

- Do not smoke
- Eat plenty of fruit and vegetables
- Moderate consumption of smoked or heavily salted foods
- Eradicate *Helicobacter pylori*

Colon and rectum

- Genetic risk factors exist (see Chapter 8)
- Long-standing severe ulcerative colitis (≥10 years) is associated with a high risk of cancerous change
- High-fat, high-red-meat, low-fibre diets appear to be associated with increased risk, although it is not clear which, if any, of these are aetiological
- Obesity, alcohol, physical inactivity (colon only) may be associated with increased risk
- Folic acid may be protective
- Non-steroidal anti-inflammatory drugs (including aspirin) appear to have a protective effect. Early results suggest that the new generation of cyclo-oxygenase II inhibitors may have a stronger colon cancer protecting effect than cyclo-oxygenase I inhibitors
- Many colon cancer specialists believe that there is emerging good evidence to support a national screening programme of regular colonoscopy supplementing faecal occult blood testing. This is not yet official policy in the UK

Liver

- Restrict alcohol consumption to moderate intake
- Avoid hepatitis B and C; immunization is available against hepatitis B

Kidney

- Do not smoke
- Obesity may increase risk

Bladder

- Do not smoke
- Certain occupations carry risk of industrial carcinogen exposure
- In the developing world, *Schistosoma haematobium* infection is a risk factor, and can be immunized against

Prostate

- Prostate specific antigen (PSA) testing in asymptomatic men has not been advised hitherto as a population screening method. At the time of writing the government is encouraging wider availability of the PSA test as part of an individual risk assessment following a consultation and history and examination
- Digital rectal examination, transrectal ultrasound, and PSA are reasonable investigations in symptomatic men

- Many more prostate cancers have been diagnosed in recent years, but it is by no means certain that therapeutic zeal is preferable to watchful waiting in patients with non-metastatic disease
- Trials are under way to establish the benefits of combined digital rectal examination and PSA

Testis

- Early detection by self-examination should be promoted as a preventative measure
- Early treatment is highly successful

Cervix

- Invasive cancer is preceded by precancerous change that can be detected by cervical smear screening
- Risk is substantially reduced in non-smokers and in smokers who stop as compared with smokers who continue
- Early commencement of sexual intercourse and possible infection with human papilloma virus 16 and 18 may be associated with increased risk
- A diet high in fruit and vegetables may be helpful in reducing risk

Ovary

- Genetic risk (see Chapter 8)

- A national screening trial is under way
- Extended use of the contraceptive pill is protective

Endometrium

- Obesity and prolonged use of unopposed oestrogen in hormone replacement therapy (HRT) increase risk
- All prolonged oestrogen HRT should now contain some progestogen
- Tamoxifen causes a small increase in incidence

Skin and melanoma

- Sunburning, particularly in children, must be avoided. There is insufficient evidence to determine whether early detection through routine skin examination decreases deaths
- Ultraviolet avoidance measures should be adopted

Lymphoma

- Previous HIV infection is a risk factor
- Previous cancer treatments or immunosuppression for a previous transplant increase risk
- The new tumour necrosis factor alpha-blocking drugs for rheumatoid disease and Crohn's disease carry a theoretical long-term increased risk of lymphoma

References and Further Reading

Doll R, Peto R. The causes of cancer. *J Natl Cancer Inst.* 1981; **66**: 1191–308.

Effectiveness Matters Vol. 3 Issue 1 March 1998.

Emery J, Murphy M, Lucassen A. Hereditary cancer: the evidence for current recommended management. *Lancet* 2000; 9–16.

Food Nutrition and the Prevention of Cancer: a Global Perspective. World Cancer Research Fund and the American Institute for Cancer Research, 1997.

Guidance on Commissioning Cancer Services. Improving Outcomes in Lung Cancer: the Research Evidence. Smoking cessation. Clinical practice guideline no. 18. Catalogue number 97CC123 June 1998. Agency for Health Care Policy and Research.

Heller T, Davey B, Bailey L (eds). *Reducing the Risk of Cancers.* Hodder and Stoughton, 1989.

IARC Handbook of Cancer Prevention, vol 1. Non-steroidal anti-inflammatory drugs. Lyon: International Agency for Research on Cancer.

Ommenn GS, Goodman GE, Thornquist MF, *et al.* Risk factors for lung cancer and for intervention effects in CARET, the beta-Carotene and Retinol Efficacy Trial. *J Natl Cancer Inst.* 1996; **88**: 1550-9.

Osborne M, Boyle P, Lipkin M. Cancer prevention. *Lancet.* 1997; **349(suppl II)**: 27–30.

Powles T, Eeles R, Ashley S, *et al.* Interim analysis of the incidence of breast cancer in the Royal Marsden Hospital tamoxifen randomised chemoprevention trial. *Lancet* 1998: **352**: 98–101.r

Pritchard KI. Is Tamoxifen effective on the prevention of breast cancer? *Lancet.* 1998; **352**: 80-1.

Sowden A, Arblaster L. Community interventions for preventing smoking in young people (Cochrane Review). In The Cochrane Library; Oxford: Update Software.

8 Heredity and Cancer

Gillian Mitchell and Ros Eeles

Introduction

Cancer is a common disease, affecting up to one-third of the population at some time during their lives. All cancer can be termed 'genetic', as cancer is caused by genetic mutations (alterations in the DNA code) that result in abnormal cellular growth and/or proliferation. The majority of these mutations are sporadic (only occur in the cancer cell) and only a small proportion of these cases (approximately 5–10%) result from the inheritance of an alteration in a cancer predisposition gene. This alteration will be present in every somatic cell and, on average, in half the gametes (a gamete contains only half of the total genes), and therefore can be passed on to a proportion of the offspring. These mutated cancer predisposition genes have a well-defined pattern of inheritance. Approximately a further 20% of cancer cases can be described as familial, that is a clustering of cancer cases within the family, but these do not show a well-defined pattern of inheritance. Such cases may arise from the chance clustering of common cancers, the inheritance of genes that are associated with only a slightly increased cancer risk, or the sharing of common environmental influences, or they can be of multifactorial origin, possibly as a result of the inheritance of genes that render an individual more susceptible to environmental influences. This chapter focuses on cancer predisposition genes and discusses patterns of inheritance, cancer risks associated with these genes, and the management of suspected gene carriers. The chapter starts with the identification of suspected mutation carriers of cancer predisposition genes and the management of individuals at increased risk of cancer in the general practitioner's (GP's) surgery and concludes with the role of cancer genetic clinics and the testing process for cancer genes.

Cancer Predisposition Genes: Inheritance and Mechanisms of Action

Cancer predisposition genes are mutated genes, the normal function of which is to regulate cell growth or the detection and/or repair of DNA damage. These are germline muta-

tions and are present in all nucleated cells and therefore can be passed onto subsequent generations. The risk that a cancer predisposition gene gives rise to the development of cancer is called the penetrance, and the fact that many of these genes do not universally result in cancer development is termed incomplete penetrance.

Cancer predisposition genes can be associated with syndromes that predominantly consist of clustering of cancers at either one or multiple associated sites (*Table 8.1*). Other genetic syndromes are associated with an increased risk of cancer in addition to other, non-malignant features of a syndrome, such as neurofibromatosis (*Table 8.2*). The ability to recognize the clustering of cancers at different sites as part of a syndrome is important in the recognition that a cancer predisposition gene may be present in a family.

Inheritance

Inheritance of germline mutations in cancer predisposition genes may be either dominant or recessive at the genetic level, or X-linked. We all carry two copies (alleles) of every gene, one copy from each parent, and as only one allele can be passed down to the next generation, there is a 50:50 chance as to which allele is inherited (*Fig. 8.1*). In dominant inheritance (*Fig. 8.2*) the presence of a single mutated allele is usually sufficient to cause the associated disease, and approximately 50% of all offspring develop the disease. In recessive inheritance (*Fig. 8.3*) the presence of a single mutated allele is not usually sufficient for disease expression, which requires two mutated alleles (i.e. both parents have to carry the disease allele to produce an affected offspring). The majority of cancer predisposition genes are recessive at the cellular genetic level. They tend to act phenotypically (the physical or biochemical effect of the genotype) in a dominant manner, as frequently a sporadic mutation occurs of the remaining normal allele in a somatic cell during the lifetime of the germline mutation-carrier (*Fig. 8.3*). In X-linked inheritance the mutated gene is carried on the X-chromosome (*Fig. 8.4*).

Mechanisms of action

Cancer predisposition genes can be oncogenes, tumour suppressor genes, or mismatch repair genes.

Table 8.1. *Syndromes associated with increased risk of malignancy in which the major feature associated with the syndrome is the development of cancer*

Syndrome name	Malignancies	Risk (%)[a]	Mode[b]	Chromosomal location[c]	Gene name
Melanoma	Melanoma	53	D	9p	CDKN2 (P16)
Familial polyposis coli	Large bowel cancer	~ 100	D	5q	APC
	Cancer of upper gastro-intestinal tract	5			
	Desmoid tumour	20			
Breast/ovary cancer syndrome	Breast	85	D	17q	BRCA1
	Ovary	60			
	Colon	6			
	Prostate	6			
Site-specific breast cancer	Breast (female)	85	D	13q	BRCA2
	Ovary	27			
	Prostate	14			
	Breast (male)	5			
	Pancreas	4			
	Other cancers, e.g. cutaneous and ocular melanoma, gall bladder, bile duct, fallopian tube, stomach	<1			
Hereditary non-polyposis colorectal cancer (HNPCC) (Lynch syndromes)			D	2p	hMSH2
				3p	HMLH1
				2p	hMLH6
				3p	TGFβ
				2q	PMS1
				7q	PMS2
Lynch type 1	Site-specific colon only	70[d]			
Lynch type 2	Colon	70–80			
	Endometrium	43			
	Ovary	9–19			
	Gastric/biliary tract				
	Transitional cell carcinoma of the renal pelvis				
	Melanoma	<10			
	Head and neck				
	Brain				
	Small bowel				
Muir–Torré syndrome	As HNPCC with skin lesions				
	Keratoacanthoma/sebaceous cysts		D	2p	hMSH2
Turcot's syndrome	Brain tumour	?	? D/R		hMSH2
	Very early onset colon cancer (<20 years) with café-au-lait patches				hMLH1
					APC
					PMS2

Table 8.1. *(contd.)*

Syndrome name	Malignancies	Risk (%)[a]	Mode[b]	Chromosomal location[c]	Gene name
Hereditary prostate cancer	Prostate	85	D/R/X-linked	1q 1p Xq 17p	HPCI, PCAP CAPB HPCX HPC2
Li–Fraumeni syndrome	Sarcoma	24 childhood cancer	D	17p	TP53
	Early-onset breast cancer Brain tumour Leukaemia Adrenocortical tumour Other cancers	Overall cancer risk, 74 in men, 95 in women			
Multiple endocrine neoplasia type 1	Parathyroid, endocrine pancreas, pituitary	70–90	D	11q	MEN1
Multiple endocrine neoplasia type 2	Medullary carcinoma of thyroid	70	D	10q	RET
	Phaeochromocytoma (type 2A)	50			
Retinoblastoma	Retinoblastoma Osteosarcoma Other cancers	90 6 8	D	13q	RB1

[a]The risk is either the 'lifetime risk', as quoted in the reference articles, or the 'risk to age 70 years' in those studies which have performed detailed age-specific calculations. Where possible, risks by set ages or a 'per site' risk is given; in the absence of such figures a 'syndrome' penetrance estimate (overall risk of cancer development) is provided. These risks are approximate and may vary between different populations with different mutation profiles.
[b]Mode of inheritance is classified as 'autosomal dominant' (D) or 'autosomal recessive' (R).
[c]Chromosomal arms: q – long arm; p – short arm.
[d]Some studies suggest a lower penetrance in women.

Oncogenes

Oncogenes are mutated normal genes (proto-oncogenes), in which mutation tends to cause a 'gain in function' effect, resulting in increased growth or proliferation of the affected cells. Most oncogenes tend to act in a dominant manner and include the *ret* oncogene in the multiple endocrine neoplasia (MEN) 2A syndrome or *met* oncogene in familial papillary renal cancer.

Tumour suppressor genes

Tumour suppressor genes are normal genes in which mutation tends to cause a 'loss of function' effect in the control mechanisms of growth and/or cellular proliferation pathways. Most cancer predisposition genes are tumour suppressor genes and are inherited as recessive genes, but express a dominant phenotype.

Mismatch-repair genes

Mismatch-repair genes [hereditary non-polyposis colorectal cancer (HNPCC) syndrome] maintain the integrity of the genome and mutations in them permit acquired genetic damage to accumulate, which results in the creation of a cancer cell.

Cancer Risks Associated with Cancer Predisposition Genes

Cancer risks depend on the specific cancer predisposition gene and penetrance (see above). Penetrance is influenced by the population under study and by the sensitivity of the mutation testing technique, and it may be confused by the pres-

Table 8.2. Some of the 'rare' genetic syndromes associated with an increased risk of malignancy and their mode of inheritance

Syndrome	Neoplasia or malignancy	Risk (%)[a]	Mode[b]	Chromosomal location[c]	Gene name
Neurofibromatosis type 1	Plexiform neurofibroma, optic glioma, neurofibrosarcoma	4–5	D	17q	NF1
Neurofibromatosis type 2	Acoustic neuroma (vestibular schwannoma)		D	22q	NF2
	bilateral	85			
	unilateral	6			
	Meningioma	45			
	Spinal tumours	26			
	Astrocytomas	4			
	Ependymomas	3			
Von Hippel–Lindau	Cerebellar haemangioblastoma	35–84	D	3p	VHL
	Retinal angioma	41–70			
	Renal cell carcinoma	25–69			
	Phaeochromocytoma	15			
	Renal, liver, and pancreatic cysts	16–50			
Ataxia telangiectasia	Lymphoma	60	R	11q	ATM
	Leukaemia	27			
Bloom syndrome	Many sites	80	R	15q	BLM
	Immunodeficiency				
Cowden syndrome	Breast cancer	30–50	D	10q	PTEN
	Thyroid cancer	15			
	Bowel cancer	?3			
	Multiple hamartomas of skin, tongue and bowel	100			
Basal cell naevus/ Gorlin's syndrome	Basal cell carcinoma	80	D	9q	PCTH
	Ovarian fibroma	17			
	Medulloblastoma macrocephaly	4			
	Falx calcification, bifid ribs,	85			

[a]Lifetime risk of neoplasia or cancer.
[b]Mode of inheritance is classified as 'autosomal dominant' (D) or 'autosomal recessive' (R).
[c]Chromosomal arms: p – short arm; q – long arm.

ence of phenocopies (the presence of cancer in a non-mutation carrier that has occurred through chance alone). Phenocopies are a particular problem in syndromes associated with common cancers such as breast cancer. Different ethnic populations tend to have a different gene penetrance, and therefore it is essential to ascertain the genetic origin of the patient before formal genetic counselling is initiated.

Tables 8.1 and 8.2 summarize the current penetrance, or risk, estimates associated with known cancer predisposition genes.

Risk assessment

This is arguably the most difficult part of cancer genetic counselling, firstly to arrive at a risk estimate and, secondly, to convey this information in the most appropriate manner to

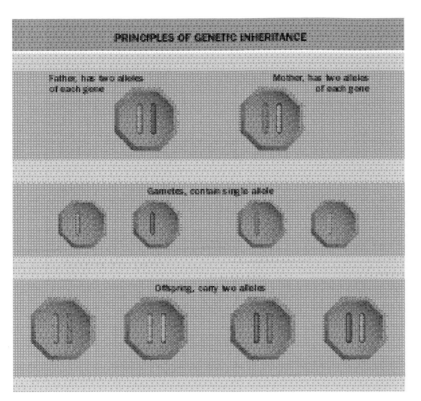

Figure 8.1. Principles of genetic inheritance.

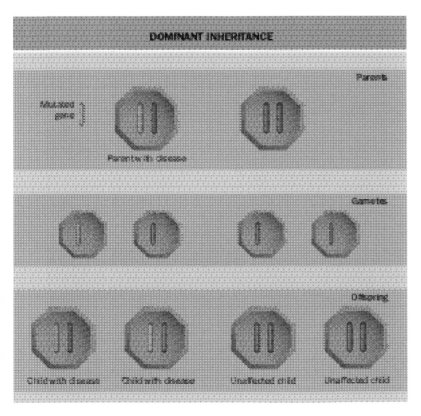

Figure 8.2. Inheritance of a dominant mutation.

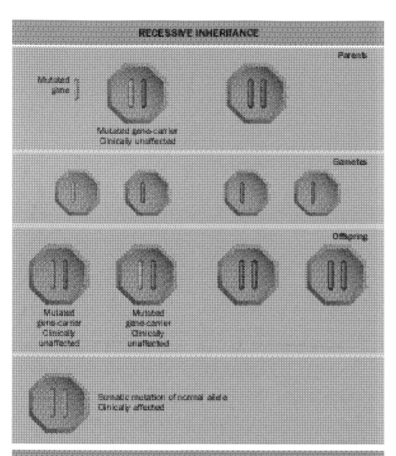

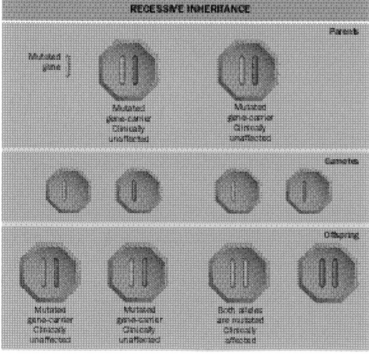

Figure 8.3. *(a) Inheritance of a recessive mutation. Only one parent carries the mutated allele. The disease phenotype is observed only if a further somatic mutation occurs in the remaining 'normal' allele. (b) Inheritance of a recessive mutation. Both parents carry a mutated allele.*

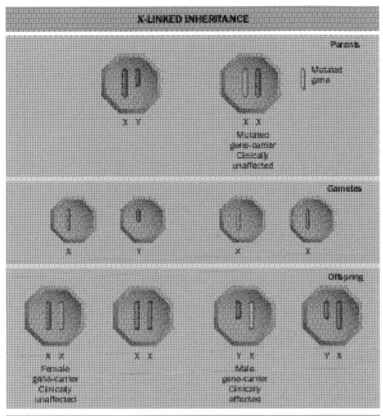

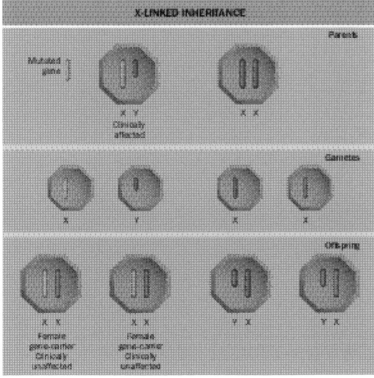

Figure 8.4. *(a) Inheritance of an X-linked mutation, mother carries the mutated allele. (b) Inheritance of an X-linked mutation, father carries the mutated allele.*

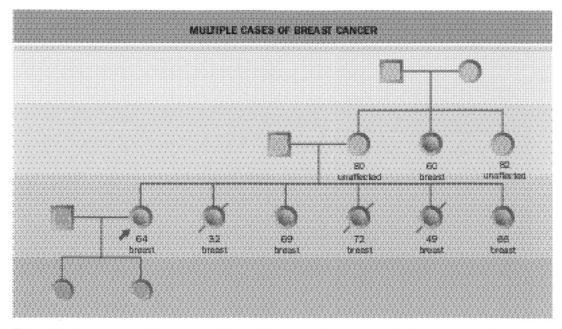

Figure 8.5. A complex family history demonstrating multiple cases of breast cancer. Numbers are age at diagnosis, or current age if unaffected.

the individual so that he or she can understand and retain the information and not be made unduly anxious about the risks.

The first risk estimation is the chance that a familial cluster results from genetic predisposition. The second estimation is the chance the individual has inherited a particular gene based upon his or her position in the family tree, whether the individual is affected by cancer, and his or her current age. The final estimate is the chance that cancer will develop if a gene has been inherited. These calculations can be complex, particularly if there are multiple generations to consider, and there may be intervening unaffected individuals between affected individuals, as demonstrated in *Figure 8.5*. Laptop computer software packages are now available for many of these calculations, but they are very model-dependent and so knowledge of any problems with the models is very important to determine whether the risks are over- or under-estimated.

Expressing these risks in a form that is meaningful for the consulting individual is difficult. It can be seen from above that risk estimation is complex and can be explained in various ways, as outlined in *Table 8.3*. The optimum format for conveying risk information is unknown. Currently, risk estimates tend to be given as a percentage risk or a '1 in x' value and followed up with a written summary to the individual of the genetics consultation, which incorporates this risk estimate.

Management of a Known or Suspected Cancer Predisposition Gene Mutation-Carrier

The general practice clinic

An individual at genetic risk must first be identified. There are many potential sources of identification, including consultations with a GP or a hospital clinic while under treatment for an associated disease, through an individual's concern of a potential genetic problem in his or her family, or through conversation with an associated professional such a practice or clinic nurse, radiographer, or doctor. Unless an individual expresses concern about his or her perceived risk, the only way an at-risk family could be identified is by systematic questioning of all patients about a family history of cancer while eliciting a general medical history, in addition to a general professional knowledge about cancer predisposition genes and disease patterns that maybe associated with them. Many surgeries take a familial history as routine assessment when registering a new patient. As a quick guideline, taking a history of all first-degree relatives only (parents, siblings, and children) and then asking if there are any cancers in other members of the family will detect 95% of familial syndromes.

Table 8.3. *Methods of presentation for cancer risk estimates*

Method of presentation	Expression of risk
Numerical	Risk per year
	Risk by certain age
	1 in *x* value or percentage format
	Relative risk corrected for age
General categorization	High/moderate/low risk
Situational analogy	A situation carrying an equivalent risk without any numerical information (e.g. the chances of picking an ace if one card is chosen at random from a card pack)
The risk figure measure	Risk of developing cancer
	Risk of not developing cancer/Risk of death from cancer (this is rarely given in clinics as it is perceived as too distressing)

It is not currently possible, or appropriate, to see all individuals with a family history of cancer in a cancer genetics clinic because of the limited availability of resources. Therefore it is important that local cancer genetics clinics provide guidelines for referral (see *Table 8.4* for the Royal Marsden Hospital NHS Trust genetics clinic referral guidelines for 2001); these will vary according to local resources for genetic and cancer services and current medical practice. The genetics clinic may also suggest appropriate management plans for individuals at increased risk of cancer, but not a sufficiently high risk to warrant referral to a specialist centre. This is particularly true for breast cancer, which is a common disease, and could result in many referrals to genetics clinics precipitated by anxious women with only a moderately increased risk of breast cancer. A GP is in an ideal situation to counsel these moderate-risk women and to initiate mammographic screening via the local breast unit. The main difficulty is for the GP to make an assessment of the level of genetic risk. Guidelines are helpful, and a number of computer software packages are now

Table 8.4. *The Royal Marsden NHS Trust familial cancer clinic referral guidelines*

Breast cancer families

- Single case <40 years if of Ashkenazi Jewish origin
- Two cases of breast cancer diagnosed under the age of 50 years
- Three cases of breast cancer diagnosed under the age of 60 years
- Four or more cases of breast cancer diagnosed at any age
- Breast cancer and ovarian cancer; this includes the case where a patient develops both cancers
- Any male breast cancer cases with a relative affected with breast cancer (male or female)

Ovarian cancer families

- Any family with two or more cases of ovarian cancer
- Any family with ovarian cancer and any of colorectal, endometrial, or breast cancer diagnosed under the age of 50 years

Colon cancer families

- Families with three or more cases of the following: colorectal cancer and either endometrial cancer and/or ovarian cancer and/or breast cancer
- Single cases of colorectal cancer diagnosed under the age of 45 years

Prostate cancer families

- Any family with two cases of prostate cancer of which one is diagnosed under the age of 65 years
- Families with three or more cases of prostate cancer at any age

Li–Fraumeni families/Li–Fraumeni-like families

- Childhood cancer or sarcoma/brain tumour/adrenocortical cancer diagnosed under 45 years with first- or second-degree relative with sarcoma/breast cancer/brain tumour/leukaemia/adrenocortical cancer at any age and another first- or second-degree relative with cancer diagnosed under 60 years
- Sarcoma at any age with two of the following in first- or second-degree relatives: breast or stomach cancer diagnosed under 50 years or brain tumour/adrenocortical cancer/prostate cancer/melanoma/germ cell tumour/leukaemia diagnosed under 60 years or sarcoma at any age

Other Families

- Any other families with an unusual pattern of cancer in the family or rare syndromes (e.g. testicular cancer in two or more relatives at any age, multiple endocrine neoplasia, von Hippel–Lindau, etc.)

available to aid risk assessment, although each has specific limitations, as outlined above.

Genetics clinics

Following the identification of an at-risk individual, referral to a specialist clinic is necessary for a formal assessment of the individual or family risk, for screening, and for management strategies, and for possibly genetic testing. Cancer genetics counselling needs to provide a simple explanation of how cancer develops (most commonly as a result of somatic mutation), the principles of genetic inheritance, an estimation of the chance that a familial cluster is due to genetic predisposition, information about the specific predisposition gene, an estimation of cancer risk, options for managing the risk, and the opportunity for genetic testing.

Clinical management

The future management of an individual depends upon the final risk estimates regarding the inheritance of a cancer predisposition gene and the potential cancer risks associated with this. In general, management strategies fall into four categories – cancer screening, lifestyle changes, genetic testing, and preventative strategies. Cancer screening and lifestyle changes can be advised for most individuals at moderately increased risk, but for individuals at the highest genetic risk, genetic testing or prophylactic or preventative measures may also be possible, such as prophylactic mastectomy or oophorectomy in *BRCA*1/2 gene carriers or colectomy in *FAP* gene carriers. *Table 8.5* outlines guidance protocols for screening in individuals with a high probability of mutations in cancer predisposition genes.

Table 8.5. *Screening protocols for family cancer syndromes (for guidance only; different clinics may have minor variations to this schema)*

Disease	Screen	Age (years) at start of screen/range for screening
von Hippel–Lindau, affected	Annual physical examination	
	Urine testing	
	Direct ophthalmoscopy	
	Fluorescein angiography	
	24-hour urinary vanillylmandelic acid (VMA)	
	Renal ultrasound	
	3-yearly MRI scan of the brain	
	CT scan of the kidneys (more frequent if multiple cysts)	
von Hippel–Lindau, at-risk relatives	Annual physical examination	5 upwards
	Urine testing	
	Direct ophthalmoscopy	5 upwards
	Fluorescein angiography	10 until 60
	24-hour urinary VMA	
	Renal ultrasound	20 until 65
	3-yearly MRI scan of the brain	15 until 40
	CT scan of the kidneys (more frequent if multiple cysts)	20 until 65
	5-yearly MRI scan of the brain	40 until 60
Familial polyposis, affected	Offer total colectomy with ileorectal anastomosis	Teenager (see below)
	Annual rectal stump screening (if conserved in surgery)	
	Upper gastrointestinal endoscopy 3 yearly	
	(annually if polyps found)	20 upwards
Familial polyposis, at-risk relatives	Offer genetic analysis if possible	11 (polyps are rare before this age) until 40
	Annual sigmoidoscopy	Perform colonoscopy when polyps found on sigmoidoscopy and arrange colectomy

Table 8.5. *Continued*

Disease	Screen	Age (years) at start of screen/range for screening
Gorlin's syndrome, affected (at-risk children usually have abnormal skull or spine radiographs by 5 years)	Annual dermatological examination 6 monthly orthopantomogram for jaw cysts Examination of infants for signs of medulloblastoma (some advocate MRI scanning *but not* CT scanning, owing to radiosensitivity)	Infants upwards
MEN Type 2	Offer genetic screening if possible; if positive perform prophylactic thyroidectomy Annual: plasma calcium, phosphate and parathormone Pentagastrin test Thyroid ultrasound Abdominal ultrasound and CT scan 24 hour urinary VMA/blood catecholamines	5 8 until 70
MEN1	Annual: symptom enquiry (dyspepsia, diarrhoea, renal colic, fits, amenorrhoea, galactorrhoea) Examination Serum calcium Parathormone Renal function Pituitary hormones (PL, GH, ACTH, FSH, TSH) Pancreatic hormones (gastrin, VIP, glucagon, neurotensin, somatostatin, pancreatic polypeptide) Lateral skull radiograph for pituitary size or MRI for pituitary adenomas	5
Wilms tumour, at-risk individuals	3-monthly renal ultrasound 6-monthly renal ultrasound	Birth to 8 years 8 until 12
Retinoblastoma (siblings and offspring of affected)	Offer genetic screening if possible Monthly retinal examination without anaesthetic 3-monthly retinal examination under anaesthetic 4-monthly retinal examination under anaesthetic 6-monthly retinal examination without anaesthetic Annual retinal examination without anaesthetic Annual examination for sarcoma	 Birth to 3 months 3 months until 2 years 2–3 years 3–5 years 5–11 years Early teens for life
Li–Fraumeni syndrome	Annual breast examination MRI scan (under investigation) Annual examination	18 until 60 Lifelong
NF1, affected	Annual examination Visual field assessment	Lifelong
NF2, at-risk relatives	Offer genetic screening if possible Annual examination Ophthalmoscopy for congenital cataracts Annual audiometry Brain-stem audiotory-evoked potentials 3-yearly MRI brain	 Childhood 10 until 40

Table 8.5. *Continued*

Disease	Screen	Age (years) at start of screen/range for screening
Lynch 1 syndrome	2-yearly colonoscopy	25 upwards
Lynch 2 syndrome	2-yearly colonoscopy	25 upwards
	Annual pelvic examination and ovarian and endometrial ultrasound and CA125	30 upwards
	Some screen for other cancers in kindred such as skin and urothelial malignancy	35 upwards
	Annual: mammography	35 upwards; its use depends on the amount of breast cancer in the family
Muir–Torré syndrome	2-yearly colonoscopy	25 upwards
Turcot's syndrome	2-yearly colonoscopy	20 upwards
Colon cancer in a single relative aged <45 years	5-yearly colonoscopy (3-yearly if polyps are found)	35 upwards
Familial melanoma	Annual skin examination General sun avoidance advice	Teenager upwards
Breast/ovarian syndrome	Annual mammography	Start from 35 upwards or 5 years younger than youngest case in the family (not less than 25–30 years)
	Annual pelvic examination	35 upwards (30 if young ovarian cancer case in family)
	Annual transvaginal ultrasound CA125 serum measurement	
Familial breast cancer	Annual mammography	35 upwards or 5 years younger than youngest case (not less than 25)
Familial ovarian cancer	Annual pelvic examination Transvaginal ultrasound CA125 serum measurement	30–35 upwards
Familial prostate cancer	Annual serum prostate specific antigen	50 upwards or 5 years young than youngest case (minimum age 40)
Familial testicular cancer	Annual digital rectal examination Regular testicular self examination	Late teens to 50

Genetic testing is possible for some cancer predisposition genes (*Table 8.6*) and requires only a simple blood sample. Genetic testing may either be diagnostic (the detection of a mutation in an individual affected by cancer) or predictive (the detection of a mutation in a clinically unaffected individual). Mutations in cancer predisposition genes often occur throughout the gene, and the vast majority of mutations so far have been observed only in limited numbers of families (except in specific ethnic groups). Hence, unless an individual is a member of such a group, the specific mutation for that family must first be identified. An affected family member is tested first because he or she is the family member most likely to have a cancer predisposing mutation. Predictive testing may then be offered to unaffected family members for the identified mutation. Unfortunately, as a result of the high penetrance of certain predisposition genes, for example *BRCA1/2*, it is not uncommon to be presented with a family with multiple cases of cancer in which all affected individuals have died from their cancer. In this difficult situation it is not currently possible to offer mutation testing to unaffected cases, and their future clinical management will depend upon their probability of having inherited a mutation. An exception is the rare circumstance of a closed ethnic group in which the suspected mutation is known to occur with a high probability.

Genetic testing should only take place following full genetic counselling to outline its implications. A recognized counselling schedule allows at least a month of reflection between two counselling sessions prior to blood being taken for mutation analysis. The personal and wider social implications of positive and negative results are issues discussed during these sessions. A positive result could have psychological implications as well as widespread repercussions involving the rest of the family. The additional social implications of the ability to purchase life and medical insurance, mortgages, and a possible effect on employment opportunities may be just as important as, if not more important than, the personal and familial implications. Currently, effects on employment are only theoretical. A negative test result may have just as serious consequences as a positive result because of the recognized 'survivor guilt syndrome', which has been documented in the setting of Huntington's disease.

For genes predisposing to adult-onset cancers, testing of young children is not advised as the age of cancer onset permits the individual to make their own decision to have genetic testing once they have reached adulthood and following full genetic counselling. Children are offered genetic testing when it may alter management, for example, in MEN 2A syndrome when thyroidectomy is offered at 5–15 years for gene carriers, as it is totally protective against medullary thyroid cancer.

Summary

Cancer is a common disease, but only a small proportion of cases can be attributed to the inheritance of specific cancer predisposition genes. However, in absolute terms, this represents a significant number of families or individuals because of the high population frequency of cancer. Only a few cancer predisposition genes have been identified, although the existence of many more is suspected. Currently, we can offer limited advice regarding risks, genetic testing, and general management of suspected gene carriers, but cancer genetics is one of the most rapidly expanding areas of medical knowledge. Any advice given regarding cancer predisposition genes may be liable to change with advances in research and knowledge, so specialists in the field of cancer genetics should facilitate the dissemination of any changes in advice to other colleagues likely to be in contact with individuals at risk.

Table 8.6. *Location of and status of genetic testing for cancer predisposition genes in 2003*

Disease	Location	Mutation analysis available
Breast/ovarian	17q21	BRCA1
Familial breast cancer/ male breast cancer	13q12	BRCA2
von Hippel–Lindau	3p25	VHL
Familial adenomatous polyposis	5q21	APC
Gorlin's syndrome	9q22	PTCH (research only)
Multiple endocrine neoplasia Type 2	10q11	RET
Multiple endocrine neoplasia Type 1	11q13	MEN1
Wilms tumour	11p13	WT1 (research only)
Retinoblastoma	13q14	RB1
Li-Fraumeni	17p13	TP53
Neurofibromatosis 1	17q11	NF1 (research only)
Neurofibromatosis 2	22q12	NF2
Lynch syndrome 1	2p22	hMLH1
Lynch syndrome 2	3p21	hMSH2

Cancer genetics for the general practitioner – an aide memoir

- Most cases needing referral will be detected by a standard family history taken at registration with a GP.
- Take a family history in first-degree relatives (parents, siblings, children) and ask if there are any cancer cases in other relatives.
- Cancer site and age at diagnosis are important.
- Consider referral along local guidelines but, in general, a family history of two cases of cancer at <50 years of age, or one case at a very young age compared with the general population's age of onset of cancer, may merit referral (for example, one case of breast cancer at <40 years of age, colon cancer at <45 years of age, or ovarian cancer at <40 years of age).

Further Reading

Dickenson DL. Can children and young people consent to be tested for adult onset genetic disorders? *BMJ*. 1999; **318**: 1063–5.

Eeles RA, Ponder BAJ, Easton DF, Horwich A eds. *Genetic Predisposition to Cancer*. London: Chapman and Hall Medical, 1996.

Foulkes WD, Hodgson SV, eds. *Inherited Susceptibility to Cancer. Clinical, Predictive and Ethical Perspectives*. Cambridge: Cambridge University Press, 1998.

Juengst ET. Caught in the middle again: Professional ethical considerations in genetic testing for health risks. *Genetic Test*. 1997/8; **1**: 189–200.

9 Screening for Cancer

Jane Melia and Sue Moss

Introduction

In the UK screening for certain diseases is regarded as an important part of the health care system. The National Screening Committee (www.doh.gov.uk/nsc) provides a remit and terms of reference for the development, evaluation, implementation, monitoring, and (if necessary) halting of screening programmes. In the White Paper *Saving Lives: Our Healthier Nation* (Secretary State of Health, 1999) screening is recognized as one of the key public health strategies to meet the target 'to reduce the death rate from cancer in people under 75 years by at least a fifth by 2010 – saving up to 100,000 lives in total'. In the document produced by the Chief Medical Officer (Update 23 Department of Health, www.doh.gov.uk/cmo/cmoh.htm), the promotion of partnership at different levels, including Primary Care organizations, was recommended as a means to improve standards in public health.

Screening for cancer aims to detect the disease at an early stage or in a precancerous phase, when treatment is most effective, and can lead to a reduction in both morbidity and mortality from the disease. It is usually offered to a target population defined by sex or age range, those with a family history of disease, or those working in certain environments. Most of the population are asymptomatic and do not have the disease. There is an ethical difference between treating a person who has sought help because of symptoms and offering screening to an apparently healthy population. This difference renders it essential that the advantages clearly outweigh the disadvantages before a population screening programme is introduced as part of the health service. Screening also needs to be cost-effective, but the balance of costs and benefits is not always easy to resolve. The potential benefits and costs are summarized in *Figure 9.1*.

The principles of evaluation are outlined below, followed by a section on current screening programmes.

The Development, Evaluation and Implementation of Screening

Certain criteria should be met before a population screening programme is introduced (*Table 9.1*). To establish these criteria for a given screening test involves three main phases of development and evaluation (*Table 9.2*). These comprise an assessment of the performance of the test in terms of its accuracy and acceptability (phase 1), evaluation studies of the effect and cost-effectiveness of screening on mortality (phase 2), and pilot studies to investigate the logistics and practicalities of implementing a national programme (phase 3). Primary Care Organizations have a key role to play in phases 2 and 3 to help develop and evaluate effective strategies.

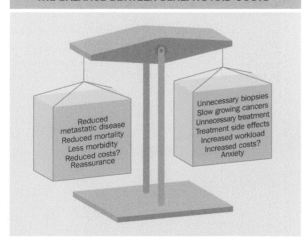

THE BALANCE BETWEEN BENEFITS AND COSTS

Reduced metastatic disease
Reduced mortality
Less morbidity
Reduced costs?
Reassurance

Unnecessary biopsies
Slow growing cancers
Unnecessary treatment
Treatment side effects
Increased workload
Increased costs?
Anxiety

Figure 9.1. *Benefits of screening must outweigh costs.*

Table 9.1. *Criteria for assessing screening*

- Prevalence of the disease known
- Natural history understood
- Safe and practical screening test
- Overall procedure ethically acceptable
- Psychosocial effects known
- Effective treatment
- Reduces mortality
- Cost-effectiveness known and acceptable

Table 9.2. *Phases required before a screening programme can be established*

Phase	Description
Phase 1	Studies on small series of patients and people who are asymptomatic to investigate the accuracy and acceptability of the screening test
Phase 2	Large-scale studies to evaluate the long-term impact of screening on mortality and the cost- effectiveness of screening; additional aims include further assessment of the performance of the screening test, the uptake rates, the psychosocial effects of screening, detection rates of cancer by stage and grade, and interval cancer rate
Phase 3	Pilot studies of the proposed screening programme in the general population to ensure that it is run as effectively and efficiently as possible

The results of evaluation studies often benefit from an artificial high-quality performance and control of the diagnostic and management processes. Pilot studies are therefore needed to test the generalizability of research findings to the setting of the health service. Aspects of the organization of screening and of quality assurance of the screening and diagnostic procedures can be reviewed and costed to ensure that any national programme is set up efficiently. Primary care teams can advise on updating patient registers and on monitoring of the uptake of screening and workload arising from the screening process and from patients subsequently diagnosed with cancer. A two-way process of information should be established, so that general practitioners (GPs) also receive feed-back on the results of screening and further diagnostic tests.

Factors Affecting the Effectiveness of Screening

Acceptability
Ideally, the uptake rate of screening in the target population should be high (70% or more) to ensure that a large proportion of cases can be detected at an early stage and that a population programme is cost-effective. Uptake of screening can be improved by a variety of factors, including raised public awareness, provision of information to the target population, the location of screening, choice of appointment times, and method of invitation. Consent must be obtained from each individual, on the basis that they are given full information about and understand clearly the nature of the screening test, and the possible benefits and disadvantages of screening. GPs and Primary Care Organizations have an important role to play in providing and discussing such information.

The performance of the screening test
The performance of the screening test is assessed using information from phases 1 and 2 of the evaluation process. The four main measures of performance (positive predictive value, negative predictive value, sensitivity, and specificity) are defined in terms of screening-test results in a (hypothetical) population for which the presence or absence of cancer is truly known (*Table 9.3*).

A positive test result does not mean that a person is 100% certain to have cancer; nor does a negative test result mean that a person definitely does not have cancer. It is important to be able to convey the implications of positive and nega-

Table 9.3. *Number of people according to results of the screening test and the true presence or absence of cancer*

	True presence of cancer	True absence of cancer	Total population
Positive screening test	a	b	a + b
Negative screening test	c	d	c + d
Total	a + c	b + d	a + b + c + d

Table 9.4. *Measures of the accuracy and performance of a screening test*

Measure	Definition	Calculation from Table 5.3
Positive predictive value	The proportion of people with a positive test result who truly have the disease	a/(a + b)
Negative predictive value	The proportion of people with a negative test result who truly do not have the disease	d/(c + d)
Sensitivity	The proportion of truly diseased people in the screened population who are identified as diseased by the screening test	a/(a + c)
Specificity	The proportion of truly non-diseased people who are so identified by the screening test	d/(b + d)

tive test results to those who are screened. The ability of the screening test to predict whether a person truly has cancer or not is measured by the positive and negative predictive values, respectively (*Table 9.4*).

The effectiveness of the screening test is also measured by the proportion of cancers in the population that are detected (sensitivity), and conversely the proportion of people who do not have the disease who have a negative test (specificity). Ideally, both sensitivity and specificity should be high, but for most screening tests there is a trade-off between the two. The higher the specificity the smaller the proportion of false positive cases, and the less the amount of workload that results from unnecessary referrals.

Detection rate of cancers by stage, size, and grade

The stage of cancer is a predictor of prognosis. Effective screening leads to an increase in the detection rate of early-stage cancer or premalignant lesions, which should be followed by a decrease in the incidence rate of late-stage cancers and, subsequently, in the number of deaths from the disease. This is likely to occur over a period of several years following one or more screens of the population.

Additional factors

The natural history of the cancer affects the proportion of cancers that progress, and their rate of progression. One of the major concerns about screening is that it leads to the diagnosis of a proportion of cancers that may not have become clinically significant. The effectiveness of treatment options for early-stage cancer affects the impact that screening has on morbidity and mortality. It is also one of the factors that influences the psychosocial effects of screening.

These need to be studied at all stages of the screening process.

The Cost-Effectiveness of Screening

The aim of a cost-effectiveness analysis is to assess the efficiency of screening by weighing up the costs and effectiveness using units such as life-years gained, cases cured, or cases of disease detected. No economic value is placed on the outcome. In phase 2, a comparison is usually made between offering population screening and not offering screening. The options are compared using a cost-effectiveness ratio such as the cost per case detected. A cost–utility analysis takes this a step further to consider the value placed on a specific health status. The most common measure used is the quality-adjusted life-year (QALY). This is particularly important in the evaluation of screening because of both the psychosocial effects associated with the early detection of disease and the false positive and false negative results from the screening test. In phase 3, comparisons can be made between different screening strategies to identify the most efficient way of delivering a programme. Direct costs associated with the organization and operation of the programme are among the most important to the health service, and they have to be weighed up against the possible cost savings associated with reducing the scale of advanced treatment.

Screening for Different Cancer Sites

For several cancers national programmes are already established or evaluation studies are under way (*Table 9.5*). For

Table 9.5. Screening status for site specific cancers in the general population

Screening status	Site specific cancer	Target population	Screening test
National programme	Breast	Women 50–65 years of age	Mammography
	Cervical	Women 25–64 years of age	Pap smear test
Pilot studies for general screening	Colorectal cancer	Men and women 50–65 years of age	Faecal occult blood test
Evaluation studies underway	Prostate	Men mainly 55–69 years of age	Prostate-specific antigen (PSA), digital rectal examination, transrectal ultrasound
Evaluation underway	Ovary	Women 50–64 years of age	Ultrasound, CA125

other cancers, such as melanoma and testicular cancer, there is considerable interest in promoting early detection by the general public, although the effectiveness of this has not been fully evaluated.

National programmes for cervical and breast cancers

Screening for cervical cancer by the Papanicolaou (Pap) test has been widely available in the UK since the 1960s, but prior to the mid-1980s it was poorly organized, which resulted in low-risk women being screened repeatedly with a large population remaining unscreened. With the introduction of systematic call and recall in the mid-1980s, the programme is now estimated to prevent up to 3900 cases of cervical cancer each year, and to save up to 1300 lives. Women of age 20–64 years should be called or recalled every 3–5 years. In 2001/2 82% of women in the age range 25–64 years had been screened at least once in the previous 5 years. One of the problems associated with cervical screening is to decide the optimum management of women when the smear result is borderline or mildly dyskaryotic. About 4.5% of women screened fall into this category, with highest percentages in the youngest age groups.

Under the NHS Breast Screening Programme, women of age 50–64 years are currently offered screening by mammograhy every 3 years, but those who are older are entitled to refer themselves for screening. Pilot studies have demonstrated the acceptability and practicality of inviting women up to 69 years of age, and the programme is now being extended to invite women up to age 70. Research is also taking place on the effectiveness of screening younger women. Of women who are 50–64 years of age, 75% accept an invitation to screening, although there is geographical variation. Approximately 8% of women screened for the first time (now mainly those who are

50–52 years of age) and 4% of those who attend for routine rescreening are recalled for further assessment, and of these approximately 8% and 13%, respectively, are diagnosed as having cancer. A proportion of these are ductal carcinoma in situ, the natural history of which is not fully understood.

As a result of the increased use of fine-needle aspiration cytology and core needle biopsy, in 2000/2001 87% of breast cancers diagnosed through the screening programme were diagnosed without the need for an open biopsy. The effects of hormone replacement therapy, both on a woman's risk of breast cancer and on the sensitivity of mammography, is unclear. These effects are currently being investigated in a large cohort study in the UK (Million Women Study Collaborative Group, 1999).

Pilot studies for colorectal cancer screening

Screening for colorectal cancer by the faecal occult blood (FOB) test is being piloted at two centers in England and Scotland. This follows the results of three randomized trials, which demonstrated a 15–21% reduction in the mortality rate from colorectal cancer in a population offered screening by the FOB test. The pilot studies offered first-round screening to 200,000 people. The Department of Health has funded an evaluation study to investigate aspects of the organization, management, patient information, acceptability of screening, uptake rates, quality assurance of the screening test, colonoscopy and pathology, and short-term outcome measures such as the detection rate of polyps and cancers. These data will be used to review the full cost implications of a national programme.

Future developments may help to refine or improve the benefits of screening for colorectal cancer. These include screening by a once-only flexible sigmoidoscopy, a method currently being evaluated, and the use of molecular markers to identify those individuals at greatest risk of developing the disease. Research is under way to investigate the proportion of cancers associated with these markers, and the risk of developing cancer in gene carriers.

Evaluation studies

In the UK there is considerable interest in the potential of screening for both prostate and ovarian cancers. Two main trials for prostate cancer screening are under way in Europe and the USA (de Koning et al, 2002). Various combinations of screening tests are being evaluated, including digital rectal examination and the prostate-specific antigen (PSA) blood test. The most promising seems to be the PSA test. It is simple, reliable, reasonably acceptable, and inexpensive to use. The first results on the effects on mortality in the European study are expected in 2008.

A randomized trial of screening for ovarian cancer by measurement of CA125 is in progress in the UK.

High-risk groups with a family history of cancer

There are no national screening policies for people with a family history of cancer, but guidelines to advise GPs about the identification and referral of high risk groups are being developed. Collaboration with specialist cancer genetic clinics is recommended to ensure the appropriate assessment of cancer risk and the best course of patient management, including screening. Screening of such groups starts at a younger age than for the general population. The same screening tests may be used for those with a family history of cancer as for the general population, but there is uncertainty about the effectiveness of tests such as mammography in younger age groups, and the frequency with which screening should take place. Patient management should include a fully informed discussion about the advantages and limitations of direct genetic testing, and screening, and the availability of different management and screening options.

References and Further Reading

Austoker J. *Cancer Prevention in Primary Care*. London: BMJ Books, 1995.

de Koning HJ, Auvinen A, Berenguer Sanchez A et al. Large-scale randomized prostate cancer screening trials: Program performances in the European Randomized Screening for Prostate Cancer trial and the Prostate, Lung, Colorectal and Ovary cancer trial. *Int J Cancer* 2002; **97**: 237–44.

Chamberlain J, Moss S. *Evaluation of Cancer Screening*. Focus on Cancer Series. London: Springer-Verlag, 1996.

Miller AB, ed. *Recent Advances in Cancer Screening*. London: Kluwer Academic Publishers, 1996.

Pas L, ed. *General Practice and Cancer Prevention in Europe: The involvement of general practitioners in cancer screening programmes*. Gent: Mys and Breesch, 1994.

Peckham C, Dezateux, eds. *Screening*. British Medical Bulletin Vol. 54 (No. 4): London: The Royal Society of Medicine Press Ltd, 1999.

Secretary State of Health. *Saving Lives: Our Healthier Nation*. London: The Stationery Office, 1999.

10 Hormones and Cancer

Irene Boeddinghaus, Stephen Johnston and Mitch Dowsett

Introduction

Hormonal manipulation is used successfully in the treatment of many cancers and it is likely that hormonal factors are involved in the development of these cancers. In some cases the evidence is compelling, while in others it is more speculative. Some cancers are thought to be caused (in part) by sex steroid hormones (e.g. oestrogen, testosterone), and these usually manifest differently in men and women. Some cancers are associated with non-steroid hormone production, and affect both sexes, such as the multiple endocrine neoplasia (MEN) syndromes. These are not dealt with here.

Female Cancers

Breast cancer

The association between female breast cancer and oestrogen was documented over 100 years ago, when bilateral oophorectomy was shown to be a successful treatment for advanced breast cancer. Anti-oestrogens (such as tamoxifen) and drugs that reduce oestrogen synthesis are given to millions of women in both the metastatic and in the adjuvant settings, in which their administration has been shown to impart a survival advantage to both pre- and postmenopausal women (*see*

Chapter 13). Recently, tamoxifen has also been shown to decrease the incidence of breast cancer in certain groups of healthy women, although it is still unclear precisely which women benefit, and whether this translates into a survival advantage. Measurement of the oestrogen receptor has become increasingly important. It is now clear that women whose cancers are oestrogen-receptor-negative (and some who appear positive but whose pathways are defective) infrequently respond to hormone treatment (*Figs 10.1* and *10.2*).

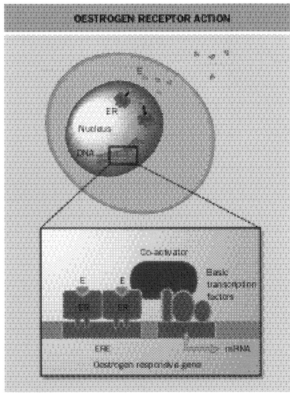

Figure 10.2. *Mechanism of action of oestrogen (E) stimulation in oestrogen-receptor (ER)-positive cells. Oestrogen receptors are positioned on the cell membrane. Binding of oestradiol causes them to dimerize and move into the nucleus. Here they bind to an area of DNA known as the oestrogen response element (ERE). This binding allows the recruitment of co-factors, which induce mRNA production by basic transcription factors.*

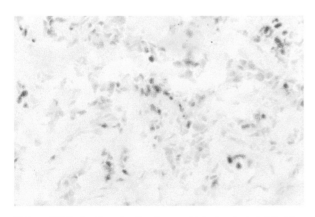

Figure 10.1. *Section showing immunohistochemical staining for oestrogen receptor in invasive breast cancer. Cells staining positively (brown) lie alongside negatively staining cells (blue).*

Table 10.1. *Hormonal factors associated with increased/decreased risk of breast cancer*

Well established	Weakly associated or under evaluation	Possible protective factors
Nulliparity	Early age at menarche	Chemoprevention
Late age at first birth	Oral contraception	Breastfeeding
Late age at menopause	Hormone replacement therapy	
	Obesity (postmenopausal women)	

A number of endogenous and exogenous hormonal factors are associated with the risk of breast cancer and might play a role in the rising incidence of breast cancer in the developed world (*Table 10.1*). Several recent prospective studies reported an association between high levels of plasma oestrogen and the risk of breast cancer development in postmenopausal women. In general, those reproductive factors associated with increased breast cancer risk are also associated with increased breast exposure to oestrogenic stimulation.

Endogenous factors

The endogenous factors of breast cancer in women are summarized in *Table 10.2* and discussed below.

Long reproductive interval

Women who start menstruating early or who have a late menopause are at an increased risk of developing breast cancer. The relative risk of breast cancer is increased by about 3% for each year older at menopause. In contrast, women who undergo bilateral oophorectomy before the age of 35 years have only 40% of the risk of breast cancer of women who have

a natural menopause. The effect of early menarche is less substantial, possibly because of the narrower age range for menarche than for menopause.

Parity

Nulliparous women are at an increased risk of breast cancer compared with parous women. In addition, there is a clear trend of falling risk with increasing parity in women of at least 45 years of age: women who have a full-term first pregnancy at 16 years of age have only 40% of the chance of developing breast cancer as those who have their first pregnancy at over 30 years of age. Late age at first birth has also been linked with a high risk of breast cancer. However, some evidence indicates that, despite the reduced incidence of breast cancer in women who have had early pregnancies, those women in this category who go on to develop breast cancer have a particularly poor prognosis.

Breastfeeding

Opinions differ as to the possible protective effect of breastfeeding. Of note, the largest prospective study to investigate this, which looked at almost 90,000 women in the US Nurses' Health Study, found no important association between breast-feeding and the occurrence of breast cancer.

Weight

In postmenopausal women the risk of breast cancer in obese women is increased. This is thought to be caused by the higher plasma oestrogen levels in these women. In contrast, a weak inverse relationship is generally reported in premenopausal women. A number of theories have been put forward to explain this seemingly paradoxical observation. One postulates that increased exposure to progesterone and oestrogen increases the risk of breast cancer more than exposure to oestrogen alone, and that obese premenopausal women have decreased levels of progesterone but similar oestrogen levels to their lean counterparts.

Table 10.2. *Summary of endogenous factors of breast cancer in women*

- Increased oestrogenic stimulation in general results in greater breast cancer risk
- Delayed menopause increases the risk of breast cancer by approximately 3% per year
- Delayed and low parity is associated with an increased risk of breast cancer
- Breastfeeding is unlikely to impact significantly on the incidence of breast cancer
- Obese, postmenopausal women have an increased risk of breast cancer

Exogenous factors

The exogenous factors of breast cancer in women are summarized in *Table 10.3* and discussed below.

Hormone replacement therapy

A large overview analysis has shown that among current users of hormone replacement therapy (HRT) or those who have ceased use in the previous 1–4 years, the relative risk of having breast cancer diagnosed increases by a multiple of between 2% and 3% for each year of use. The relative risk is 1.35 for women who have used HRT for 5 years or longer, but 5 or more years after cessation of HRT use there is no significant excess of breast cancer overall or in relation to duration of use (*Table 10.4*). The risks appear to be greatest for women of low weight, and no evidence indicates that they vary between the HRT preparations used. Importantly, the excess risk of breast cancer incidence arises mainly from tumours with good prognostic features, and there is no evidence that death from breast cancer is increased by HRT usage. Although very few data are available on the use of

HRT in women who have a diagnosis of breast cancer, its use is not routinely advocated. In some women, the advantages outweigh the theoretical disadvantages, such as those women whose tumours are oestrogen-receptor-negative (and therefor do not rely on oestrogenic stimulus as a growth factor), and those whose quality of life is severely affected by menopausal symptoms (especially if they are receiving tamoxifen).

Combined oral contraceptive pill

During usage of the combined oral contraceptive pill (COCP), and in the first 10 years after stopping it, there is a small increase of between 1.07 and 1.24 in the relative risk of having breast cancer diagnosed. This is related neither to the formulation of the contraceptive, nor to the duration of use. In nulliparous women, the pattern of risk is the same as that for parous women, irrespective of whether oral contraceptive use began before or after the birth of the first child. The additional cancers tend to be localized to the breast at presentation, and there is no evidence of increased risk 10 or more years after cessation of use (*Fig. 10.3*). Women who have had a diagnosis of breast cancer are usually advised to use a non-hormonal form of contraception.

Ovarian cancer

Clear risks and benefits exist as regards risk of ovarian cancer for women with various hormonal and/or reproductive manipulations (*Table 10.5*). Clear trends of decreasing risk

Table 10.3. *Summary of exogenous factors of breast cancer in women*

- The small increased risk of breast cancer associated with hormone replacement (HRT) use disappears by 5 years after cessation
- In some special cases it is possible for a woman with a diagnosis of breast cancer to take HRT
- The small increased risk of breast cancer associated with combined oral contraceptive pill use disappears by 10 years after cessation

Table 10.4. *Risk of breast cancer for duration of hormone replacement therapy use*

Duration of use and time since last use	Average annual risk
Never user	Standard
Last use <5 years before diagnosis	
Duration 5–9 years	Increase 2–3fold
Duration 10–14 years	Increase 2–3 fold
Last use ≥ 5 years before diagnosis	
Duration 5–9 years	Standard

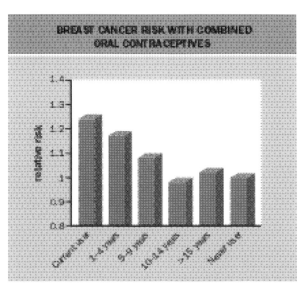

Figure 10.3. *Risk of breast cancer by time since last use of combined oral contraceptives relative to never users.*

Table 10.5. *Summary of risks for ovarian cancer*

- Pregnancy and breastfeeding decrease the risk of ovarian cancer
- Use of the combined oral contraceptive pill leads to a marked decrease in the incidence of ovarian cancer
- Use of hormonal replacement therapy for 10 years or more is associated with a significantly increased risk of ovarian cancer
- Hormonal therapy may sometimes be used in the treatment of ovarian cancer

Table 10.6. *Summary of risks for endometrium cancer*

- Obesity and low parity are associated with an increased risk of endometrial cancer
- Unopposed oestrogens result in a increased risk of endometrial cancer
- Tamoxifen 20 mg daily for 5 years increases the risk of endometrial cancer 2–3-fold
- Progestins may be used to treat endometrial cancer

have occurred with increasing numbers of pregnancies (regardless of outcome) and increasing duration of breastfeeding. Use of the COCP also protects against ovarian cancer. The common factor in this protective effect is the temporary cessation of ovulation, which is considered to be the most likely mechanism, although there may be a direct antiproliferative effect of progestins in oral contraceptives. The degree of protection afforded by oral contraceptives is striking. All studies in which the duration of use is evaluated show a protective effect equivalent to approximately a 40% decrease in risk after 2 years or more of oral contraceptive use. Longer durations of use are associated with even greater protection: approximately a 50% reduction at 4 years and a 60–80% reduction at 7 years or more.

The benefits derived are greatest for those women at highest risk (i.e. low parity) and persist for many years after cessation of oral contraceptive use. Risk of ovarian epithelial cancer appears to be increased three-fold among women who have used fertility drugs. No consistent trend is seen with age at menarche or menopause. More recent studies have addressed whether HRT is associated with an increased risk of gynaecological malignancy. A recent meta-analysis reviewing over 300 publications in the past 30 years showed that the relative risk of ovarian cancer among ever users of HRT was 1.15 (95% CI 1.05–1.27). This study, in particular, showed that only 10 years or more of HRT is associated with a significant increased risk. Once again it remains unclear as to whether this is a true association, or whether confounding factors such as differences in parity or increased surveillance of HRT users are responsible.

There is evidence for the expression of hormone receptors in ovarian cancers, and numerous small studies have been carried out of tamoxifen in women with stage III/IV ovarian cancer that has relapsed or is refractory to chemotherapy. A recent systematic review showed an overall objective response rate of 10.4%, although the response rate may be higher in untreated patients. Up to 30% of patients may benefit from stable disease. Other hormonal agents may show less evidence of activity, but progestins are sometimes used for their other palliative benefits.

Endometrial cancer

Endometrial cancer has also been shown to be a hormonally regulated disease, and (among other risk factors) obesity and low parity have been shown to be associated with a higher incidence (*Table 10.6*). Nulliparous women have also been shown to have a poorer 5-year survival than parous women, with a hazard ratio of 2.81 (95% CI 1.55–5.06) after adjustment for traditional risk factors. Any condition that increases exposure to unopposed oestrogen increases the risk of endometrial cancer (e.g. oestrogen replacement therapy without progestin, and oestrogen-secreting tumours are risk factors). In the recent tamoxifen prevention study, the rate of endometrial carcinoma was increased in the tamoxifen group by a factor of 2.53 (95% CI 1.35–4.97). This increased risk occurred predominantly in women older than 50 years of age, all the cancers detected were stage 1, and there were no resultant deaths. This is thought to be caused by the agonist effects of tamoxifen on the endometrium. Relative to women who never use hormones, women who take unopposed oestrogens have a 4–9-fold increased risk of endometrial cancer. Women who use combined therapy with oestrogen and cyclic progestin have an increased risk of approximately 1.5 compared to non-users. Use of less than 10 days of added progestin per cycle gives an intermediate risk (*Table 10.7*). Endometrial cancer can be treated with hormones, and for many years progestins have been used with an overall response rate of 34% plus 13% stable disease.

Male Cancers

Hormonal causes of cancer in men are summarized in *Table 10.8*, and discussed below.

Table 10.7. *Influence of number of days of progestin use per cycle of hormone replacement therapy (HRT) on the odds ratio of developing endometrial cancer*

Progestin use	Number of cases	Number of controls	Adjusted odds ratio
Never used HRT	270	593	1.0
<10 days progestin/month	25	26	3.1
10–21 days progestin/month	25	64	1.3

Table 10.8. *Summary of hormonal causes of cancer in men*

- Male breast cancer is rare, and often successfully treated with tamoxifen
- Androgen deprivation is the mainstay of treatment for metastatic prostate cancer
- Adverse effects of anabolic steroid abuse are difficult to quantify
- Vasectomy does not appear to be linked with prostate or testicular cancer
- Increased serum testosterone is seen in patients with prostate cancer, but not in patients with testicular cancer

Breast cancer

Cancer of the male breast does occur, although at a far lower incidence than female breast cancer (less than 1%). Male breast cancers have a strikingly high rate of oestrogen-receptor positivity (±80–90% versus 60–70% in females), and the majority respond to anti-oestrogen treatment.

The effects of endogenous oestrogens present in the environment (phyto-oestrogens) and of exogenous testosterone administration on the incidence of male breast cancer have been studied, but as yet no evidence indicates that these substances are important in the aetiology of male breast cancers. Testosterone replacement therapy is contraindicated in male patients with breast cancers.

Prostate cancer

Prostate cancer is the most common cancer in Caucasian men. Serum levels of free testosterone appear to be slightly higher in men with prostate cancer compared with healthy, age-matched controls. Early initiation of androgen deprivation therapy is the mainstay of treatment in metastatic disease, and its use now appears to be warranted in locally advanced disease also. The addition of androgen ablation

therapy to radiotherapy alone in lymph-node positive disease improves the overall 10-year survival from 60% to 83%. The efficacy of combined androgen blockade compared with gonadal androgen deprivation alone remains unclear.

Case reports of body builders who take anabolic steroids and who have gone on to develop prostatic cancers have been published, but it remains extremely difficult to quantify the associated risks. Worryingly, use of 17-alkylated androgens such as methyltestosterone or fluoxymesterone (which are considered obsolete in conventional treatment but are still available on the black market) has been associated with raised liver enzymes, cholestasis, peliosis of the liver, and liver tumours. While one early report showed a strong positive association between vasectomy and prostatic cancer, this has not been borne out by numerous other studies, including one by the authors who originally reported the association.

Testicular cancer

A certain amount of testosterone is vital for the pubertal development of the male testis, and for the maintenance of spermatogenesis in adults. However, high doses of testosterone suppress gonadotropin secretion from the pituitary via a negative feedback mechanism, which results in a drastic decrease in sperm concentration (azoospermia) in the ejaculate, and a decrease in testis size of approximately 30%. The effects appear to be completely reversible, even after massive doses. No evidence indicates a causal effect between serum testosterone levels and testicular cancer. Exposure to environmental oestrogens has been proposed as a potential risk factor for subsequent testicular disease (including neoplasia), and some studies have found an association between early puberty and the subsequent development of testicular cancer. Vasectomy does *not* cause testicular cancer, and does not accelerate the growth or diagnosis of pre-existing testicular neoplasms.

Further Reading

Bagatell CJ, Bremner WJ. Androgens in men – uses and abuses. *N Engl J Med*. 1996; **334**: 707–14.

Colditz GA. Hormones and breast cancer: evidence and implications for considerations of risks and benefits of hormone replacement therapy. *J Wom Health*. 1999; **8**: 347–57.

Kelsey JL, Gammon MD, John EM. Reproductive factors and breast cancer. *Epidemiol Rev*. 1993; **15**: 36–47.

McPherson K, Steel CM, Dixon JM. ABC of breast diseases. Breast cancer – epidemiology, risk factors and genetics. *BMJ*. 1994; **309**: 1003–6.

1Whittemore AS, Harris R, Itnyre J. Characteristics relating to ovarian cancer risk: collaborative analysis of 12 US case-control studies. II. Invasive epithelial ovarian cancers in white women. Collaborative Ovarian Cancer Group. *Am J Epidemiol*. 1992; **136**: 1184–203.

11 Mechanisms of Cancer Therapy

Ian Judson and Gillian Ross

Introduction

For those tumours that are localized and amenable to complete resection, the most effective treatment is undoubtedly surgery. Radiotherapy may also be used to treat local disease and may be curative, as in some cases of Hodgkin's disease. However, it is now understood that cancer is often a systemic disease and in such cases we need to treat the whole patient.

Chemotherapy

Principles of chemotherapy

The majority of current anticancer drugs kill dividing cells (cytotoxic drugs), or at least limit their ability to grow (cytostatic drugs). It is not true that cytostatic drugs do not shrink tumours. Tumours are in an equilibrium between cell death and cell division, with the latter predominating (*Fig. 11.1*). If you switch off cell division in a tumour with a high rate of cell loss (a common situation in aggressive cancers) the tumour will shrink.

Unfortunately, most chemotherapy drugs are poorly selective for cancer cells and also result in damage to healthy dividing tissues such as the bone marrow, gut lining, and hair follicles. This can lead to infection, diarrhoea, and hair loss. It is for this reason that the majority of treatment schedules involve intermittent dosing to allow the recovery of normal tissues between treatments. Reasons for the selective killing of cancer cells that sometimes occurs are unclear, but include the fact that tumours have a higher proportion of dividing cells, which are more susceptible to damage. In some cases there may be an increased tendency for that damage to lead to cell death rather than growth arrest.

Types of chemotherapy drug

Chemotherapy drugs can be grouped in different ways but the simplest classification is based on their target in the cell (*Table 11.1* lists some but is by no means exhaustive).

DNA damaging agents

The first DNA-binding agents to be developed were the classic alkylating agents (e.g. cyclophosphamide). They cause chemical cross-links between the two strands of the DNA molecule. Not only does this in itself halt the process of DNA replication, but the distortion caused is recognized by repair enzymes. In the process of removing the bound drug, or adduct, some DNA is lost and this, or the damage caused by adduct formation, may lead to the initiation of programmed cell death, or apoptosis.

The platinum anticancer drugs act somewhat differently. Cisplatin, a simple molecule with one platinum atom at its core, binds mainly to a single strand of DNA to produce intrastrand cross-links. Different processes are involved in the recognition and repair of these adducts, but the end result is the same. It is the differences in the precise nature of DNA damage and the timescale of its formation that are responsible for the tumour selectivity of the different drugs.

Agents that inhibit replication or repair processes

A group of enzymes called topoisomerases is responsible for the unfolding of DNA required to allow the strands to be copied

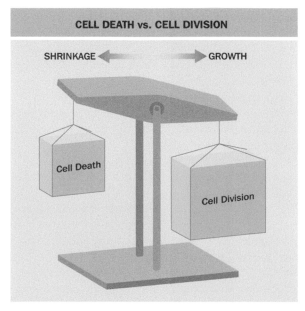

Figure 11.1. *Cell division predominates over cell death in tumours.*

Table 11.1. *Mechanisms of action of cytotoxic drugs*

DNA damage	DNA replication and repair	Mechanics of cell division	Metabolic processes involved in cell growth
Cyclophosphamide	Etoposide	Vincristine	5-Fluorouracil
Carmustine	Doxorubicin (adriamycin)	Vinblastine	Methotrexate
Chlorambucil	Epirubicin	Vinorelbine	Cytosine arabinoside
Cisplatin	Irinotecan	Paclitaxel	Cladribine
Carboplatin	Topotecan	Docetaxel	Pentostatin
Mitomycin C			6-Mercaptopurine
Temozolomide			6-Thioguanine
Bleomycin			
Busulphan			

or to allow access to repair enzymes in the event of damage. DNA is packaged in the cell in a highly coiled form. These 'supercoils' can be relaxed by a process of nicking and rejoining the DNA strands; it is this process that is performed by topoisomerases.

Inhibitors of these enzymes may either bind to the DNA and then interfere with the process indirectly, or bind to the enzyme itself. Some DNA-binding agents (e.g. doxorubicin) slot between the base pairs, a process called intercalation. In addition to inhibiting topoisomerase II (topo II), doxorubicin has a number of other actions, including the production of free radicals that damage DNA. Etoposide is a topo II inhibitor that does not intercalate DNA and has a relatively selective action against the enzyme. In the process of topo II inhibition, the DNA is locked in a state in which breaks occur at the points where the enzyme is bound, but rejoining does not occur, which results in double-strand breaks. This damage is recognized and may lead to apoptosis (cell death).

Inhibitors of topoisomerase I produce single-strand breaks and in the process halt DNA replication, a process called chain termination.

Agents that interfere with the mechanisms of cell division

The process of cell division involves the chromosomes being replicated. They are lined up in pairs and pulled apart by the mitotic spindle, which consists of tiny hollow fibres, or microtubules, formed from a protein called tubulin. A group of drugs derived from the Madagascan periwinkle, called vinca alkaloids (e.g. vincristine), cause the microtubules to disaggregate and block the cell in mitosis. The taxanes (paclitaxel and docetaxel) cause abnormal aggregation of tubulin

by interfering with the constant remodelling that is necessary for the normal function of microtubules. These agents are also natural products and are derived from varieties of yew. Initially, it was necessary to kill the trees to obtain the basic material from the bark. However, these chemicals can now be obtained from renewable sources, such as the leaves of yew trees.

Agents that interfere with metabolic processes

Inhibitors of enzymes crucial for the production of the basic building blocks of DNA, RNA, and protein were among the very first anticancer drugs. Methotrexate remains in use for the treatment of acute lymphoblastic leukaemia, breast cancer, and osteosarcoma. Methotrexate mimics the vitamin folic acid and prevents its utilization by the cell, which interferes with many processes including the production of thymidine for DNA synthesis and purines for DNA and RNA synthesis.

Drug combinations

The use of anticancer drugs in combination brought great advances because of the synergy between different agents and the additive effect against cancer of drugs with non-overlapping toxicities. This brought about the first cures in diseases such as Hodgkin's disease and non-Hodgkin's lymphomas. However, the design of such combinations remains largely empirical, and satisfactory laboratory models have proved hard to find.

Drug resistance

Currently, one of the most serious problems in the treatment of common solid tumours is the development of resistance, which may be acquired through selection or mutation. There are also pharmacological problems to do with the enhanced efflux of drug from the cancer cell, a common problem with drugs derived form natural products, and with altered DNA repair capacity. Such problems might be amenable to improvements in drug design, and analogue development has been successful in broadening the spectrum of action of a number of useful drugs. However, more fundamental problems may affect the ability of a cell to respond to damage by entering apoptosis. If the machinery for apoptosis is lost (and it is defective in many cancers), then the cell may be resistant to a wide variety of different treatments.

New targets

The current move is away from drugs that are crudely cytotoxic towards the development of drugs that have specific molecular targets, in the hope of designing drugs with enhanced selectivity for cancer cells. An improved understanding of cancer biology has resulted in an explosion of potential new targets for cancer therapy.

For example, to invade locally the tumour cells have to break down tissue barriers, which may involve the release of matrix metalloproteinases (MMPs) such as collagenase, and generate the growth of new blood vessels (angiogenesis). Inhibitors of MMPs and angiogenesis are currently in clinical trial, although their potential remains unclear.

The most widely reported angiogenesis inhibitors, angiostatin and endostatin, are related to natural substances produced by tumours and appear to be very effective in laboratory models of cancer.

Cancer cells signal to each other and to the adjacent normal cells, setting up what are referred to as autocrine or paracrine growth loops. The mechanisms by which signalling molecules or growth factors result in tumour cell growth are now well understood. These signalling pathways consist of the binding of ligand to a cell surface receptor and the resultant chemical reactions set up within the cell. Some of these signalling pathways can be blocked by antibodies [e.g. trastuzumab for breast cancer (c-erbB2), rituximab for lymphoma] or by small molecule drugs, of which there are many currently in development. Two inhibitors of receptor tyrosine kinases are of particular note. Imatinib (Glivec) is highly effective in the treatment of chronic myeloid leukaemia and a rare sarcoma of the gut called gastrointestinal stromal tumour (GIST) and ZD 1839 (Iressa) has been shown to have activity in the treatment of non-small cell lung cancer.

Radiotherapy

What is radiotherapy and how does it work?

Radiotherapy is the use of ionizing radiation to kill or suppress the growth of cancer cells selectively, while minimizing the effects on healthy surrounding tissues. It is a very focal therapy, but is highly reliant on a thorough understanding of anatomy, and on the availability of modern, high-resolution diagnostic imaging, such as contrast-enhanced computed tomography or magnetic resonance imaging. Modern equipment can deliver therapy X-ray beams to an accuracy of within millimetres, with little day-to-day variability. High-energy X-rays, or photons, are generated by machines called 'linear accelerators', and are used to treat deep-seated tumours. The same equipment can also produce electron beams commonly used for skin cancer. These beams can be directed and shaped to individual patients in a process called treatment planning (*Fig. 11.2*). The various radiotherapy techniques are outline in *Table 11.2*.

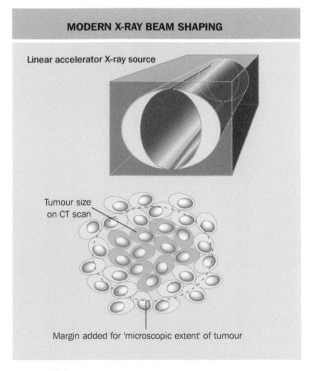

MODERN X-RAY BEAM SHAPING

Linear accelerator X-ray source

Tumour size on CT scan

Margin added for 'microscopic extent' of tumour

Figure 11.2. Modern shaping of X-ray beams.

Table 11.2. Radiotherapy techniques

Technique	Description
Conformal radiotherapy	The radiotherapy beam is 'customized' by metal shielding devices (multileaf collimators), which alter the shape of the beam
Stereotactic radiotherapy (gamma knife)	This technology is used for several beams, which permits high doses to be 'focused' onto small areas
Intensity-modulated radiotherapy	The X-ray output from a linear accelerator is varied and combined with conformal techniques; this allows further 'shaping' of the field in three dimensions
Continuous hyperfractionated accelerated radiotherapy (CHART)	CHART shortens the time between fractions of treatment; patients are treated three times a day, which can partly overcome the problem of tumour repopulation between fractions while keeping toxicity to a minimum
Radiosensitizes	Radiotherapy can be made more effective by combining it with various agents including breathing carbogen (O_2 + 5% CO_2) and chemotherapy (chemoradiation)
Brachytherapy	This places the radioactive source close to the tumour – solid sources can be inserted into a body cavity (e.g. vagina or bronchus) through hollow tubes placed at surgery (after loading) or implanted via radioactive needles

EFFECT OF IRRADIATION ON CANCER CELLS

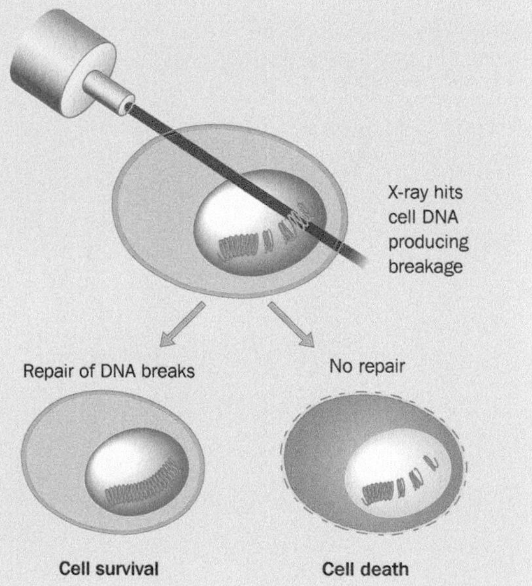

X-ray hits cell DNA producing breakage

Repair of DNA breaks

No repair

Cell survival

Cell death

Figure 11.3. Effect of inability of cancerous cells to repair radiation damage.

Table 11.3. Curative and palliative treatment of cancers

Cancers often treated with high-dose 'curative' radiotherapy

Breast cancer, postlumpectomy, or after mastectomy
Squamous cancers of cervix, head and neck, lung
Skin cancers (e.g. basal cell, squamous)
Muscle-invading bladder cancer, prostate cancer
Upper gastrointestinal tract, colorectal
Hodgkin's disease
Non-Hodgkin's lymphoma

Palliative treatments of cancer

Bone pain from metastatic disease (e.g. breast, prostate, lung)
Spinal cord compression by tumour
Superior vena cava compression (e.g. lung cancer)

The cancer cell 'kill effect' is produced by these X-rays generating DNA damage. Normal cells have very efficient DNA repair processes that eradicate radiation damage within a few hours. By contrast, malignant cells fail to activate normal DNA 'house-keeping' processes and continue to try to divide, with the radiation damage persisting. This results in cell death (*Fig. 11.3*), which is in proportion to the dose given. One of the principles behind giving radiotherapy in small daily doses over 5–6 weeks is to exploit these differences between the recovery potentials of normal and malignant cells after radiotherapy (so-called 'dose-fractionation'). Each such treatment session takes minutes, and hence most patients attend on an out-patient basis.

Another method of delivering radiotherapy is the implantation or temporary insertion of radioactive material directly into the tumour area under general anaesthesia, so-called brachytherapy. This is a vital part of the treatment of cancers of the cervix, endometrium, and some types of head and neck tumours.

Which cancers benefit from radiotherapy?

If radiotherapy is used with curative intent, instead of surgery, to treat a tumour, the clinician must be able to delineate the tumour extent by a combination of examination and imaging, and then design treatment beams that target this area with an appropriate margin of 'normal' tissue, to allow for microscopic tumour extent. If a tumour has been resected, in certain circumstances radiotherapy as 'adjuvant' therapy may be given to the region to eradicate microscopic disease. Radiotherapy is also commonly given at much lower doses to locally advanced or metastatic disease to control symptoms, often referred to as 'palliative therapy'. Examples of common uses of curative and palliative treatments are summarized in *Table 11.3*.

New developments in radiotherapy include much more sophisticated ways to shape beams to tumour site, which reduces the extent of healthy tissue treated unnecessarily. This should reduce short-term and long-term side-effects. Importantly, it may create opportunities to increase tumour radiotherapy doses while keeping side-effects at acceptable levels, with a potential for higher cure rates.

Further Reading

A great deal of material is available on the Internet concerning new treatments for cancer. However, readers should be aware of the fact that some exciting new developments prove disappointing or never make it to the market place. Reliable information can be obtained from the National Cancer Institute CancerNet website

http://cancer.gov/cancerinformation, from the Cancer Research UK CancerHelp website
www.cancerhelp.org.uk and from the cancer patients charity BACUP
www.cancerbacup.org.uk

Specific Types
of Cancer

12 Lung Cancer

Kate Gregory and Mary O'Brien

Incidence

Lung cancer is the most commonly occurring cancer world-wide; in the UK over 40,000 new cases are diagnosed annually and of these 30,000 deaths each year are recorded. On average 1 in 14 men and 1 in 33 women develop the disease, although the incidence in women is rising, largely because of a change in the smoking habits of the population. Mesothelioma is less common, with 1000 cases per annum currently diagnosed in the UK, but this is expected to rise to a peak of 3000 cases in the year 2020, when it will account for approximately 1% of all male cancer deaths. Lung cancer is uncommon before 40 years of age, and patients over 65 years of age account for over half of newly diagnosed cases. Various statistics relating to lung cancer are shown in *Figure 12.1*.

Pathology

Lung cancers are of two main types – approximately one quarter are small cell carcinomas and the remainder are non-small cell carcinomas, including adenocarcinomas, squamous carcinomas, and large cell carcinomas. The histological subtypes are detailed in *Table 12.1*. Mesothelioma is a tumour of the pleura, although abdominal peritoneal mesothelioma can occur in both primary and secondary forms.

Aetiology

The major risk for the development of lung cancer is smoking, since 90% of patients who develop lung cancer are or have been smokers. In the UK, the smoking epidemic among men began at the turn of the 20th century and reached a peak in the 1940s, when two-thirds of all men smoked, and remained high through the early 1970s. Since then the rate of smoking has fallen steadily and now only 28% of adult men smoke. In women smoking only really became established after World War II, reached a peak of 40% in 1948–1980, since when the rate has declined and currently 25% of adult women smoke. Worryingly, in recent years the

Table 12.1. *Histological types of invasive carcinoma of the lung*

Histological type	Frequency (%)
Small cell carcinoma	25
Non-small cell carcinoma	75
squamous cell carcinoma	50
adenocarcinoma	15
large cell carcinoma	10

trend for teenage girls to smoke has increased. Other risk factors include exposure to certain carcinogens such as arsenic and radon gas.

Mesothelioma is particularly associated with exposure to asbestos, which may be difficult to document because the duration of exposure may have been short and the exposure may have occurred up to 40 years previously and may have been indirect in nature (e.g. a woman may have been exposed through contact with her husband's clothing).

Clinical presentation

The signs and symptoms of lung cancer are detailed in *Table 12.2*. The main presenting symptoms of lung cancer are often attributable to a chest infection or exacerbation of a pre-existing lung condition (e.g. cough and shortness of breath). Other non-specific symptoms, such as fatigue and weight loss, are often present. Small cell lung cancers in particular can present with confusion, deranged biochemistry, and paraneoplastic syndromes. Occasionally, patients present asymptomatically with an abnormal chest radiographic performed pre-operatively or as part of a medical check-up.

Screening

Currently, routine screening for carcinoma of the lung is not undertaken. Several studies investigated the role of chest

LUNG CANCER STATISTICS

New lung cancers

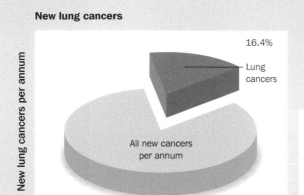

New lung cancers per annum

16.4%

Lung
cancers

All new cancers
per annum

New cases per annum	40260
Males rank	1
Females rank	3
Deaths per annum	34855

Incidence

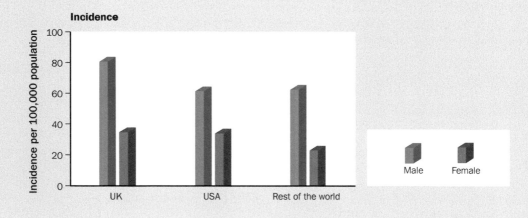

Incidence per 100,000 population

UK USA Rest of the world

Male Female

Survival rate

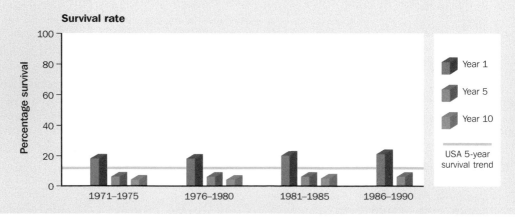

Percentage survival

1971–1975 1976–1980 1981–1985 1986–1990

Year 1
Year 5
Year 10
USA 5-year
survival trend

Figure 12.1. *Statistics relating to lung cancer.*

Table 12.2. *Presenting signs and symptoms of lung cancer*

Common
Persistent cough
Chest pain
Haemoptysis
Continual or non-resolving chest infections
Weight loss
Fatigue
Shortness of breath (pleural effusion, collapse, endobronchial disease)
Confusion (low serum sodium and high serum calcium levels, cerebral metastases)
Bronchorroea (bronchioalveolar carcinoma)
Finger clubbing

Rare
Ear pain
Chest wall deformity
Swelling of the breast (lymphangitic obstruction in mesothelioma)
Dysphagia
Wheeze
'Stopping smoking'

with prolonged or repeated chest infections should have radiographs taken and sequential comparisons made.

Hospital

For patients who present with an abnormal radiograph, cytological or histological confirmation of the disease type is required. Depending on the location of the abnormality this can be done by bronchoscopy, CT-guided lung biopsy, or if lymphadenopathy is present by fine needle aspiration of the affected nodes. In patients who present with a pleural effusion, pleural fluid should be sent for cytological evaluation and a pleural biopsy performed. Histological confirmation of mesothelioma is particularly important for patients seeking industrial compensation for asbestos exposure. All patients with a diagnosis of lung cancer should have a staging CT scan of the thorax and upper abdomen to assess stage, operability, radiotherapy planning, and any other palliative procedures, as well as to help with the prediction of prognosis. In some cases sampling of the mediastinal nodes is required to establish operability or involvement of these structures. Some centres routinely perform a CT scan of the brain on patients who present with small cell lung cancer, which is certainly indicated if the patient has suspicious neurology. Other routine investigations include full blood count and biochemistry, looking in particular for hyponatraemia, hypercalcaemia, and deranged liver function tests. Bone scans are not performed routinely, but are indicated if bone pain is a presenting symptom.

radiographs in screening for this disease and failed to demonstrate a significant reduction in mortality. Other studies used sputum cytology as the screening tool but again failed to demonstrate any benefit with this approach. More recently, studies reported a high detection of early stage carcinomas with computed tomography (CT) scanning compared with chest radiographs in the same group (Lam and Shibuya, 1999). It is as yet too early to say whether this will result in a survival benefit, but the advent of the new millennium will show a renewed interest in screening with spiral CT scans and new molecular markers in sputum.

Investigations

General practice

In patients who present with signs and symptoms suggestive of carcinoma of the lung, the initial investigation of choice is a chest radiograph. If the patient has a productive cough a sputum sample should also be sent for cytology. Smokers

Stage and 5-Year Survival

The staging system for non-small cell carcinoma of the lung, which forms the basis for planning treatment, is outlined in *Tables 12.3* and *12.4*. CT scans form the basis of the system, although sometimes mediastinal node sampling is required to confirm nodal involvement in this area. Positron emission tomography (PET) scanning may become useful in patients who appear on CT scan to have operable disease. For small cell carcinomas of the lung, stage is referred to as limited (confined to the thorax) or extensive (metastatic). Survival figures according to stage are given in *Table 12.5*.

Management of lung cancer

Patients with carcinoma of the lung or mesothelioma should be managed by a multidisciplinary team to ensure all the treatment options are explored. Ideally, this should include a consultant radiologist, respiratory physician, clinical oncologist, medical oncologist, thoracic surgeon, palliative care specialist, and a specialist nurse.

Table 12.3. Tumour, node, metastasis (TNM) classification for non-small cell lung cancer (1995)

Tx	Tumour cannot be assessed, or tumour proved by the presence of malignant cells in sputum or bronchial washings, but not visualized by imaging or bronchoscopy
T0	No evidence of primary tumour
Tis	Carcinoma in situ
T1	Tumour 3cm in diameter or less surrounded by lung or visceral pleura, without bronchoscopic evidence of invasion more proximal than the lobar bronchus
T2	Tumour with any of the following features: 3–5cm in greatest dimension involves main bronchus >2cm distal to the carina invades the visceral pleura
T3	Tumour of any size that directly invades chest wall, diaphragm, mediastinal pleura, or parietal pericardium or that is centrally placed (i.e. within 2 cm of the carina)
T4	Tumour of any size that invades any of the following: mediastinum, trachea, heart, vertebral body, oesophagus, carina or a tumour with a pericardial or pleural effusion or with satellite within the ipsilateral primary tumour lobe of the lung
N0	No regional lymph node metastasis
N1	Metastasis to ipsilateral peribronchial and/or ipsilateral hilar nodes
N2	Metastasis to ipsilateral mediastinal and/or subcarinal nodes
N3	Metastasis to contralateral mediastinal, contralateral hilar, ipsilateral or contralateral scalene or supraclavicular nodes or arm oedema
M0	No distant metastases
M1	Metastases present

Table 10.4. Stages based on TNM classification for non-small cell lung cancer (1995)

Stage	Tumour	Node	Metastasis
IA	T1	N0	M0
IB	T2	N0	M0
IIA	T1	N1	M0
IIB	T2	N1	M0
	T3	N0	M0
	T3	N1	M0
IIIA	T1–3	N2	M0
IIIB	Any T	N3	M0
	T4	Any N	M0
IV	Any T	Any N	M1

Table 12.5. 5-year survival for lung cancer

Cancer	Stage	5-year survival (%)
Non-small cell lung cancer	Stage I	69
	Stage II	40
	Stage III	13
	Stage IV	7.5
Small cell lung cancer	Limited	15–20
	Extensive	5

Management of patients with small cell lung cancer

The initial treatment of choice for patients with small cell lung cancer is chemotherapy, which should commence as soon as possible once the diagnosis has been made, as these patients can deteriorate rapidly. Small cell lung cancer is relatively chemosensitive, with response rates in the region of 65–85%. Chemotherapy regimens commonly used are platinum or carboplatin and etoposide (PE or CE), or doxorubicin (Adriamycin) or ifosfamide plus cyclophosphamide and etoposide (ACE or ICE). Other regimens used are cyclophosphamide, doxorubicin, and vincristine (CAV), alternating PE and CAV, and oral etoposide is still used in selected situations. Patients normally receive between four and six cycles of treatment.

Intensive regimens are still under investigation and may show survival benefits for some patients, such as young fit patients with limited disease. The initial course of treatment can be stormy for the patient in terms of neutropenia and sepsis, and prophylactic broad spectrum antibiotics (e.g. ciprofloxacin) are often given to cover the expected period of neutropenia (days 7–14).

On completion of chemotherapy, patients with limited stage disease should be referred for consolidation radiotherapy to the mediastinum and brain [prophylactic cranial irradiation (PCI)], because this reduces the risk of recurrence and prolongs survival.

Patients with extensive stage disease are incurable and treatment is given with palliative intent. Consolidation radiotherapy or PCI is not routinely given after chemotherapy. In this group of patients radiotherapy is usually reserved for symptom relief.

Patients who relapse following the initial treatment can be rechallenged with chemotherapy, with some durable symptomatic responses.

Management of patients with non-small cell lung cancer
Surgery, neoadjuvant, and adjuvant therapy
Surgery is the treatment modality in lung cancer that offers the greatest likelihood of cure. Unfortunately, the vast majority of patients are not suitable for this approach because of either advanced disease at presentation or concurrent medical conditions. Patients who, after the staging investigation, have stage I or II disease and selected patients with stage IIIA disease should be discussed with a thoracic surgeon. The number of patients who reach surgery may be increased by the use of induction chemotherapy, and patients deemed inoperable at the start of chemotherapy could become operable after chemotherapy. The role of neoadjuvant chemotherapy (treatment prior to surgery) in patients with operable tumours is still being tested in clinical trials and may lead to survival benefits as a result of the earlier treatment of micrometastases.

Following complete resection of T1–2N0 tumours, postoperative radiotherapy does not improve either local control or survival. In patients with N2 tumours, radiotherapy may reduce the incidence of locoregional recurrence, but data to support this are limited. Patients with macroscopic or microscopic residual disease after surgery should be considered for postoperative radiotherapy. Postoperative (i.e. adjuvant) chemotherapy with cisplatin-containing regimens is also the subject of clinical trials as the data are still limited. The current recommendation is that patients should be considered for postoperative chemotherapy in the context of a clinical trial.

Radical radiotherapy
Some patients have technically operable disease but are not suitable for surgery because of either intercurrent medical problems (e.g. because of poor cardiac or respiratory function) or refusal to undergo an operation. These patients should be considered for radical radiotherapy. Similarly, patients with locally advanced tumours downstaged by chemotherapy may still not be suitable for surgery, but could receive radical radiotherapy as consolidation treatment. Published 5-year survival rates for patients treated with this approach range from 6 to 32%. Survival rates may improve with the use of continuous hyperfractionated regimens in which patients receive two or three fractions of radiotherapy daily, including weekends, as opposed to conventional daily treatment (continuous hyperfractionated accelerated radiotherapy – CHART).

Palliative radiotherapy
Radiotherapy also has a major role in the palliative management of haemoptysis, cerebral metastases, bone metastases, and symptoms caused by progression of the primary tumour. A single fraction or a more prolonged course can be administered on an outpatient basis.

Palliative chemotherapy
The majority of patients who receive chemotherapy for non-small cell lung cancer do so in the palliative setting, either at presentation or on relapse following primary surgery or radical radiotherapy. Platinum-based combination chemotherapy is the treatment of choice and the same regimens are used in the adjuvant and neoadjuvant settings. Commonly used combinations include mitomycin C, vinblastine, and cisplatin (MVP), mitomycin C, ifosfamide, and cisplatin (MIC), and more recently vinorelbine or gemcitabine with cisplatin (NP). Patients with impaired renal function, pre-existing neurological abnormalities, or deafness may have carboplatin substituted for cisplatin. Objective response rates for all these combinations are in the order of 30–40%, although up to 70% of patients may have a symptomatic response. Maximum benefit seems to be gained with three courses. In patients who fail on first-line chemotherapy or who have relapsed following an initial response to treatment, second-line agents are of use to help control symptoms and prolong life. However, these new drugs are relatively expensive, and work is ongoing on the health economics of this and other situations in lung cancer.

Management of mesothelioma
Surgery is rarely an option in the treatment of mesothelioma, although if disease is localized or if pain is a problem there may be a role for debulking. This approach will be explored further in national clinical trials. Adequate management of recurrent pleural effusions is particularly important in patients with this disease. This is usually best achieved by thoracoscopic talc pleurodesis under the care of a thoracic surgeon. Following this procedure or, indeed, any drainage procedure or pleural biopsy, consideration should be given to drain-site radiotherapy to prevent the development of exit-site nodules. Patients with symptomatic disease or rapidly progressing disease may benefit from palliative chemotherapy. This is usually combination chemotherapy similar to that given for non-small cell carcinoma of the lung. Radiotherapy may also have a role in the palliation of the disease, particularly if there is chest wall invasion or development of superior vena caval obstruction (SVCO).

Key points: lung cancer

Age	Only 1% of cases occur before 40 years
	85% of cases occur over 60 years
Risk factors	About 90% of patients are smokers or ex-smokers
Predominant symptoms at presentation	Cough
	Dyspnoea
	Haemoptysis
	Weight loss
	Chest and/or shoulder pain
	Hoarseness

More than 90% of patients are symptomatic at the time of diagnosis

Chest radiography findings are abnormal in the vast majority of symptomatic patients; however, a normal chest radiograph does not exclude a diagnosis of cancer

In most cases it is appropriate for a GP to request a chest radiography as an initial investigation, with referral to a chest physician if the chest radiograph is suggestive and/or suspicious of lung cancer

In a limited number of circumstances, urgent referral to a chest physician is appropriate without requesting a chest radiograph.

Sputum cytology is rarely indicated and should not routinely be requested prior to referral for a specialist opinion

Reproduced from England Department of Health Cancer Referral Guidelines Consultation Document May 2000.

Guidelines for urgent referral: lung cancer

Urgent referral to a chest physician

Any of the following conditions:

Chest radiograph suggestive and/or suspicious of lung cancer.

Signs of superior vena caval obstruction (swelling of face and/or neck with fixed elevation of jugular venous pressure).

Persistent cervical and/or supraclavicular lymphadenopathy (NB consider referral to a head and neck specialist, particularly in younger patients).

Stridor (consider emergency referral).

Features suggestive of metastasis (e.g. brain, liver, bone, or skin).

Urgent referral for chest radiography

Haemoptysis

Unexplained or persistent (more than 3 weeks):

   cough

   chest and/or shoulder pain

   weight loss

   chest signs

   dyspnoea

   hoarseness

   finger clubbing (that is not hereditary)

Reproduced from England Department of Health Cancer Referral Guidelines Consultation Document May 2000.

Referral proforma: lung cancer

Demographics

Age:			
Current or ex-smoker	Yes	No	
History of chronic obstructive pulmonary disease	Yes	No	

Symptoms

Haemoptysis:	None	Once	More than once
Unexplained or persistent (>3 weeks):	Yes	No	
cough			
breathlessness			
wheeze			
chest and/or shoulder pain			
weight loss			
hoarseness			

Clinical examination:

chest signs			
signs of superior vena cava obstruction			
cervical lymph nodes			
stridor			
signs of metastases			
finger clubbing			

Chest radiograph:

not done			
abnormal, follow-up recommended			
abnormal, suspicious of cancer			
abnormal, other			

Comments/other reasons for requesting urgent referral:

Reproduced from England Department of Health Cancer Referral Guidelines Consultation Document May 2000.

Management of superior vena caval obstruction

SVCO can occur with any histological type of lung cancer and requires assessment and prompt treatment; emergency treatment is not usually needed. Patients are usually commenced on high-dose corticosteroids. As small cell lung cancer is chemosensitive it is usually treated with chemotherapy, but radiotherapy can be used if there is no response or for consolidation of response. Patients who do not respond to chemoradiotherapy should be considered for superior vena caval stenting. Patients with non-small cell lung cancer and mesothelioma can also develop SVCO and are usually treated with radiotherapy, but chemotherapy can be tried first if the degree of obstruction is not major and the patient is fit for chemotherapy. Again, stenting is usually kept for resistant cases, but it is expensive and operator dependent.

Palliative Care

Most patients with carcinoma of the lung present with advanced disease and treatment is palliative in intent from the outset. Early referral of all such patients should be made to the local Macmillan care team or local hospice to enable the optimal symptom control and support.

Patients whose symptoms relate to the primary tumour may benefit from palliative radiotherapy or chemotherapy if they are fit enough. Pain caused by bony metastases can respond to chemotherapy or radiotherapy in at least 50% of patients, and can also respond to intravenous bisphosphonates. In patients with recurrent pleural effusions, referral for thoracoscopic pleurodesis or pleuroperitoneal shunt should be considered. Pleural effusions are a major cause of breathlessness, but worsening dyspnoea can also result from lymphangitis, development of SVCO, collapse of a lung secondary to endobronchial disease, or compression of the bronchi caused by worsening lymphadenopathy. Symptoms from lymphangitis respond somewhat to corticosteroids, morphine preparations, and domicillary oxygen. Patients with symptomatic endobronchial disease may derive benefit from stenting or laser treatment. Cerebral metastases are common in patients with both small cell and non-small cell carcinoma, and both histological types may respond to palliative radiotherapy and corticosteroids. Occasionally, cerebral metastases are associated with an obstructive hydrocephalus, and these patients should be discussed with a neurosurgeon and considered for stenting. Similarly, a solitary non-small cell lung cancer brain metastasis can be resected in appropriate situations.

Lung cancer has hitherto had a dismal prognosis, but survival figures for small cell lung cancer have improved. With combined modality and earlier treatments, we are optimistic about the outcome for non-small cell lung cancer and we are only now beginning to manage mesothelioma actively.

References and Further Reading

Ellis PA, Smith IE, Hardy JR, *et al*. Symptom relief with MVP (mitomycin C, vinblastine and cisplatin). *Br J Cancer*. 1995; **71**: 366–71.

Ihde DC. Chemotherapy for lung cancer. *N Engl J Med*. 1992; **12**: 1434–41.

Lam S, Shibuya H. Early diagnosis of lung cancer. *Clin Chest Med*. 1999; **354**: 99–105.

Lung Cancer Study Group. The benefit of adjuvant treatment for resected locally advanced non-small cell lung cancer. *J Clin Oncol*. 1998; **6**: 9–17.

Mountain CF. Revisions in the international staging system for lung cancer. *Chest*. 1997; **111**: 1710–17.

Non-small Cell Lung Cancer Collaborative Group. Chemotherapy in non-small cell lung cancer: a meta-analysis using updated data on individual patients from 52 randomised clinical trials. *BMJ*. 1995; **311**: 899–909.

Saunders M, Dische S, Barrett A, *et al*. Continuous hyperfractionated accelerated radiotherapy (CHART) versus conventional radiotherapy in non-small cell lung cancer: a randomised multicentre trial. *Lancet*. 1997; **350**: 161–5.

13 Breast Cancer

Kate Gregory and Ian Smith

Incidence

Breast cancer is the most common cancer in women, and the lifetime risk of developing this disease for women in the UK is 1 in 12. Breast cancer is responsible for 15,000 deaths per annum in the UK and is the leading cause of death in women 35–50 years of age. Despite this statistic it is important to remember that 80% of all breast cancers are diagnosed in postmenopausal women. Various statistics relating to breast cancer are shown in *Figure 13.1.*

Pathology

Histological types of carcinoma of the breast are detailed in *Table 13.1.* The majority of breast carcinomas are invasive ductal carcinomas and are graded I, II, or III on the basis of tubule formation, nuclear pleomorphism, and mitotic count. This grading has prognostic significance and is an important guide in the selection of appropriate adjuvant therapies. The rarer or so-called special-tumour types (tubular, medullary, and adenoid cystic) tend to be slow growing and have a very good prognosis.

In situ carcinoma of the breast may be ductal, lobular, or mixed. Ductal carcinoma in situ (DCIS) may present as a mass in the breast, but more commonly it is detected as a result of mammographic screening. Indeed, this condition has become much more common as a result of mass screening and now represents around 15% of all newly diagnosed breast cancers.

Up to 50% of patients who present with a symptomatic breast cancer are found to have axillary nodal involvement at surgery.

Aetiology

A number of risk factors have been identified for the development of breast cancer, of which the most important are outlined in *Table 13.2.* In addition, approximately 5% of all breast cancers are genetic in origin (see below). Endocrine factors that relate to lifetime exposure to oestrogens have also

Table 13.1. Histological types of invasive carcinoma of the breast

Histological type	Frequency (%)
Ductal	75
Lobular	10
Tubular	5
Adenoid cystic	5
Medullary	4
Papillary	1

Table 13.2. Risk factors for the development of breast cancer

Factor	Relative risk
Age at first pregnancy >30 years	2–4
Early menarche	1–1.9
Late menopause	1–1.9
First-degree relative aged <50 years with breast cancer	>4
Any first-degree relative with breast cancer	2–4
Past history of breast cancer	>4

been identified. No strong evidence links use of the oral contraceptive pill with the development of breast cancer, but some studies showed that the long-term use of hormone replacement therapy (HRT) for 10 years or more appears to increase the risk of developing breast cancer by about 20–30%. Recent evidence suggests that this increase is predominantly in good prognosis, oestrogen-receptor positive tumours and so the benefits of HRT may well outweigh this risk.

Hereditary breast cancer

Current evidence suggests that only about 5% of breast cancers are truly inherited. The genes currently known to be associated with this condition are *BRCA* (breast cancer-associated

BREAST CANCER STATISTICS

New breast cancers

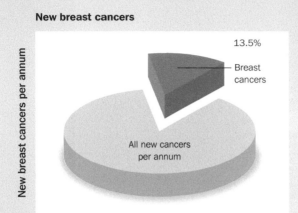

New cases per annum	33240
Males rank	18
Females rank	1
Deaths per annum	13475

Incidence

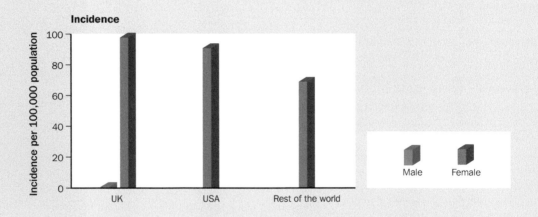

Survival rate

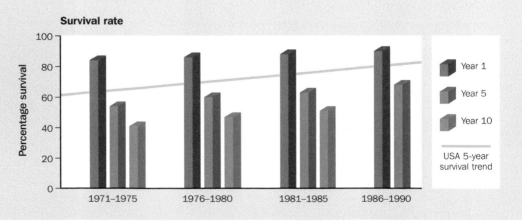

Figure 13.1. *Statistics relating to breast cancer.*

gene) 1 and 2, but it is clear that other genes are yet to be cloned. It is now possible to screen members of an affected family for the presence of these genes, but to do so it is necessary to have a DNA sample from at least one affected family member.

The presence of a mutation in the *BRCA*1 gene is associated with an 85% lifetime risk of developing carcinoma of the breast. The *BRCA*2 gene also increases the risk of developing ovarian carcinoma. Women found to be carriers of these genes require support and it is recommended that they should be counselled by a cancer geneticist before undergoing testing. For those women who test positive the options for prevention are limited. Retrospective studies suggest that prophylactic mastectomy seems to be associated with a reduction in the risk of developing the disease, although prospective data are not yet available. The psychological consequences of the procedure can be considerable and there remains a small risk of developing breast cancer in residual tissue in the axillary and subareolar areas. The other option for prevention was thought to lie in the use of anti-oestrogens as chemopreventative agents. Studies using tamoxifen in high-risk women in the USA showed a significant reduction in the risk of developing breast cancer, but this has not been borne out by European studies and most oncologists in the UK use tamoxifen as a preventative agent only in the setting of a clinical trial. Women who are carriers certainly require extensive surveillance under the care of a specialist, with annual clinical examinations. Regular mammography also has an important role, although the optimum age and frequency remain uncertain.

With increasing publicity about genetic risks in breast cancer, more and more patients are requesting referral for screening. As yet there are no national guidelines for the management of these women, although the referral of patients at moderate or high risk to a local breast clinic would seem appropriate. Criteria for women at moderate and high risk are given in *Table 13.3*.

Table 13.3. Guidelines for referral for breast screening – women at moderate or high risk

First-degree relative diagnosed with breast cancer at under age 40 years of age
First- or second-degree relative diagnosed with breast cancer under 60 years of age or with ovarian carcinoma at any age
First- or second-degree relatives with breast or ovarian cancer
First-degree relative with bilateral breast cancer

Clinical Presentation

The majority of women present with a palpable breast lump or after mammographic screening. Other suspicious features are nipple retraction, blood-stained nipple discharge, and tethering of the skin. Inflammatory carcinomas are very rare, but can present as an erythematous, swollen, hot, and usually painful breast without the presence of a discrete lump; suspicion should be high in those women who present as such and who fail to respond to antibiotics. Breast cancers are usually but not always painless. Occasionally, women present with metastases as the main clinical finding. Bone metastases from breast cancer are common and women who present with pathological fractures should always be examined to exclude a breast primary.

Screening

Population-based breast cancer screening using mammography for women aged between 50 and 65 years has been in place in the UK for some years. Current practice is to screen women in this age group every 3 years. Cancers detected by screening mammography are more likely to be small (50% are <15mm), node negative (65%), and of a histological type with good prognosis. Population-based screening in women over 50 years of age reduces 10-year mortality from breast cancer by 30%. However, the role of screening in younger women is much less clear, for two main reasons:

- breast cancer is rare in this age group; and
- difficulty occurs in detecting breast cancer mammographically in menstruating women with denser breast tissue – it may be that other forms of imaging, such as magnetic resonance imaging (MRI), are sensitive for selected high risk women in this age group.

Investigations

Patients with a breast lump should be referred directly to a specialized multidisciplinary breast clinic for investigation. Many hospitals now run a one-stop clinic for these patients, although the perceived benefits of this remain debatable. Basic investigations include a family history, clinical examination, mammography (if the patient does not present via the screening service), ultrasound of any palpable mass, and fine needle aspiration cytology of such a mass. For screen-detected lesions, a needle localization biopsy may be required. For systemic staging, most centres simply perform a chest radiograph and routine blood tests unless there is a clinical indication for more extensive staging, as in those patients with inflammatory or locally advanced tumours or with suspicious systemic symptoms (e.g. bone pain).

Stage and 5-Year Survival

The most important prognostic factor in breast carcinoma is the status of axillary lymph nodes. Patients who are node-negative have a 75% 10-year survival compared with only 20% for those with eight or more involved lymph nodes. Histological grade also carries prognostic significance, with 5-year survival rates about 90% for grade I tumours, 55% for grade II tumours, and 48% for grade III tumours. Vascular invasion and clinical tumour size are other important factors. The staging and 5-year survival according to the main prognostic variables are set out in *Tables 13.4–13.6*.

Management

Carcinoma in situ

DCIS is a proliferation of malignant epithelial cells confined to the mammary ducts and lobules without evidence of inva-

sion. It accounts for approximately 25% of mammographically detected lesions. The mainstay of treatment for DCIS is adequate surgical excision. Mastectomy is curative, but represents overtreatment for many women. The challenge is to identify those who can be successfully treated with conservative surgery. Many patients require further excisions to ensure clearance and frequently mastectomy is required for those with extensive or multifocal disease. Conservative surgery alone is associated with a local recurrence rate of around 20%, and approximately half of these recurrences occur as invasive disease. Radiotherapy does seem to reduce the risk of recurrence to about 10%, and overall survival is not affected. One study suggested that adjuvant tamoxifen

Table 13.5. Stages based on TNM classification for breast cancer

Stage	Tumour	Node	Metastasis
I	T1	N0/N1a	M0
II	T0	N1b	M0
	T1	N0,1a,1b	M0
	T2	N0,1a,1b	M0
III	T1	N2	M0
	T2	N2	M0
	T3	N0/1/2	M0
IV	T4	Any N	Any M
	Any T3		Any M
	Any T	Any N	M1

Table 13.4. Tumour, node, and metastasis (TNM) classification for breast cancer

Category	Description
T1	Tumour <2cm diameter:
a	without fixation to underlying muscle
b	with fixation to underlying muscle
T2	Tumour between 2 and 5cm diameter
T3	Tumour >5cm diameter
T4	Tumour of any size fixed to chest wall or skin
N0	Nodes impalpable
N1	Mobile nodes:
a	clinically uninvolved
b	clinically involved
N2	Nodes involved and fixed
N3	Supraclavicular or infraclavicular nodes or arm oedema
M0	No distant metastases
M1	Metastases present

Table 13.6. 5-year survival for breast cancer according to histological grade, tumour size, and nodes involved

Prognostic factor	5-year survival (%)
Histological grade	
I	85
II	60
III	40
Tumour size	
<2cm	90
>5cm	70
Nodal status	
0	75
1–3	50
>4	40

is of benefit following local treatment and another study has suggested that tamoxifen may further reduce local recurrence, although recent data suggest that the benefit is likely to be small.

Early breast cancer

Patients should be managed by a multidisciplinary team that involves both surgeons and oncologists. The majority of patients require multimodality therapy, including surgery, chemotherapy and/or tamoxifen, and radiotherapy.

If tumours are operable at presentation the usual treatment plan is surgical excision followed by appropriate adjuvant therapy. Trials have consistently shown that mastectomy has no advantage over breast-conserving surgery for small cancers. Most surgeons still favour axillary surgery of some form, although the prognostic information obtained is of less significance now because adjuvant chemotherapy is being advised for increasing numbers of women irrespective of their nodal status. However, some form of treatment to the axilla is important, except in low-risk women; if axillary surgery is not performed and the axilla is considered at risk, the patient should receive radiotherapy to this site. Interest is increasing in the role of sentinel node biopsy (i.e. the first lymph node into which the breast lymphatics drain) in breast cancer surgery since as it may reduce the morbidity from an axillary node dissection, and many centres are conducting studies in this. Patients who have multifocal disease or large primaries usually require mastectomy.

Many breast surgeons offer breast reconstruction either at the time of mastectomy or at some later stage. The reconstruction procedure offered depends upon the expertise of the surgeon and the size of the woman's breasts. Options include latissimus dorsi (LD) reconstruction (in which the LD muscle is freed and rotated round onto the chest), a Becker implant (in which a saline-filled bag is inserted as an implant with a port allowing for the implant to be expanded to give a shape comparable to the remaining breast), and a transcutaneous rectus abdominus myocutaneous flap (TRAM-flap) reconstruction (in which the abdominal muscle and subcutaneous fat are rotated up onto the chest).

The role of chemotherapy is usually in the adjuvant setting. Overview analyses of clinical trials worldwide confirmed the benefit of adjuvant chemotherapy in both node-negative and node-positive patients up to the age of 70 years, but the amount of benefit decreases with age. The overall benefit of polychemotherapy at 10 years is about 10% for recurrence-free survival and 15% for overall survival. Guidelines as to who

Table 13.7. *Guidelines for prescribing adjuvant chemotherapy in carcinoma of the breast*

All patients <70 years of age with node positive disease
Node negative patients unless good prognosis by all of the following criteria:
tumour <1cm
grade I histology
age >35 years
Oestrogen receptor positive
No vascular/lymphatic invasion

should receive adjuvant chemotherapy vary between hospitals. Recommendations from a recent consensus meeting on adjuvant chemotherapy are outlined in *Table 13.7*. Current evidence suggests a modest increase in survival benefit for anthracycline-based chemotherapy over the more traditional cyclophosphamide, methotrexate, and 5-fluorouracil (CMF) combination. This is generally given on an outpatient basis and patients usually receive six cycles in total at 3-week intervals.

Over recent years interest has increased in the use of chemotherapy before surgery in the neoadjuvant setting to downstage locally advanced or large tumours and thus make conservative surgery possible. Several studies showed a marked reduction in the mastectomy rate with this approach. Efforts are now under way to develop methods of using the primary tumour as an in vivo measure of response to treatment; the hope is that this could become an early surrogate marker for survival benefit.

Adjuvant tamoxifen is recommended for all patients who are oestrogen-receptor-positive. Currently, the recommendation is for 5 years of tamoxifen in the adjuvant setting, although there are ongoing trials to investigate the optimum duration of treatment. Additional benefit may be found in the use of luteinizing hormone releasing hormone (LHRH) antagonists in premenopausal patients to achieve ovarian ablation, although this may be associated with significant toxicity in terms of menopausal symptoms.

Adjuvant radiotherapy is recommended for all patients after conservative surgery to maximize local control. In addition, in post-mastectomy patients with nodal involvement there may be benefits in radiotherapy to the chest wall and supraclavicular fossa. Fractionation schedules vary between hospitals, but generally speaking treatment extends over 6–7 weeks.

After completion of primary treatment patients are followed up predominantly by clinical examination and annual

Key points: breast cancer

Age	Incidence increases with age; 5% of cases occur before 40 years of age and only 2% before 35 years of age
Incidence	A general practitioner with a list of 2000 patients can expect to see one new patient with breast cancer per year, but will see a considerably larger number of women with benign breast problems

Other breast problems include:	
diffuse nodularity	Common in all age groups up to 50 years of age
fibroadenoma	Peak range at 20–30 years of age
cysts	Peak range 40–60 years of age
breast pain and/or mastalgia	Pain alone is a very uncommon presentation of breast cancer

Presenting features of symptomatic cases of breast cancer:	
lump	90%
painful lump	20%
nipple change	10%
nipple discharge	3%
skin contour change	5%

Reproduced from England Department of Health Cancer Referral Guidelines Consultation Document March 2000.

Guidelines for urgent referral: breast cancer

Urgent referrals

Patients with a discrete lump in the appropriate age group

Definite signs of cancer such as:
   ulceration
   skin nodule
   skin distortion

Conditions that require referral – but not necessarily urgently

Lump	Discrete lump in a younger woman (eg age <30 years)
	Asymmetrical nodularity that persists at review after menstruation
	Abscess
	Persistently refilling or recurrent cyst
Pain	Intractable pain not responding to reassurance, simple measures such as wearing a well-supporting bra, and common drugs
Nipple discharge	<50 years of age with bilateral discharge sufficient to stain clothes
	<50 years of age with bloodstained discharge
	>50 years of age with any nipple discharge

Nipple retraction or distortion, nipple eczema

Referral proforma: breast cancer

Age:

Symptoms	Yes	No	
Patient aware of lump			
Pain			
Change in shape of breast			
Nipple change			
Nipple discharge			

Previous history	Yes	No	
Benign breast problems			
Breast cancer			

Family history	Yes	No	
Breast cancer			

Clinical examination	Yes	No	
Discrete lump			
If yes, size:............cm			
If yes, right and /or left			
Ulceration of breast			
Skin nodule			
Skin distortion			
In-drawn nipple			
Visible nipple discharge			
Nipple eczema			
Asymmetrical nodularity			
Axillary lymphadenopathy			

Comments/other reasons for urgent referral, plus diagram of breasts

These guidelines for urgent referral of patients with suspected breast cancer are based on those set out in Guidelines for Referral of Patients with Breast Problems, second edition (1999), prepared by Joan Austoker and Robert Mansel under the auspices of the NHS Breast Screening Programme and the Cancer Research Campaign.

mammography. Systemic screening has no role unless there is clinical suspicion. Likewise, the tumour marker CA15–3 does not have a role in routine follow-up.

Many women suffer menopausal symptoms following adjuvant chemotherapy and endocrine therapy. In some cases these symptoms can be severe and can significantly impair quality of life. If simple treatments such as oil of evening primrose (at a dose of >1000mg daily) fail to help alleviate the symptoms, consideration should be given to commencement of HRT. Current dogma states that HRT should not be given to women with a history of breast cancer on the basis that it will increase the risk of recurrence. In reality, no convincing evidence supports this dogma and the use of HRT remains unclear. If there is a detrimental effect at all, it is likely to be a very small one, and it has to be balanced against the proved long-term benefits of HRT as a protection against cardiovascular disease and osteoporosis. In addition, the short-term benefits, both physical and psychological, are very important for many women. It is our current practice in many centres to put these arguments to patients who are considering HRT, and to encourage them to go ahead with this treatment if they so wish. There is a current national study to investigate the role of HRT in women treated for breast cancer.

Pregnancy-related breast cancer

Pregnancy-related breast cancer was traditionally thought to carry a particularly bad prognosis. However, when matched for age and stage the outlook is no different from that for cancers that arise in non-pregnant women. There is no indication that continuing with the pregnancy jeopardizes the health of the mother and hence no medical indication for therapeutic abortion. Surgery is performed in the first instance, followed by adjuvant chemotherapy if indicated in the second or third trimesters; contrary to clinical instinct, this does not appear to be associated with an increase in foetal abnormalities. Radiotherapy should be delayed until after the baby is delivered.

Metastatic breast cancer

Although the majority of patients present with apparently localized disease, 80% subsequently relapse with metastatic spread. At this stage treatment is not curative, but useful remissions can be obtained with chemotherapy and endocrine manoeuvres. The management of the disease depends on the site of metastases and the symptoms that the patient is experiencing.

Bone metastases are common in women with breast carcinoma. Bony metastatic disease is usually diagnosed on plain radiographs and bone scintogram, but MRI scans may be required if these preliminary investigations are equivocal. Increasing evidence indicates that bisphosphonate therapy can prevent the complications of bony metastases, including pain, fractures, and hypercalcaemia. In the absence of other systemic disease further treatment usually consists of endocrine therapy. Aromatase inhibitors are the treatment of choice for postmenopausal women, and LHRH antagonists for premenopausal women. Palliative radiotherapy can also have analgesic benefit when a solitary metastasis is causing pain. In addition, surgical stabilization is occasionally required when a lytic lesion threatens the integrity of a bone. If bone disease progresses despite the measures outlined above, chemotherapy can sometimes be very effective.

Other systemic disease is usually treated with chemotherapy or endocrine therapies as described previously. Patients who are chemo-naïve usually receive an anthracycline-containing regimen, whereas patients who have previously received this in the adjuvant setting are considered for therapy with a taxane. In the context of metastatic disease some patients may find these treatments difficult to tolerate and in these situations treatment with a single-agent such as vinorelbine (a vinca-alkaloid) may be more appropriate. New therapies are constantly emerging, including the recent development of the monoclonal antibody trastuzumab, which is directed against the cell surface receptor coded by the oncogene HER-2. This oncogene is known to be associated with poor prognosis and relative resistance to chemotherapy. Preliminary studies in the USA showed encouraging results with this agent given as a single agent and in combination with chemotherapy. This drug is now available for routine use in the UK – either as a single agent or in combination with taxanes.

In the case of brain metastases the treatment of choice is whole-brain radiotherapy, usually given in 10 fractions. Chemotherapy can also sometimes be helpful in the treatment of brain metastases in association with systemic disease. Meningeal disease can occur in breast carcinoma and is usually treated with weekly intrathecal methotrexate. It is worth noting that patients with central nervous system disease who are otherwise well may achieve remissions that measure years rather than months with the appropriate treatment.

Palliative care

Patients with breast cancer may develop many problems in the latter stages of their disease. Pain from bony metastases can be debilitating so adequate analgesia and the oncological interventions outlined above are vital in maintaining quality of life. Locally advanced disease can be particularly distressing with burning pain caused by skin infiltration, ulceration, infection, and bleeding. The involvement of specialist nurses is crucial to the management of this problem. The pain may respond to anti-epileptic drugs, the bleeding to tranexamic acid, and metronidazole gel is useful in controlling superficial infection and the smell, which can be particularly distressing to patients. Lymphangitis is common with dyspnoea and cough; patients who are not suitable for further treatment may be helped by corticosteroids, oral morphine solution, or methadone linctus.

Further Reading

Breast cancer metastatic: Breast cancer non-metastatic. In: *Clinical Evidence*. London: BMJ Publishing Group, Issue 7, June 2002: 1579–63.

Carter CL, Allen C, Henson DE. Relation of tumor size, lymph node status, and survival in 24,740 breast cancer cases. *Cancer* 1989; **63**: 181–7.

CRC Breast Cancer Factsheet 1996.

Early Breast Cancer Triallists Group. Effects of radiotherapy and surgery in early breast cancer: an overview of the randomized trials. *N Engl J Med* 1995; **333**: 1444–55.

Early Breast Cancer Triallists Group Collaborative Group. Polychemotherapy for early breast cancer: an overview of the randomized trials. *Lancet* 1998; **352**: 930–42.

14 Gastrointestinal Cancer

Kate Sumpter and David Cunningham

Introduction

Overview

- Gastrointestinal cancers are common
- They account for 25–30% of European cancer deaths
- Management depends on anatomical site
- Management is multidisciplinary

Figure 14.1 shows the 10 most common causes of cancer death in the UK. Tumours that arise from the gastrointestinal tract are common and in many instances fatal, accounting for between 25 and 30% of European cancer deaths. The management of these tumours is increasingly multimodality-based, but it also varies greatly depending on the anatomical site of the tumour. In this chapter the various tumours that comprise the gastrointestinal tract are reviewed in turn, beginning proximally, with particular emphasis on the presentation, diagnosis, and management of patients with these tumours. In the case of colorectal cancer (CRC) we also discuss the issue of screening high-risk individuals and relatives with the diagnosis.

Oesophageal Cancer

Key points: oesophageal cancer

- Pathologically divided into squamous cell carcinoma and adenocarcinoma
- Careful staging is imperative, including computed tomography scan and transoesophageal ultrasound
- Poor survival rate with surgery
- Increasing use of chemotherapy and radiotherapy for localized disease

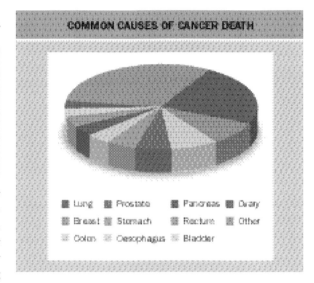

Figure 14.1. *Ten most common causes of cancer death in the UK.*

Incidence

Oesophageal carcinoma is the ninth most common cancer worldwide and in the UK it accounts for approximately 2% of cancer deaths annually. Various statistics related to oesophageal cancer are shown in *Figure 14.2*. There is a wide geographical variation in the incidence of oesophageal carcinoma worldwide, with parts of China and Iran having a particularly high incidence. In such areas the aetiology is thought to be micronutrient deficiencies. In Western Europe and North America world smoking and alcohol consumption are aetiologically linked to the development of the disease.

Pathology

Tumours of the oesophagus can be divided pathologically into squamous cell carcinomas (which account for 80% of all tumours of the oesophagus) and adenocarcinomas (the

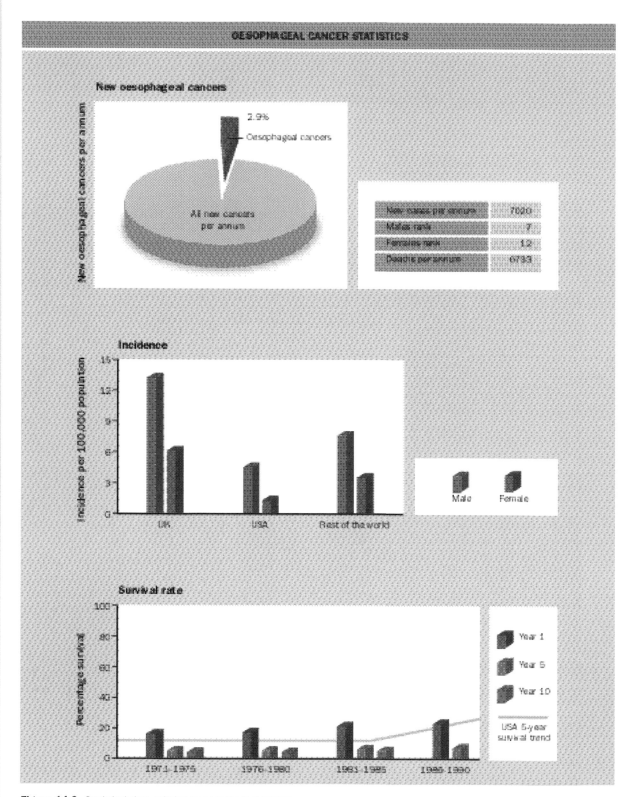

Figure 14.2. Statistical data relating to oesophageal cancer.

incidence of which is rising). Adenocarcinomas arise predominantly within the lower third of the oesophagus and may develop within an area of Barrett's oesophagus. Rarer tumours of the oesophagus include leiomyosarcoma, melanomas, lymphomas, and Kaposi's sarcoma.

In addition to pathological subdivision, tumours of the oesophagus are often divided, according to their anatomical site, into four subtypes:

- cervical (tumours arising from the cricoid cartilage to the thoracic inlet);
- upper thoracic (thoracic inlet to the tracheal bifurcation);
- mid-thoracic [tracheal bifurcation to half way to the oesophagogastric junction (OGJ)]; and
- lower thoracic (half way to extending to the OGJ).

Approximately 50% of oesophageal tumours arise in the mid-thoracic region.

Staging and diagnosis

Staging is based on the Union Internationale Contre le Cancer (UICC) and tumour, nodes, and metastases (TNM) system. Accurate staging of oesophageal tumours is important predominantly because management is, to a large extent, dependent upon the stage of the disease at presentation, but also because survival is strongly linked to the stage of disease (*Table 14.1*).

Patients with oesophageal tumours most commonly present with progressive dysphagia, initially to solids, which extends over time to an intolerance of softer substances and ultimately to fluids. Other common presenting symptoms include epigastric or chest pain, weight loss, anorexia, and haematemesis.

Diagnosis is usually made from either a barium swallow or an endoscopy (which is required to establish a histological diagnosis). Following a diagnosis of oesophageal carcinoma, patients need to be staged clinically. The initial investigations should include a computed tomography (CT) scan of the chest, abdomen, and pelvis predominantly to delineate whether there is metastatic spread, but also to assess the nodal and local status of the tumour. CT scanning is not a very sensitive technique for the T staging of oesophageal lesions and, with the development of transoesophageal ultrasound scanning, which should become more widely available in the future, radiological T staging will improve dramatically. If the tumour appears operable, the use of positive emission tomography (PET) scanning can be considered to further ensure that there is no evidence of metastatic disease.

Table 14.1. *Tumour, nodes, and metastases (TNM) and Union Internationale Contre le Cancer (UICC) staging systems for oesophageal carcinoma and the 5-year survival figures following surgical resection*

UICC staging group	TNM	5-year survival postsurgical resection (%)
Stage I	T1, N0, M0	66
Stage IIA	T2/3, N0, M0	40
Stage IIB	T1/2, N1, M0	19
Stage III	T3, N1, M0	16
	T4, Any N, M0	16
Stage IV	Any T, Any N, M1	2

Management

Surgery for patients with operable disease (i.e. clinically operable tumours in patients who are fit for surgery) has been generally considered the optimal treatment. The use of postoperative chemotherapy in oesophageal cancer is complicated by the prolonged recovery period that usually follows an oesophagectomy. This delay tends to conflict with the aims of adjuvant chemotherapy, so postoperative chemotherapy should only be used within the context of a clinical trial.

However, surgical resection for patients with stage II or III disease is associated with poor survival rates of only 15%. In view of this there is increasing interest in the use of preoperative chemotherapy and radiotherapy to improve the long-term survival figures in this group of patients. The rationale behind the combined modality approach is both to optimize local control of the disease and to deliver a systemic treatment to control micrometastatic disease. Neoadjuvant chemoradiation has been shown to result in tumour downstaging, with a survival advantage seen in two studies (Urba *et al.* 1995, Walsh *et al.* 1996). A meta-analysis of neoadjuvant chemoradiation studies demonstrated a 31% 3-year survival for chemoradiation compared to 22% in surgery alone (odds ratio survival 1.62, 95% CI 1.17–2.26). A randomized MRC study has shown a survival advantage for the use of pre-operative cisplatin and 5FU in patients with operable oesophageal cancers and this is now considered standard treatment. *Figure 14.3* illustrates our recommended algorithm for treatment of oesophageal cancer.

For locally advanced disease the combination of chemotherapy and radiotherapy is superior, both in terms of response rates and survival, to radiotherapy alone and this should be the treatment of choice.

In the case of metastatic oesophageal carcinoma, no randomized trials have evaluated the role of palliative

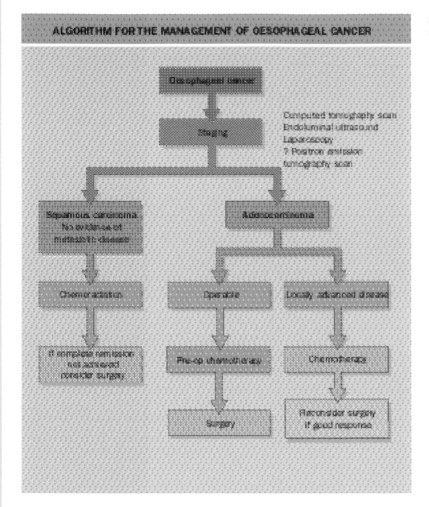

Figure 14.3. Algorithm for the management of oesophageal cancer.

chemotherapy. However, in the multicentre UK study in advanced oesophagogastric cancer (Allum 1995), oesophageal tumours derived the same benefit from palliative chemotherapy as those of tumours of the OGJ or stomach. Chemotherapy regimens frequently used include 5-fluorouracil (5FU) and cisplatin, often in combination with either epirubicin or mitomycin C (MMC). Response rates in the order of 40–60% can be achieved with combination regimens.

Our current standard treatment regimen at the Royal Marsden Hospital is with epirubicin, 5FU, and cisplatin (ECF) chemotherapy – the 5FU is administered as a protracted venous infusion via a Hickman line. Current interest focuses on the development of more effective regimens, using newer chemotherapeutic agents such as the taxanes in combination with established agents such as 5FU and cisplatin.

Gastric Cancer

Key points: gastric cancer

- Worldwide increasing incidence, and in the UK an increase in oesophagogastric junction tumours
- Accurate staging vital, with computed tomography scanning, endoluminal ultrasound, and laparoscopy before surgery
- Ongoing trials of preoperative chemotherapy for operable disease
- Palliative chemotherapy improves survival and quality of life

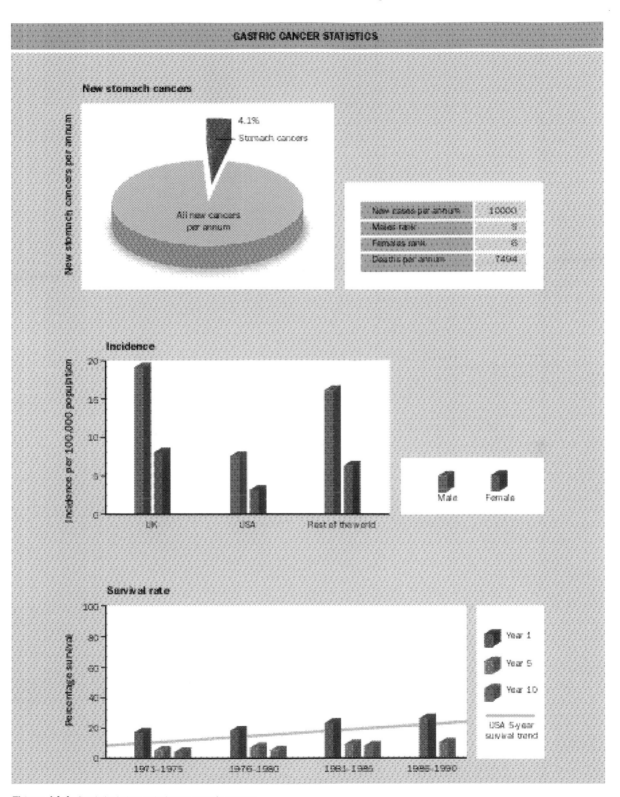

Figure 14.4. Statistical data relating to gastric cancer.

Incidence

In the UK gastric cancer is the sixth commonest cancer in men and the seventh in women, but globally it is the second commonest cancer. Various statistics related to gastric cancer are shown in *Figure 14.4*. There is a wide geographical variation in its incidence, with particularly high rates occurring in Japan, China, and Eastern Europe. Worldwide, the incidence of gastric cancer is decreasing, but in the UK there has been a recent increase in carcinomas of the OGJ. In Japan, as a result of the prevalence of the disease, screening is performed with barium meal and gastroscopy. This has lead to an increase, by 30–40%, in the number of early gastric cancers diagnosed. In the UK, screening of asymptotic individuals is not practical because of the low incidence of the disease.

Pathology

Over 90% of gastric carcinomas are adenocarcinomas; the remainder are mainly lymphomas and leiomyosarcomas. Classification can be further divided into an intestinal type, in which the neoplastic cells form glandular structures (these usually present as an ulcer) and a diffuse type, in which there is no cohesion between the neoplastic cells (these infiltrate and thicken the stomach wall without forming a discrete mass). Of these the intestinal type is more common, accounting for approximately 70% of all tumours. A number of risk factors have been identified for the development of gastric cancer, including atrophic gastritis, pernicious anaemia (associated with a 2–3-fold increased risk), and gastrectomy for peptic ulcer disease (a three-fold increased risk after a latency period of between 15–20 years). Among first-degree relatives of an affected individual there is a 2–3-fold increased risk of developing the disease.

Diagnosis and staging

Gastric cancer is staged according to the TNM staging system, shown in *Table 14.2*. As one would expect, survival is very much stage-dependent, but the overall 5-year survival figures are poor, in the range 5–10%.

The most common presenting symptoms are dyspepsia, epigastric pain, weight loss, upper intestinal bleeding, and symptoms related to anaemia. The diagnosis is usually established with either a barium meal or a gastroscopy (the latter is necessary for a histological diagnosis). CT scanning should then be performed to detect the spread of tumour to regional lymph nodes and distant metastases. As with oesophageal carcinoma, endoluminal ultrasound helps to assess the depth of invasion of the primary tumour and also the presence of local lymphadenopathy.

Table 14.2. *Staging of gastric cancer*

Stage	TNM	5-year survival (%)
Stage 0	Tis, N0, M0	
Stage IA	T1, N0, M0	85
Stage IB	T1, N1, M0	65
	T2, N0, M0	
Stage II	T1, N2, M0	45
	T2, N1, M0	
	T3, N0, M0	
Stage IIIA	T2, N2, M0	20
	T3, N1, M0	
	T4, N0, M0	
Stage IIIB	T3, N2, M0	15
	T4, N1, M0	
Stage IV	T4, N2, M0	5
	Any T, Any N, M1	

For patients with operable disease, after CT scanning a laparoscopy should be performed to confirm operability, as this is the most sensitive way to exclude peritoneal metastases. Other useful investigations include measurement of serum carcinoembryonic antigen (CEA), which is raised in a proportion of patients with gastric carcinoma.

Management

The management of gastric carcinoma depends upon whether the disease is operable or not. In reality, only 20–25% of tumours are surgically resectable, and for these surgery is the standard treatment. As a result of the high rates of relapse following surgery the use of adjuvant chemotherapy has been studied in this disease. In 1993 a meta-analysis of 11 small randomized trials that compared surgery plus adjuvant chemotherapy to surgery alone was reported (Hermans *et al.*, 1993). No significant survival benefit was found in association with adjuvant chemotherapy. This meta-analysis was, however, subsequently criticized for not including two studies. When these were included in the analysis, the common odds ratio for survival was 0.82 (CI 0.68–0.98) in favour of chemotherapy. In Japan, adjuvant chemotherapy is recommended on the basis of two randomized studies, but in the UK most patients are not offered adjuvant chemotherapy outside the context of a clinical trial.

There is also a potential role for the use of preoperative chemotherapy, given the high numbers of patients who are deemed inoperable at either laparoscopy or laparotomy. The Medical Research Council (MRC) Adjuvant Gastric Infusions Chemotherapy (MAGIC) study has randomized patients to either three courses of neoadjuvant chemotherapy (ECF) followed by surgery and then a further three courses of ECF chemotherapy to surgery alone. The results are awaited.

For locally advanced and metastatic disease, treatment is predominantly with chemotherapy. Gastric cancer is one of the most chemosensitive solid tumours; the most commonly used drugs in this disease are 5FU, cisplatin, MMC, and more recently irinotecan and docetaxol. Four randomized studies were carried out to compare chemotherapy with best supportive care in gastric carcinoma, three of which demonstrate improved survival with the use of palliative chemotherapy (Murad *et al.*, 1993, Glimelius *et al.*, 1994, Pyrhonen *et al.*, 1995).

The ECF regimen was developed at the Royal Marsden Hospital, and compared with 5FU, adriamycin, and methotrexate (FAMTX), the previous standard treatment, ECF shows improved response rates and survival. In addition, quality of life was also improved with ECF. This is currently the standard treatment for gastric cancer.

In the case of locally advanced disease, re-staging following chemotherapy is required to establish if the tumour has been sufficiently downstaged to consider surgery.

Carcinoma of the Pancreas

Key points: pancreatic cancer

- Increasing incidence and poor survival (<10% 1 year)
- Commonly asymptomatic until locally advanced
- Poor survival even after surgery
- Palliative chemotherapy gives survival and quality of life advantage in patients with good performance status

Incidence, aetiology, and pathology

Pancreatic cancer has a relatively high incidence worldwide, and in Western Europe it is increasing in incidence. Currently, over 30,000 new cases are diagnosed per year in

Europe. Various statistics relating to pancreatic cancer are shown in *Figure 14.5*. The prognosis of the disease is poor and 1-year survival rates are <10%. The majority (over 95%) of pancreatic tumours arise from the exocrine pancreas, and the remainder arise from islet cells. The vast majority are adenocarcinomas. Smoking and diabetes mellitus are two known factors that predispose to this disease.

Diagnosis and staging

Pancreatic carcinomas classically remain asymptomatic until they have reached a relatively advanced stage. Common presenting symptoms include epigastric pain, abdominal bloating, and symptoms related to obstructive jaundice, such as steatorrhoea, dark urine, and pruritus.

Investigations to establish the diagnosis should include an ultrasound scan if there is clinical or biochemical evidence of jaundice, and a CT scan of the chest, abdomen, and pelvis to delineate the extent of the disease. An endoscopic retrograde cholangiopancreatogram (ERCP) and biliary stenting are necessary in the event of obstructive jaundice. Histological diagnosis can sometimes be obtained from brushings performed at an ERCP, but it can often to be difficult to obtain a histological diagnosis from the primary tumour. Ultrasound- or CT-guided biopsies of pancreatic masses may be required. Approximately 65% of pancreatic tumours are associated with a raised serum Ca19–9 tumour marker.

Management

At diagnosis, over 90% of patients have inoperable disease, in which case the main aim of treatment should be symptom control. For those patients with operable disease, surgery remains the standard of care and 2-year survival rates of 20–30% can be achieved with careful patient selection. Long-term cure, however, is rare.

Three randomized studies have been performed to compare the use of chemotherapy with best supportive care in advanced pancreatic cancer. The chemotherapy regimens used differed, but they all included 5FU. In all three trials, a statistically significant advantage was found in terms of survival for the chemotherapy-treated patients, with the median survival increasing from approximately 3 to 9 months. Patient selection for palliative chemotherapy is extremely important. Often, by the time patients are seen by a medical oncologist, they have a poor performance status. In this situation, if the patients are treated with cytotoxic agents they are more likely to experience severe toxicity, and any

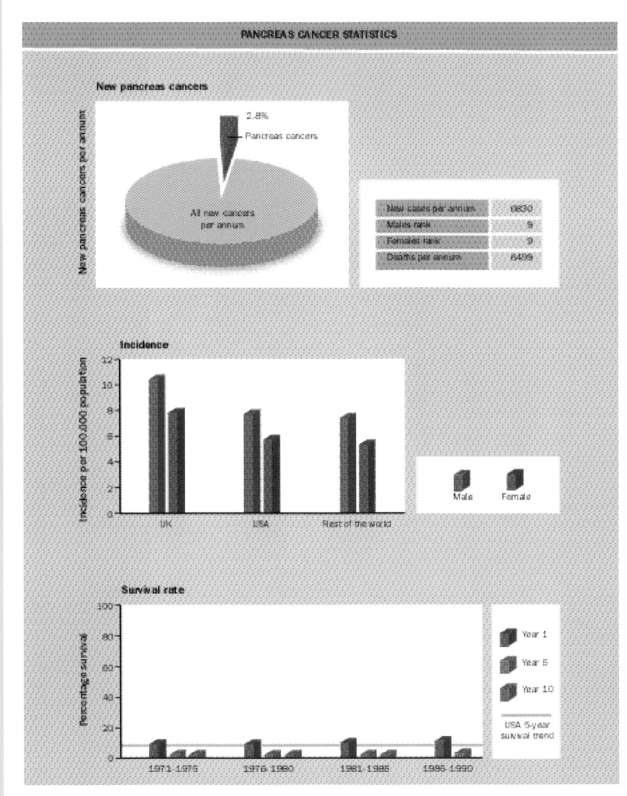

Figure 14.5. *Statistical data relating to pancreatic cancer.*

potential benefits of chemotherapy are far outweighed by the toxicity risk. The patients who do benefit from palliative chemotherapy are those with a good performance status, for whom treatment should begin as soon as possible to prevent a deterioration.

For locally advanced tumours, combined modality treatments with chemotherapy and radiotherapy can be considered, although their role has not yet been fully established.

Gemcitabine and 5FU are the main cytotoxic drugs used in pancreatic cancer.

Tumours of the Biliary Tract

Incidence and aetiology
Tumours of the biliary tract encompass both cholangiocarcinomas and carcinomas of the gall bladder. In Western Europe they are rare, accounting for only 4% of gastrointestinal malignancies. Various statistics related to biliary tract cancers are shown in *Figure 14.6*. Inflammation of the biliary tract is felt to be important in the pathogenesis and, supporting this, the incidence is increased in patients with ulcerative colitis and sclerosing cholangitis. In the Far East, as a result of liver fluke infestation, cholangiocarcinoma is a much more common entity.

Key points: tumours of the biliary tract

- Rare in Europe
- Aetiologically linked to inflammation (e.g. sclerosing cholangitis and liver fluke infestation)
- Usually present with obstructive jaundice
- Surgery is the treatment of choice
- Combination chemotherapy for inoperable disease shows survival benefit

Diagnosis and management
Patients often present with obstructive jaundice, and a definitive diagnosis is usually made through a combination of either ultrasound or CT imaging and ERCP.

Surgery remains the treatment of choice for the small number of tumours that are resectable. Patients with inoperable tumours and good performance status should be considered for chemotherapy. 5FU, doxorubicin, and MMC

are agents that have been shown to have activity in this disease. A trial that compared the benefits of palliative chemotherapy with best supportive care showed both a survival and quality of life benefit in association with chemotherapy.

Hepatocellular Carcinoma

Key points: hepatocellular carcinoma

- Rare in the UK, but very common worldwide
- Risk factors: viral hepatitis, aflatoxin, and haemochromatosis
- Surgery is the optimal treatment
- Systemic or local chemotherapy can be used

Incidence and aetiology
Hepatocellular carcinoma is rare in the UK, but global estimates of its incidence are 250,000–12,000,000 new cases each year. The highest incidence is found in parts of Asia and sub-Saharan Africa. The most widely recognized risk factors include viral hepatitis, haemochromatosis, and aflatoxin ingestion. Tumours may be uni- or multifocal, and in 80% of cases the liver is cirrhotic at diagnosis. Typically, the tumours are locally invasive.

Management
Less than 10% of patients with hepatocellular carcinoma are suitable for resection or orthotopic transplantation, but these remain the only curative options in this disease. Even in these cases, long-term results are poor. Other treatment options include cryosurgery and percutaneous intratumoural injections of alcohol and radiolabelled antibodies. Interferon and tamoxifen have not been shown to have a demonstrable benefit in this disease.

The results of systemic chemotherapy are generally disappointing, with response rates <20% and responses typically being of short duration. Anthracyclines remain the most widely used agents, but 5FU, etoposide, and cisplatin are also used. Hepatic artery infusions can be used for chemotherapy. An alternative approach has been chemoembolization of the tumour followed by the administration of chemotherapy, but this is associated with hepatotoxicity.

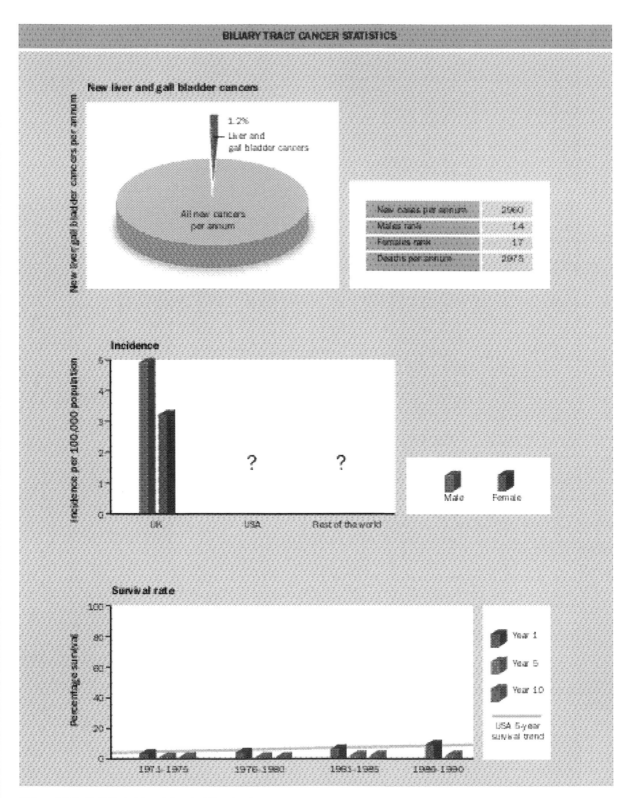

Figure 14.6. Statistical data relating to biliary tract cancer.

Colorectal Cancer

Key points: colorectal cancer

- Common in the UK, and usually occurs in sixth and seventh decades
- There is a genetic component, but the majority remain sporadic
- Surgery to treat primary tumours
- Role of adjuvant chemotherapy for Dukes C and selected cases of Dukes B tumours is proven
- Palliative 5-fluorouracil chemotherapy survival advantage is proven
- Irinotecan has a proven role as a second-line agent

Incidence and aetiology

CRC is the fourth commonest cancer worldwide. In Europe approximately 130,000 new cases are diagnosed each year. Various statistics related to CRC are shown in *Figure 14.7.* Most tumours of the large bowel arise within pre-existing polyps or adenomas. In the general population, in western Europe the incidence of either polyps or adenomas is approximately 30%. Aetiological factors felt to be involved in the development of CRC can be divided into a genetic predisposition and environmental factors:

- environmental factors include a diet low in fibre, vegetable, and folate, and one that is high in fat, red meat, and alcohol (tobacco smoking is also linked); and
- increasingly the genetic component of CRC is being recognized, with two main inherited syndromes that predispose to the disease – familial adenomatous polyposis (FAP) and hereditary nonpolyposis colorectal cancer (HNPCC).

Despite recognition of the genetic aspect, the vast majority of CRCs arise sporadically. A number of genetic events are described by Vogelstein *et al.* (1988) in what is probably a multistep process along an 'adenoma–carcinoma sequence'. These events include oncogenic transformation of *K-ras*, loss of the tumour suppressor genes such as deleted in colorectal cancer (*DCC*), *p53*, and adenomatous polyposis coli (*APC*).

Familial adenomatous polyposis

Familial adenomatous polyposis (FAP) is an autosomal-dominant disorder in which multiple adenomatous polyps develop in the colon, usually during an individual's second or third decade. The risk of developing CRC is almost 100% by 40 years of age. The Adenomatous Polyposis Coli gene (*APC*) causes FAP and is located on the long arm of chromosome 5. It can be detected in family members with a high sensitivity rate. For individuals with the disorder, prophylactic proctocolectomy is performed with ileoanal anastomosis.

Hereditary non-polyposis colorectal cancer

Hereditary non-polyposis colorectal cancer (HNPCC) is also an autosomal-dominant condition, and accounts for up to 6% of cases of CRC. It can be further subdivided into two syndromes – firstly, those associated with colon tumours only, and secondly those associated with tumours in the ovary, endometrium, stomach, and hepatobiliary tract. HNPCC should be suspected if three or more family members have CRC, with one of the cases being a first-degree relative of two of the others. Cases usually arise over two or more generations and one or more cases usually occurs at under 50 years of age.

Staging and survival

In 1932 Cuthbert Duke first described a staging system for rectal carcinoma. Since then a number of modifications have occurred, including the addition of colon cancer. The most widely used version currently is the Astler–Coller modification. The Gunderson–Sosin classification includes a B3 and C3 category depending on whether the tumour involves other structures that are still removable en bloc at the operation. Five-year survival is, as one would expect, stage-dependent. The staging classifications and survivals are given in *Table 14.3.*

Diagnosis

Tumours that arise from the left side of the colon typically present with either rectal bleeding, tenesmus, or a change in bowel habit. Tumours of the right side of the colon, particularly the caecum, are often asymptomatic and are discovered at investigations for an iron-deficiency anaemia. *Figure 14.8* shows the distribution of tumours by site within the large intestine.

Investigations should include a full blood count, serum urea and electrolyte, liver function tests, and serum CEA. The diagnosis is established most commonly with either barium enema or colonoscopy. Preoperatively, liver imaging with either an ultrasound or CT scan is performed to establish whether or not metastatic disease is present.

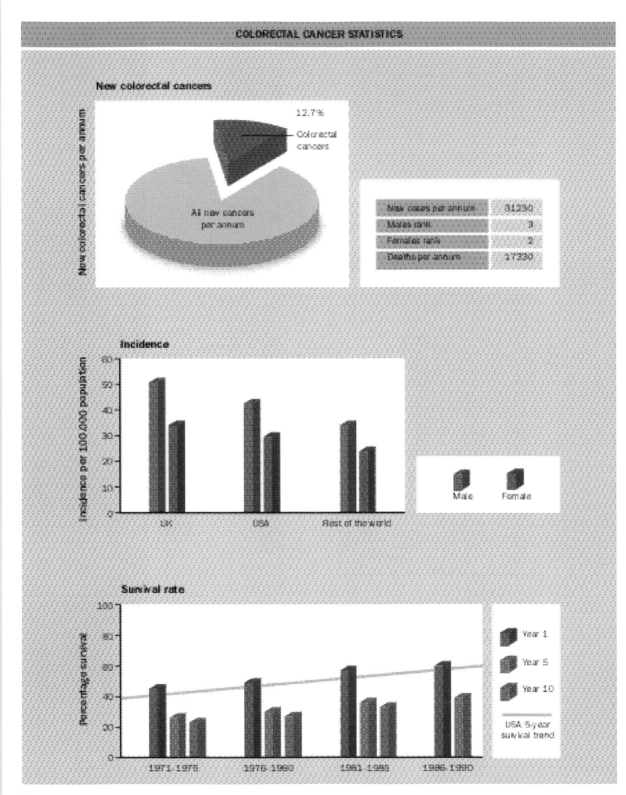

Figure 14.7. Statistical data relating to colorectal cancer.

Table 14.3. Staging of colorectal cancer

Gunderson–Sosin stage	TNM	UICC group staging	5-year survival (%)
A	T1, N0, M0	Stage I	95
B1	T2, N0, M0		85
B2	T3, N0, M0	Stage II	70
B3	T4, N0, M0		
C1	T1–2, N1–3, M0	Stage III	55
C2	T3, N1–3, M0		40
C3	T4, N1–3, M0		
D	Any T, Any N, M1	Stage IV	5

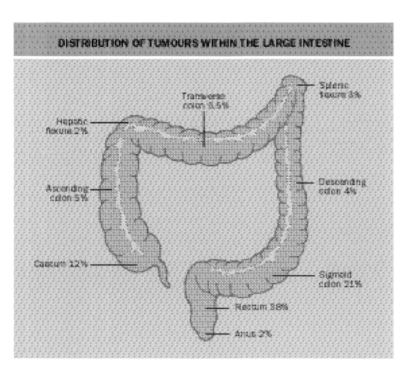

DISTRIBUTION OF TUMOURS WITHIN THE LARGE INTESTINE

Figure 14.8. Distribution of tumours by site within the large intestine.

Management
Surgically resectable disease

At presentation 50% of patients have disease that can be cured by an operation. However, half of these subsequently relapse, either locally or at a distant site. While surgery remains the mainstay of treatment for operable tumours of both the colon and rectum, adjuvant chemotherapy has become important to improve further on survival figures. Following resection of the tumour, there is a period of compensatory growth in any malignant cells remaining and it is

during this time, because of the increase in proliferation rates, that micrometastases are most susceptible to chemotherapy.

In colon cancer four control trials have clearly shown a survival benefit for the use of adjuvant chemotherapy in patients with Dukes C carcinoma of the colon (Wolmark *et al.*, 1988, 1993, Moertel *et al.*, 1990, 1995, IMPACT Investigators, 1995). For Dukes B tumours, a meta-analysis of the National Surgical Adjuvant Breast and Bowel Projects (NSABP) showed an equivalent reduction in mortality for

Key points: upper gastrointestinal cancers

Incidence: The incidence of stomach cancer is decreasing, whereas the incidence of oesophageal cancer is increasing; tumours at the junction between the stomach and oesophagus are increasing particularly rapidly

Age: For all three tumour types 99% of cases occur in patients over 40 years of age and 95% in those over 50 years of age

Risk factor: Smoking

Alcohol

Common symptoms in cancer patients

Any upper gastrointestinal cancer	Weight loss	60%
	Anorexia	50%
	Anaemia	50%
	Vomiting	25%
Oesophagus	Heartburn	80%
	Reflux	50%
	Dysphagia	85%
Stomach	Epigastric Pain	90%
	Dysphagia	40%
Pancreas	Jaundice	80%

Dysphagia is a relatively uncommon symptom in a community and/or general practice setting. Patients with difficulty swallowing food should always be referred for further investigation.

Dyspepsia is an extremely common problem in a community and/or general practice setting. The index of suspicion of cancer is very considerably raised if dyspepsia is combined with an 'alarm' symptom (weight loss, anorexia, anaemia). In patients over 55 years of age, the recent onset of dyspepsia and/or continuous symptoms is associated with an increased risk of cancer.

Local arrangements should be made to determine whether patients who require urgent assessment are seen in a clinic setting or are directly referred for endoscopy.

Reproduced from England Department of Health Cancer Referral Guidelines Consultation Document May 2000.

Guidelines for urgent referral: upper gastrointestinal cancers

Dysphagia: food sticking on swallowing (any age)

Dyspepsia at any age combined with one or more of the following 'alarm' symptoms:

  weight loss

  anaemia

  anorexia

Dyspepsia in a patient 55 years of age or older with at least one of the following 'high-risk' features:

  onset of dyspepsia less than 1 year previously

  continuous symptoms since onset

Dyspepsia combined with at least one of the following known risk factors:

  family history of upper gastrointestinal cancer in more than two first-degree relatives

  Barrett's oesophagus

  pernicious anaemia

  peptic ulcer surgery over 20 years previously

  known dysplasia, atrophic gastritis, intestinal metaplasia

Jaundice

Upper abdominal mass

Referral proforma: upper gastrointestinal cancers

Age:

Symptoms:	Yes	No	
Dyspepsia			
Anorexia			
Dysphagia			
Weight loss			
Vomiting			
Symptoms of anaemia			

Nature of dyspepsia:

Duration:...............weeks/months/years

Continuous   Yes ☐   No ☐

Risk factors:	Yes	No	
Family history of upper gastrointestinal cancer			
Pernicious anaemia			
Barrett's oesophagus			
Previous peptic ulcer surgery			
Known dysplasia, atrophic gastritis or intestinal metaplasia			
Clinical examination:			
Epigastric mass			
Hepatomegaly			
Jaundice			

Comments and/or other reasons for referral:

Reproduced from England Department of Health Cancer Referral Guidelines Consultation Document May 2000.

patients with Dukes B and Dukes C tumours (Mamounas *et al.*, 1999). In contrast, the IMPACT group failed to show a statistically significant benefit for adjuvant chemotherapy in Dukes B tumours in their meta-analysis, although there was a trend towards it. Based on the results of the NSABP analysis, we recommend adjuvant chemotherapy in all medically fit patients with Dukes C tumours and selected cases with Dukes B.

When discussing adjuvant chemotherapy, tumours of the rectum should be considered separately from those of the colon, because of the anatomical differences, as rectal tumours by definition lie below the peritoneal reflection. Hence the expansion of rectal tumours to the surrounding structures is more common than in colon cancers. A survival advantage has been shown with postoperative radiotherapy for patients with Dukes B and C tumours.

Key points: colorectal cancers

Age: 99% >40 years of age

95% >50 years of age

Primary symptoms:

rectal bleeding

change in bowel habit – most commonly increased frequency and/or looseness of stool (alternating constipation and

diarrhoea is rare, as is true constipation)

abdominal pain

Systemic symptoms:

weight loss

symptoms of anaemia

pain from metastases

Clinical examination:

abdominal mass

rectal mass

signs of obstruction and/or perforation

Note:

Rectal bleeding in association with anal symptoms is less likely to be the result of cancer than rectal bleeding alone

For patients with rectal bleeding and anal symptoms but no change in bowel habit or palpable anorectal mass the likelihood of having cancer is

very low

Reproduced from England Department of Health Cancer Referral Guidelines Consultation Document May 2000.

Guidelines for urgent referral: colorectal cancer

Rectal bleeding and persistent change in bowel habit for at least six weeks

Rectal bleeding persistently with no anal symptoms in patients over 65 years of age (with no obvious external evidence of benign anal disease)

Change of bowel habit of recent onset to looser stools and/or increased frequency of defecation, persistent for more than 6 weeks

Iron deficiency anaemia without an obvious cause and Hb <10g/dl

An easily palpable abdominal or rectal mass

Furthermore, other groups have shown a survival advantage with postoperative combined modality treatment (chemotherapy and radiotherapy). A Swedish rectal cancer trial showed a survival advantage with the use of preoperative radiotherapy alone (Swedish Rectal Trial, 1997). Currently, we recommend the use of postoperative combined modality therapy for patients with Dukes B or C rectal cancer, unless the local recurrence rates of the institution are <10%. In this case radiotherapy can be reserved for patients with B3 or C3 tumours, those with positive lateral margins, or those with a local recurrence.

Management of advanced disease

The use of chemotherapy in metastatic CRC is well established. Four trials with palliative 5FU-based chemotherapy clearly demonstrated both a survival advantage and an improvement in quality of life over best supportive care (Nordic Gastrointestinal Tumour Adjuvant Therapy Group, 1992, Scheithaeur et al., 1993, Bretta et al., 1994, Allen-Mersh et al., 1994). Evidence from one of the studies indicates that the early use of chemotherapy, rather than a delay in treatment until symptoms develop, is beneficial. The main agent used in CRC is 5FU, which can be administered in a

Referral proforma: colorectal cancer

Age:

Primary symptoms:	Yes	No	
Abdominal pain			
Change in bowel habit:			
increased frequency or looseness			
other			
Anal symptoms			

Systemic symptoms:	Yes	No	
Weight loss			
Tiredness and/or weakness			
Symptoms of anaemia			
Other, please state......................................			

Investigations:	Yes	No	
Haemoglobin..................g/dl			
Other, please state......................................			

Reproduced from England Department of Health Cancer Referral Guidelines Consultation Document May 2000.

number of ways – bolus, short infusion, or protracted venous infusion (via a Hickman line). When administered as a bolus, response rates are improved approximately two-fold when the biochemical modulator leucovorin (LV) is used concurrently.

MMC is another agent used in the management of metastatic CRC. A trial performed at the Royal Marsden Hospital showed that the administration of PVI 5FU with MMC yielded superior response rates and survival when compared to PVI 5FU alone (Ross *et al.*, 1997).

Over recent years newer agents (including irinotecan, oxaliplatin, and raltitrexed) have been developed that show encouraging results in this disease. Irinotecan has been shown to have a clear benefit on both survival and quality of life in patients who have failed on 5FU. In addition to its role as a second-line agent in the disease, data indicate that a combination of 5FU and irinotecan as a first-line treatment of metastatic CRC is superior to 5FU/LV alone (Douillard *et al.*, 2000, Saltz *et al.*, 2000).

Oxaliplatin is a third-generation platinum compound. As a single agent response rates of 10% are observed, but when combined with 5FU/LV these can be improved to 30%. The combination of 5FU/LV and oxaliplatin has been trailed against 5FU/LV alone as a first-line treatment for metasta-

tic disease. While the combination was shown to improve progression-free survival, no overall survival advantage has been documented.

NICE guidance 2002 states that 5FU is the first line agent for metastatic CRC, with the combination of oxaliplatin and 5FU reserved for patients with liver only disease in whom downstaging for surgery may be possible. Irinotecan should be reserved for second line treatment.

Surgery in metastatic disease

Surgery is being used increasingly for individuals with metastatic disease. Liver and lung metastases are the most common sites considered for resection. Depending on the number of lesions and their site, 5-year survival figures in the order of 30% can be achieved with surgery for liver or lung metastases. Careful patient selection is necessary, as the strongest predictors for survival are few lesions and clear postsurgical margins. Patients need to be preoperatively assessed with magnetic resonance imaging and, often, positron emission tomography.

All patients with metastatic disease should be considered for surgical resection, as this offers a potential for cure and in cases of doubt a surgical opinion should be sought.

Screening for colorectal cancer

The role of population screening for CRC has been much discussed. CRC is a common disease that is curable when detected at an early stage. Screening has been studied in three randomized control trials that showed a reduction in mortality in populations offered faecal occult blood testing (Hardcastle *et al.*, 1996, Mandel *et al.*, 1993, Kronborg *et al.*, 1996). The National Colorectal Cancer Screening Programme is currently planning a pilot study to further evaluate this issue. The proposed programme will involve biennial, home FOB testing for patient's aged between 50 and 69 years of age. Screening will be by invitation from general practitioners and completed tests are to be returned to the screening centre. Investigations will be performed at the cancer unit when indicated and will involve colonoscopy plus or minus barium enema.

Currently screening with a colonoscopy is recommended to high-risk individuals:

- those with a first-degree relative who developed the disease at younger than 50 years of age;
- those with inflammatory bowel disease;
- those with a known genetic predisposition, such as FAP; and
- those with a history of polyps or previous bowel cancer.

Conclusion

Tumours of the gastrointestinal tract are common and a high cause of morbidity and mortality in the UK. They are curable only when diagnosed at early stages and hence much emphasis needs to be placed on prompt referral for investigation when suggestive symptoms present. In the case of CRC, screening is likely to become more widespread in the next decade.

Management of these tumours is increasingly multimodality based, and hence the importance of a multidisciplinary approach involving surgeons and medical and clinical oncologists from an early stage in the management planning of these patients. The development of newer chemotherapeutic drugs provides further scope for the treatment of these conditions.

Further Reading

Allen-Mersh G, Earlem S, Fordy C, *et al.* Quality of life and survival with continuous hepatic artery floxuridine infusion for colorectal liver metastases. *Lancet.* 1994; **344**: 1255–9.

Allum W. Combination chemotherapy with epirubicin, cisplatin and 5-fluorouracil for the palliation of advanced gastric and oesophageal adenocarcinoma. The MRC Gastric Cancer Working Party and the British Stomach Cancer Group. *Br J Surg.* 1995; **82**: 565.

Anonymous. Efficacy of adjuvant fluorouracil and folinic acid in colon cancer. International Multicentre Pooled Analysis of Colon Cancer Trials (IMPACT) investigators. *Lancet.* 1995; **345**: 939–44.

Anonymous. Expectancy or primary chemotherapy in patients with advanced asymptomatic colorectal cancer: a randomized trial. Nordic Gastrointestinal Tumour Adjuvant Therapy Group. *J Clin Oncol.* 1992; **10**: 904–11.

Anonymous. Improved survival with preoperative radiotherapy in resectable rectal cancer. Swedish Rectal Trial. *N Engl J Med.* 1997; **336**: 980–7.

Beretta G, Bollina R, Martingnoni G, *et al.* Fluorouracil and folates (FUFO) as standard treatment for advanced/metastatic gastrointestinal carcinomas (AGC) (abstract). *Ann Oncol.* 1994; **5(suppl 8)**: 239.

Douillard JY, Cunningham D, Roth AD, *et al.* Irinotecan combined with fluorouracil compared with fluorouracil alone as first-line treatment for metastatic colorectal cancer: a multicentre randomised trial. *Lancet.* 2000; **355**: 1041–7.

Dukes CE. The spread of cancer of the rectum. *Br J Surg.* 1930; **12**: 643–8.

Glimelius D, Hoffman K, Haglund U, *et al.* Initial or delayed chemotherapy with best supportive care in advanced gastric cancer. *Ann Oncol.* 1994; **5**: 189–90.

Hardcastle JD, Chamberlain JO, Robinson MH, *et al.* Randomised controlled trial of faecal-occult blood screening for colorectal cancer. *Lancet.* 1996; **348**: 1472–7.

Hermans J, Bonenkamp JJ, Boon MC, *et al.* Adjuvant therapy after curative resection for gastric cancer: meta-analysis of randomized trials. *J Clin Oncol.* 1993; **11**: 1441–7.

Kronborg O, Fenger C, Olsen J, *et al.* Randomised study of screening for colorectal cancer with faecal-occult-blood test. *Lancet.* 1996; **348**: 1467–71.

Mamounas E, Wieands S, Solmark N, *et al.* Comparative efficacy of adjuvant chemotherapy in patients with Dukes' B versus Dukes' C colon cancer: results from four National Surgical Adjuvant Breast and Bowel Project adjuvant studies (C-01, C-02, C-03, and C-04). *J Clin Oncol.* 1999; **17**: 1349–55.

Mandel JS, Bond JH, Church TR, *et al.* Reducing mortality from colorectal cancer by screening for fecal occult blood. Minnesota Colon cancer Control Study. *N Engl J Med.* 1993; **328**: 1365–71.

Moertel CG, Fleming TR, Macdonald JS, *et al.* Levamisole and fluorouracil for adjuvant therapy of resected colon carcinoma. *N Engl J Med.* 1990; **322**: 352–8.

Moertel GC, Fleming TR, Macdonald JS, *et al.* Fluorouracil plus levamisole as effective adjuvant therapy after resection of stage III colon carcinoma: a final report. *Ann Intern Med.* 1995; **122**: 321–6.

Murad AM, Santiago FF, Petroianu A, *et al.* Modified therapy with 5-fluorouracil, doxorubicin and methotrexate in advanced gastric cancer. *Cancer.* 1993; **72**: 37–41.

Pyrhonen S, Kuitunen T, Nyandoto P, *et al.* Randomised comparison of FEMTX plus supportive care with supportive care alone with non-resectable gastric cancer. *Br J Cancer.* 1995; **71**: 587–91.

Ross P, Norman A, Cunningham D, *et al.* A prospective randomised trial of protracted venous infusion 5-fluorouracil with or without mitomycin C in advanced colorectal cancer. *Ann Oncol.* 1997; **8**: 995–1001.

Scheithauer W, Rosen R, Kornek G, *et al.* Randomised comparison of combination chemotherapy plus best supportive care with supportive care alone in patients with metastatic colorectal cancer. *BMJ.* 1993; **306**: 752–5.

Urba S, Orringer M, Turrisi A, *et al.* A randomized trial comparing transhiatal esophagectomy to preoperative concurrent chemoradiation followed by esophagectomy in locoregional esophageal carcinoma. *Proc Annu Meet Am Soc Clin Oncol.* 1995; **14**: A475.

Vogelstein B, Fearon ER, Hamilton SR, *et al.* Genetic alterations during colorectal tumour development. *N Engl J Med.* 1988; **319**: 525–32.

Walsh T, Noonan H, Hollywood D, *et al.* A comparison of multimodal therapy and surgery for esophageal adenocarcinoma. *N Engl J Med.* 1996; **335**: 462–7.

Wolmark N, Fisher B, Rockette H, *et al.* Postoperative adjuvant chemotherapy or BCG for colon cancer: results from NSABP protocol C-01. *J Natl Cancer Inst.* 1988; **80**: 30–6.

15 Prostate Cancer

Christopher Nutting and David Dearnaley

Incidence

Prostate cancer incidence rises with increasing age, with 85% of cases diagnosed in men over the age of 65 years. Autopsy studies show microscopic foci of well-differentiated prostatic adenocarcinoma in 30–40% of men aged 75 years and over. In North America and Europe the incidence continues to increase, currently accounting for 14% of cancer deaths in men.

The incidence has been dramatically changed by early detection of disease using prostate-specific antigen (PSA) testing, particularly in North America. The annual number of men diagnosed per year rose from 115 per 100,000 in 1980 to 196 per 100,000 in 1992. The incidences have now fallen back towards that prevailing before PSA testing. This 'surge' in diagnosis corresponded to the detection of clinically 'silent' cases, some of which would have presented clinically in later years. The result has been a 'stage shift', with early localized diseased (T1C/T2A), which is potentially curable, now being the predominant form of presentation and advanced localized or metastatic disease becoming uncommon. Mortality has remained steady at approximately 37,000 per year, although it is possible this has peaked and a falling trend is now apparent. Between 1991 and 1995 there was a 6% fall in the mortality rate. In the UK, PSA testing is only just beginning to have an impact; incidences have risen from about 15,000 to 20,000 men per year, but with a relatively high mortality of approximately 10,000 per annum, which reflects the advanced localized or metastatic presentations that remain the most common in the UK.

Various statistics relating to prostate cancer are shown in *Figure 15.1*.

Pathology

Adenocarcinoma accounts for the vast majority of prostate cancers. The Gleason system is used to grade tumours based on the appearance of the two most common histological patterns. Each is given a score between 1 and 5, and these are added to a sum score of 2–10 (2–4 well differentiated, 5–7 moderately differentiated, and 8–10 poorly differentiated). Rarely, tumours can be very poorly differentiated and show the pathological features and clinical behaviour of small cell carcinoma. In many men, benign prostatic hypertrophy (BPH) coexists with prostate carcinoma, although the two are not related. Prostatic intraepithelial neoplasia (PIN) is a premalignant condition that shows histological features of carcinoma-in-situ. The natural history of this condition is uncertain, but a proportion of men progress to invasive cancer, and so close follow-up is required.

Aetiology

The highest incidences of prostate cancer are seen in the USA and Scandinavia, and the incidence is particularly high in African–Americans. Lowest levels are seen in Far Eastern populations, but migrant studies show an increased risk for populations moving to a 'Western' environment. Interestingly, microfocal autopsy-defined 'latent' prostate cancer has roughly the same incidence in Japan and North America, which strongly suggests that environmental factors act as promotional agents in the development of clinically relevant cancer. The most convincing correlations are with a high-fat diet (positive) and a diet rich in yellow and green vegetables (inverse), which may act on the prostate through modifications of circulating sex hormones. However, the precise dietary mechanisms involved are as yet unknown, although in time these might suggest methods for primary prevention. Prostate cancer also has a strong familial component, with a four- to tenfold increased risk for first-degree relatives of index cases. An active search for these genetic changes is under way, but the two cancer genes so far reported are responsible for a small proportion of familial cancer and confined to families who have a large number (four or more) of affected members.

Clinical Presentation and Diagnosis

In the UK, localized prostate cancer is most commonly diagnosed during investigation for symptoms of prostatism. Bone pain is usually the presenting feature of metastatic disease.

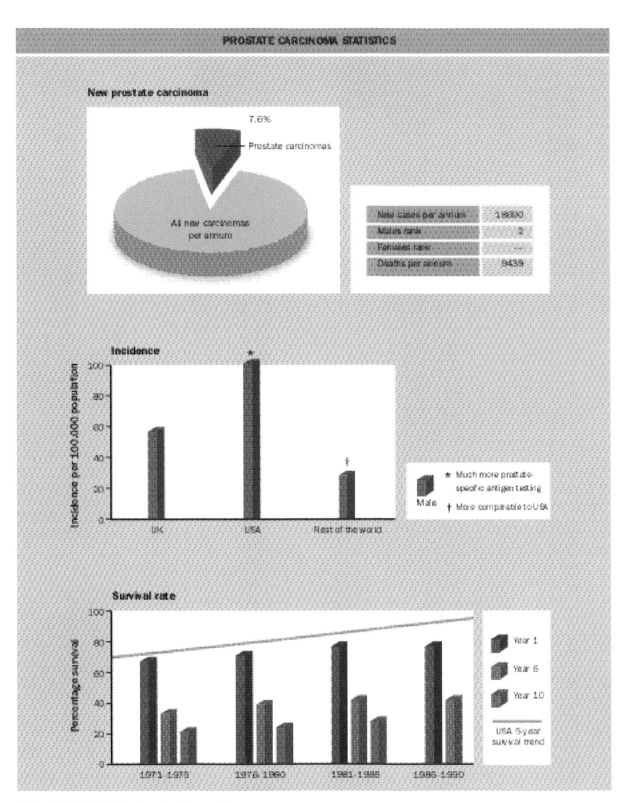

Figure 15.1. *Statistical data relating to prostate cancer.*

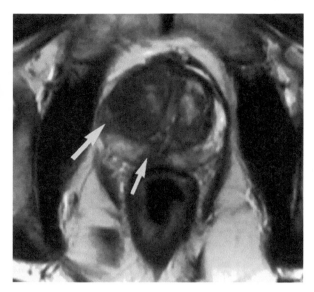

Figure 15.2. *Transaxial magnetic resonance imaging scan showing a prostatic cancer. The arrows identify a prostate cancer in the peripheral zone of the left lobe of the prostate.*

Early localized disease may be detected by digital rectal examination (DRE) or, more commonly in current practice, by PSA estimation. Disease usually develops in the peripheral zone of the prostate (*Fig. 15.2*) and does not produce symptoms unless there is progression into the central zone (to cause compressive symptoms) or considerable extension outside the prostate (to involve adjacent pelvic structure, lymph nodes, or bone).

Currently, in North America the majority of prostate cancers are diagnosed in asymptomatic men by the finding of an elevated PSA level during 'routine' medical checks, and the suspicion of prostate cancer is raised by the finding of raised PSA levels in symptomatic men with lower urinary tract symptoms.

Men who present with prostatism should be assessed initially by DRE and PSA estimation. If the PSA is raised above normal levels (>4ng/ml) or the prostate is irregularly enlarged, referral for assessment and biopsy is appropriate. PSA concentrations can also be mildly raised in prostatitis and BPH. Transrectal ultrasound may define small (up to 5mm) clinically impalpable tumours, and can be used to guide transrectal biopsy accurately. In the absence of a visible abnormality, sextant biopsies are recommended. In patients who present with a combination of very high PSA values and obvious metastatic disease, biopsy may not be necessary. After confirmation of the diagnosis of prostate cancer, a radionuclide bone scan and computed tomography of the abdomen and pelvis may be undertaken to exclude metastatic disease.

Staging systems for prostate cancer are shown in *Table 15.1*. T1 and T2 cancers are often called early localized disease; T3 and T4 cancers are often called advanced localized disease.

Screening

Whether it is useful to screen asymptomatic men with PSA measurement and DRE is unclear because of both the uncertain natural history of untreated prostate cancer and the lack of unequivocal evidence as to the effectiveness of treatment of localized disease. This reflects the lack of adequate data on which to base the treatment decisions, so this remains an area of intense research activity. The Department of Health currently does not recommend routine population screening because, as yet, it is unclear whether early detection of prostate cancer will make an impact on mortality from the disease. However, guidelines from the UK specialist professional groups recommend that PSA testing be available for men who request it, provided that adequate counselling has been given. Counselling information is available for widespread distribution and use in primary care (available from the Department of Health; e-mail-doh@prolog.uk.com; tel-08701 555455).

Treatment of Localized Prostate Cancer

Patient selection

Decisions on the management of men with prostate cancer are complicated by the wide spectrum of natural history. This ranges from patients who have rapid disease progression and death from metastatic disease, to a high prevalence of localized (incidental) tumours, especially in elderly men. Treatment options need to balance the probability of disease progression and death from prostate cancer against competing causes of death.

For apparently localized disease, potential curative treatment options are radical radiotherapy or nerve-sparing radical prostatectomy. Alternatively, a watchful waiting policy may be adopted, in which patients are monitored with PSA and DRE and treatment is reserved until the time of clinically relevant disease progression. This has the advantage of avoiding treatment-related morbidity, but risks the development of subsequent, possibly incurable, disease.

Tumour stage, initial PSA level, and tumour grade (Gleason score) can be used to select patients with a high probability of disease progression for whom radical treatment may be most appropriate. The selection process also

Table 15.1. Stages of prostate cancer: a comparison of the tumour, node, and metastasis (TNM) and Whitmore–Jewett systems

Stage[a,b]	Whitmore–Jewett[b,c]	Definition
		Tumour found incidentally, usually during transurethral resection of the prostate and:
T1a	A1	<5% of tissue is prostate cancer
T1b	A2	>5% of tissue is prostate cancer
T1c	B0	Tumour identified during prostate-specific antigen (PSA) test, with no other clinical signs
		Tumour detectable by digital rectal examination, but confined within the prostate and with involvement of:
T2a	B1	no more than one-half of a single lobe
T2b	B2	more than one-half of a single lobe
T2c	B3	both lobes
		Tumour extends through and beyond the prostate capsule, with:
T3a	C1	unilateral extracapsular extension
T3b	C2	bilateral extracapsular extension
T3c	C2–3	invasion of one or both of the seminal vesicles
		Tumour localized to the pelvic region, but:
T4a		invades bladder neck and/or external sphincter and/or rectum
T4b		invades levator muscles and/or fixed to pelvic wall
N+	D1	Prostate cancer evident in pelvic lymph nodes or extends into the rectal area
	D1.5	Rising PSA level after failed local therapy
M+	D2	Prostate cancer evident outside the pelvic area, usually as metastases
	D2.5	Rising PSA after a nadir induced by adequate hormonal therapy
	D3	(Tumour no longer responsive to hormonal therapy)

[a]The T stage describes the primary tumour within the prostate; the N stage describes the status of the pelvic lymph nodes; the M stage describes the degree of metastasis.

[b]There is no D3 equivalent in the TNM system and no T4 equivalent in the Whitmore–Jewett systems

[c]The Whitmore–Jewett stage cited is the most similar to the TNM stage described.

has to take into account the life expectancy of the patient based on age at diagnosis and concurrent illnesses. At present it seems reasonable to offer radical treatment to men judged to have a life expectancy of 10 years or more, or 5 years if histology shows poorly differentiated disease.

Prostatectomy or radical radiotherapy?

Nerve-sparing radical prostatectomy is associated with 10-year survival rates of approximately 90% for TI tumours and 50–70% for T2 tumours, but it is not appropriate for more advanced disease stages, for which the probability of either incomplete tumour excision or the development of distant metastases is high. Erectile impotence occurs in most patients. Standard management protocols for erectile dysfunction may be appropriate. Some degree of urinary incontinence occurs in 20% of patients. Operative mortality is

very low (<1%) provided that surgery is restricted to fit men, usually less than 70 years of age.

External beam radical radiotherapy remains the most commonly used treatment modality in the UK. The outcome of treatment for T1 and T2 tumours is equivalent to that of surgery (*Tables 15.2* and *15.3*), and in addition more advanced tumours can be treated if appropriate. Daily treatment lasting 6–7 weeks is typical and may cause temporary diarrhoea, proctitis, and bladder irritability. In the long term, intermittent mild rectal bleeding or mild urinary symptoms occur in 30–40% of men, but serious side effects that need surgical intervention occur in <2% of patients.

Conformal radiotherapy, in which the rectum and bladder are shielded by shaping the radiation beam, was recently shown in a randomized study to reduce the incidence of significant proctitis by two-thirds (grade ≥2, side effects are

Table 15.2. *Relative and cause-specific survival of men with localized carcinoma of the prostate compared to age-matched population using different treatment approaches (cause-specific survival shown in brackets)[a]*

Type		Watch and wait	Radiotherapy	Prostatectomy
Well differentiated	10 year	1.01 (93%)	1.17 (90%)	1.17 (94%)
Moderately differentiated	10 year	0.78 (76%)	0.93 (76%)	1.11 (87%)
Poorly differentiated	10 year	0.35 (45%)	0.63 (53%)	0.87 (67%)
	5 year	0.61 (66%)	0.92 (85%)	0.98 (87%)

[a]SEER (Statistics, epidemiology, end results) database for outcomes of 59,876 men with prostate cancer.

Data from Lu-Yao and Yau, 1997.

Table 15.3. *Relative risk of failure compared to prostatectomy[a]*

	Low-risk disease	Intermediate-risk disease	High-risk disease
External beam radiotherapy	1.1	0.8	0.9
Radiotherapy implant	1.1	3.1 (p = 0.006)	3.0 (p = 0.0002)
Radiotherapy implant and androgen deprivation	0.5	1.6	2.2 (p=0.02)

[a]Based on actuarial freedom from PSA failure after radical treatment of 1872 men with stage T1c–T2b prostate cancer.

[b]Low risk: T1c or T2a, or Gleeson sum score ≤ 6, or PSA ≤ 10[11].

[c]Intermediate risk: T2b, or Gleeson sum score 7, or PSA 10–20[11].

[d]High risk: T2b, or Gleeson sum score ≥ 8, or PSA >20[11].

Data from D'Amico, 1998.

reduced from 15% to 5%) and should be considered standard practice. Recent randomized studies showed improved local tumour control following short-term neoadjuvant androgen deprivation, which shrinks the tumour before radiotherapy.

For patients with locally advanced (T3 or 4) tumours who have a high risk of distant metastasis, a contemporary study reported that the use of adjuvant luteinizing hormone releasing hormone (LHRH) agonists for 3 years after radiotherapy is associated with prolonged local control and survival. In this patient group the benefit of radiotherapy is uncertain and is the subject of a current Medical Research Council (MRC) trial.

Implantation of the prostate gland with radioactive seeds (brachytherapy) is another treatment option for carefully selected patients with T1 and T2 prostate cancers; it delivers a higher dose of radiation to the prostate gland over several months. Bladder side effects may be more pronounced

than with external beam radiotherapy, but rectal effects are uncommon. Any superiority over external beam radiotherapy has yet to be demonstrated.

Treatment of Metastatic Prostate Cancer

Androgen suppression or blockade induces prostate cancer cell death and is the mainstay of disease control in patients with metastatic disease (*Fig. 15.3*). Orchidectomy or treatment with a luteinizing hormone releasing hormone (LHRH) agonist (e.g. goserelin) is associated with a subjective response rate of 80–90%, although the median duration of response is only 12–24 months. The duration of response is considerably longer when locoregional disease is treated. Considerable uncertainty exists as to whether the addition of an anti-androgen (such as flutamide, bicalutamide, or

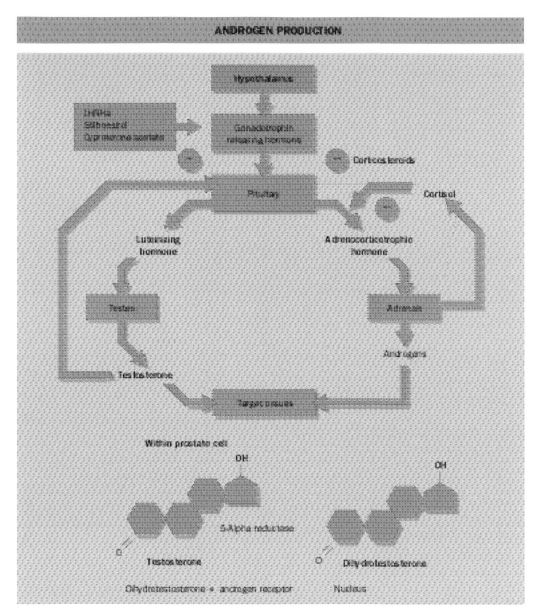

Figure 15.3. *Androgens are produced by the testes and to a lesser extent by the adrenal glands. Luteinizing hormone releasing hormone agonists (LHRHa) suppress luteinizing hormone (LH) and therefore testosterone levels. Anti-androgens such as flutamide, bicalutamide, and cyproterone acetate can block residual androgen activity. Stilbestrol and cyproterone acetate (partially) also suppress LH levels. Corticosteroids inhibit adrenocorticotrophic hormone (ACTH) stimulation of adrenal androgens*

cyproterone acetate) to block the effects of adrenal andro-gens (maximal androgen blockade) confers benefit over the use of orchidectomy or LHRH agonists alone. A recent meta-analysis showed at best a 3% benefit in favour of total androgen blockade, but this is associated with additional toxicity and financial cost. However, anti-androgens do have an important role in blocking the testosterone 'flare' that is seen within 2 weeks of the first LHRH antagonist injection. Recently, bicalutamide has been shown to be as effective as maximal androgen blockade for treatment of locoregional disease but slightly less effective for bone metas-tases.

Until recently, when to initiate hormone treatment for metastatic prostate cancer was the subject of considerable debate; some investigators favoured the immediate introduction of hormonal treatment at the time of diagnosis of metastatic prostate cancer, while others preferred to wait until the development of symptomatic disease progression. A recent randomized MRC study has gone some way towards answering this important question. In this study, patients treated at diagnosis gained a small survival benefit, but more importantly they benefited from:

- improved quality of life,
- fewer episodes of pathological fracture,
- fewer cases of spinal cord compression, and
- fewer courses of palliative radiotherapy for painful bone metastases,

compared with patients in whom treatment was delayed until symptomatic disease progression.

Treatment of relapsed disease

For hormone-resistant metastatic prostate cancer the prognosis is poor. Testosterone should be kept at castration levels, and:

- if anti-androgens have been used, they should be withdrawn (approximately 30% response rate);
- prednisolone or anti-androgens (if not previously given) may be given in addition to LHRH agonist or orchidectomy (response rate is about 30%, but the benefit is usually short-lived); and

- oestrogens (e.g. stilbestrol) have a response rate of 25–50%, but are associated with gynaecomastia and a prothrombotic (clotting) tendency – for the former breast bud irradiation and for the latter aspirin are used to reduce these effects.

Systemic cytotoxic chemotherapy has a limited role, with response rates between 10 and 20%, but single-agent mitozantrone has been shown to have palliative benefit in about 30% of patients.

Radiotherapy remains the most valuable single option for the palliation of bone pain, with an 80% response rate to a single fraction of treatment. More widespread bone metastases can be treated with hemi-body irradiation or systemically administered metastasis-seeking radioisotopes (e.g. strontium-89). Spinal cord compression remains the most common emergency in this patient population and careful neurological examination should be performed on all cancer patients who present with new back pain.

Bisphosphonates are currently being evaluated in two MRC trials to asses the impact on the development and progression of bone metastasis in prostate cancer patients.

Future Directions

The major challenge is to define which cancers, particularly those detected by PSA testing, require radical treatment. It will be many years before the results of ongoing trials of screening and intervention are available.

Considerable evidence is emerging to suggest that radiotherapy dose escalation increases the probability of eradicating localized prostate cancer. To deliver the higher

Key points: prostate cancer

99% of cases occur in men >50 years of age

Over 25% of cases present in men <70 years of agewhen life expectancy is long

Presenting features include raised prostate specific antigen (PSA), an abnormal rectal examination, bone pain, and (occasionally) spinal cord compression

Lower urinary tract symptoms are common in the normal population – over 30% of men 50 years of age have some lower urinary symptoms, rising to over 60% of men 70 years of age.

Lower urinary symptoms alone are not a reason to suspect prostate cancer; early curable prostate cancer is rarely the cause of lower urinary tract symptoms

Early prostatic cancers are either impalpable or have only a small nodule and a PSA that <20mg/1.

Reproduced from National Institute for Clinical Excellence document September 2002. *Guidelines on Cancer Services: Improving Outcomes on Urological Cancers.*.

Referral proforma: urology cancer

Age:

Suspected cancer:

Prostate	☐	Kidney	☐
Bladder	☐	Testis	☐

Other...

Symptoms:	Yes	No	
Macroscopic haematuria			
Loin pain			
Testicular swelling			
Bone pain			
Lower urinary tract symptoms (e.g., hesitancy, poor stream, etc.)			

Other, please state..............................

Clinical examination:	Yes	No	
Renal mass			
Pyrexia			
Swelling in the body of the testis			
Prostate feels malignant on rectal examination			

Other, please state...................................

Investigations:	Yes	No	
Prostate-specific antigen..................ng/ml			
Haemoglobin.................................g/dl			
Microscopic haematuria			
Mass detected on imaging			

Comments/other reasons for urgent referral

doses required, conformal treatment methods are essential if severe rectal and bladder side effects are to be avoided. In the UK (MRC RT01 Trial), Europe, and the USA randomized studies to test this hypothesis are under way, although because of the long natural history of the disease it will be several years before the results are mature.

Many questions remain unanswered as to the optimal timing and duration of hormone treatment. Neoadjuvant and adjuvant hormone therapy are currently being assessed in combination with prostatectomy and radiotherapy. The treatment of biochemical (PSA) recurrence in asymptomatic patients following local treatment is now a major new clinical problem and novel approaches, such as intermittent hormone treatment, are under investigation.

Current research is providing a deeper understanding of prostate cancer biology and the genetic changes associated with carcinogenesis. In particular, the identification of genetic markers that predict the natural history of the disease in individual patients may help in the selection of optimal treatments.

Conclusions

Careful initial assessment and staging of men who present with localized prostate cancer is essential to select the appropriate treatment. Prostatectomy, radical radiotherapy, and a careful observation policy are all acceptable methods and should be the subject of ongoing clinical trials.

Adjuvant androgen deprivation is indicated for men with locally advanced tumours treated with radiotherapy.

In patients with metastatic disease, early hormonal therapy reduces the risk of serious complications. For hormone-resistant prostate cancer new approaches to maximize quality of life are required.

Further Reading

COIN Guidelines. Guidelines on the management of prostate cancer. *Clin Oncol.* 1999; **11**: S55–88.

D'Amico AV, Whittington R, Kaplan I, et al. Equivalent biochemical failure-free survival after external beam radiation therapy or radical prostatectomy in patients with a pretreatment prostate specific antigen of >40–20 ng/ml. *Int J Radiat Oncol Biol Phys.* 1992; **37**: 1053–8.

Dearnaley DP, Melia J. Diagnosis and management of early prostate cancer. Report of the British Association of Urological Surgeons Working Party. *Br J Urol.* 1999; **83**: 18–33.

Lowe BA, Listrom MB. Incidental carcinoma of the prostate: an analysis of the predictors of progression. *J Urol.* 1998; **140**: 1340–4.

Lu-Yao, Yau SL. Population-based study of long-term survival in patients with clinically localised prostate cancer. *Lancet.* 1997; **349**: 966–910.

Royal College of Radiologists' Clinical Oncology Information Network, British Association of Urological Surgeons. Guidelines on the management of prostate cancer. *Clin Oncol.* 1999; **11**: S53–88.

Appendix

Guidelines for urgent referral: urological cancers

Macroscopic haematuria in adults

Microscopic haematuria in adults over 50 years

Swellings in the body of the testis

Palpable renal masses

Solid renal masses found on imaging

Elevated age-specific prostate specific antigen (PSA) in men with a 10 year life expectancy

A high PSA (>20ng/ml) in men with a clinically malignant prostate or bone pain

Any suspected penile cancer

16 Bladder Cancer

Paula Wells and Robert Huddart

Incidence

Bladder cancer accounts for about 4% of male and 2% female cancer deaths, with almost 5000 deaths registered in the UK each year. Considerable national and regional variations in incidence exist, for example, in the USA the frequency in Caucasians is half that in African–Americans and is higher in urban than rural areas. This difference has led to the search for environmental factors that may contribute to the development and progression of disease. The incidence rises steeply after the fifth decade of life and is considerably greater than the mortality, with only half the patients dying of their disease. Various statistics relating to bladder cancer are shown in *Figure 16.1*.

Aetiology

Carcinogens or their metabolites that are excreted in the urine, are believed to act directly on the urothelium. Although the exact site of action of the carcinogen is not known, several have been shown to leave molecular fingerprints on specific sites of the host DNA. The latency period from exposure to development of a urothelial tumour is a median of 18 years, which makes it difficult to establish a definitive 'causative' relationship between the putative carcinogen and development of disease. However, it has been estimated that occupational exposure accounts for approximately 25% of Caucasian and 10% of non-white cases in the US. Cigarette smoking is the most important risk factor, contributing towards 50% of cancers in men and 33% in women, with a two- to fourfold increased risk in smokers. Discontinuing smoking reduces the risk, but a higher risk remains for up to 10 years after smoking cessation. The known aetiological factors are indicated in *Table 16.1*.

Some data suggest a proportion of risk may be genetic. In particular, interest has focused on polymorphisms in the metabolite pathway of carcinogens. Arylamines are metabolically activated and detoxified in the liver, and recent studies showed that individuals with fast oxidator or slow acetylator phenotypes harbour an increased risk of bladder cancer. Dietary factors have also been associated with a greater risk, including consumption of large quantities of fried meat and fat, while vitamin A is protective.

Oncogenes and growth factors

It has been suggested that deletions at chromosome 9q are associated with superficial bladder tumours (Ta–T1) and deletions at 3q, 5q, and 17q are associated with invasive tumours (T2–4). Mutations in other genes [e.g. retinoblastoma (*Rb*) gene and *p53*] have been associated with progression and poor prognosis. Epidermal growth factor is excreted

---

Table 16.1. Known aetiological risk factors for bladder cancer

Chemical carcinogens	Chronic inflammation
Aniline dyes	Schistosomiasis
Rubber industry	Bladder diverticulae
β-naphthylamine and	Chronic urinary tract
related compounds	infections
Cigarettes	Squamous cell carcinoma
Drugs (e.g.	increased with chronic
cyclophosphamide,	bladder stones or indwelling
phenacetin)	catheters (e.g. in
	paraplegics)

Incidence, key points

- Bladder cancer accounts for about 4% of male and 2% female cancer deaths, with almost 5000 deaths registered in the UK each year.
- Incidence increases after the fifth decade and is considerably greater than its mortality, as only half the patients die of their disease.
- Cigarette smoking is the most important risk factor, contributing towards 50% of cancers in men and 33% in women, with a two- to fourfold increased risk in smokers.
- Bladder cancer is associated with increased levels of growth factors and chromosome abnormalities

BLADDER CANCER STATISTICS

New bladder cancers

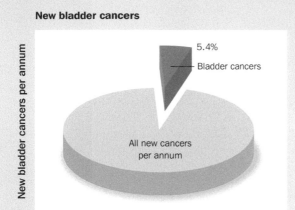

New cases per annum	13170
Males rank	4
Females rank	7
Deaths per annum	5102

Incidence

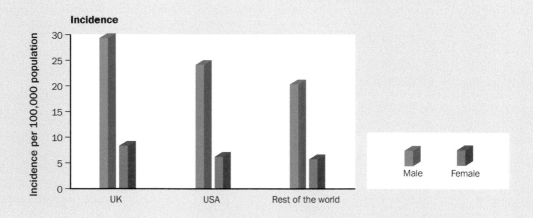

Survival rate

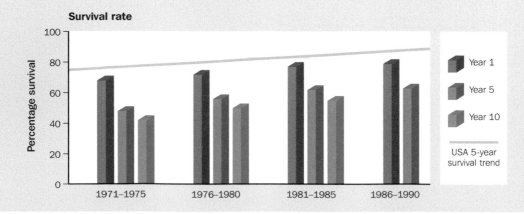

Figure 16.1. Statistical data relating to bladder cancer.

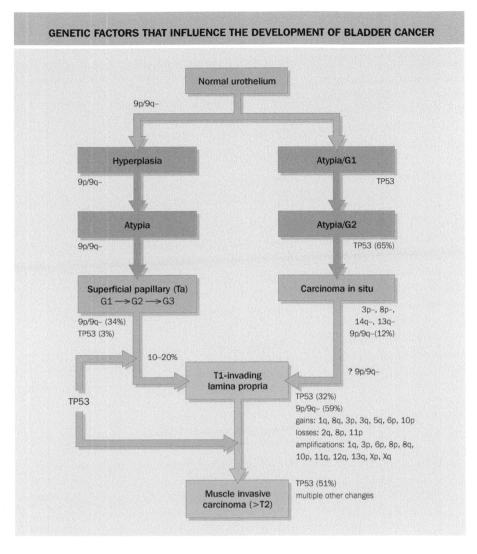

GENETIC FACTORS THAT INFLUENCE THE DEVELOPMENT OF BLADDER CANCER

Normal urothelium

9p/9q–

Hyperplasia

9p/9q–

Atypia

9p/9q–

Superficial papillary (Ta)
G1 → G2 → G3

9p/9q– (34%)
TP53 (3%)

Atypia/G1

TP53

Atypia/G2

TP53 (65%)

Carcinoma in situ

3p–, 8p–,
14q–, 13q–
9p/9q–(12%)

10–20%

T1-invading
lamina propria

? 9p/9q–

TP53

TP53 (32%)
9p/9q– (59%)
gains: 1q, 8q, 3p, 3q, 5q, 6p, 10p
losses: 2q, 8p, 11p
amplifications: 1q, 3p, 6p, 8p, 8q,
10p, 11q, 12q, 13q, Xp, Xq

Muscle invasive
carcinoma (>T2)

TP53 (51%)
multiple other changes

Figure 16.2. *A proposed model for the genetic factors that influence the development of bladder cancer.*

in increased amounts in the urine early in tumour development and has been identified as a promoter of the disease. Increased levels of vascular permeability factor, which enhances the nutritional status of the tumour, have also been isolated. A summary of these genetic abnormalities is presented in *Figure 16.2*.

Pathology

Tumour stage and grade are the most important predictive factors for recurrence and survival, and they determine the natural history of the disease. More than 90% of invasive bladder tumours are transitional cell carcinomas (TCCs).

Squamous carcinomas (SCCs) make up 5% of tumours, except in areas where the incidence of schistosomiasis is high, in which case they account for 50% of bladder malignancy. Adenocarcinomas are rare, and usually arise from urachal remnants or occur at the site of anastomosis of a uterosigmoidostomy. Other tumours include sarcomas (leiomyosarcoma in adults and rhabdomyosarcoma in children), phaeochromocytomas, lymphomas, or metastatic disease.

Two-thirds of bladder cancers are papillary tumours that developed from normal or hyperplastic mucosa. These superficial tumours are generally low grade, run an indolent course, and (although they have a tendency to recur locally) only 10% of low-grade lesions show evidence of muscle invasion at 10 years. High-grade tumours behave more aggressively, with 50–80% of patients progressing within 5 years. Patients who have multiple recurrences over many years at various sites throughout the urinary tract are considered to have a diffusely unstable or tumourigenic urothelium.

Carcinoma in situ (CIS) is a different pathological entity. It is a flat, usually high-grade lesion of the urothelium that is often found adjacent to infiltrating TCCs. Primary CIS, occurring in isolation, is rare but 50–80% progress to invasive disease in 5 years. CIS is most frequently multifocal, and attempts to eradicate the disease from one site in the urothelium are frequently frustrated by its reappearance at another site.

Stage and 5-year survival

The staging system for bladder cancer is based on depth of tumour invasion, which has a direct correlation with survival. Two staging classifications are described for each site. The clinical or pretreatment classification, designated TNM (tumour, node, and metastasis), is based on physical examination, imaging, endoscopy, biopsy, surgical exploration, and other investigations used to classify the tumour before definitive treatment. The pathological staging, designated pTNM, is based on the evidence from surgery and the pathological samples following cystectomy (*Fig. 16.2*).

The major division is between superficial tumours confined to the mucosa and submucosa (Ta and T1), and tumours invading into (T2) or through the muscle wall (T3). The presence of lymph node metastasis has a further negative impact on survival (5-year survival, 10–20%). Major sites of haematogenous metastasis include liver, lungs, and bone. TNM and the 5-year survival rates for each stage are shown in *Table 16.2* and illustrated in *Figures 16.3* and *16.4*.

Table 16.2. *Tumour (T), node (N), and metastasis (M) staging and 5-year survival of patients with bladder cancer*

Stage	Description	5-year survival (%)
Ta	Non-invasive papillary	95
Tis	In-situ 'flat tumour'	
T1	Invades subepithelial connective tissue	75
T2	Invades muscle	
T2a	Inner half	50
T2b	Outer half	
T3	Extravesical extension	25
T3a	Microscopically	
T3b	Extravesical mass	
T4	Invades surrounding structures	15
T4a	Prostate, uterus, and vagina	
T4b	Pelvic and abdominal wall	
N1	Single <2cm	
N2	Single >2cm to 5cm, multiple <5cm	
N3	>5cm	

Pathology, key points

- More than 90% of invasive bladder tumours are transitional cell carcinomas.
- Two-thirds of bladder cancers are papillary tumours that arise from normal or hyperplastic mucosa, and recur locally but run a benign course.
- High-grade tumours behave more aggressively, with 50–80% of patients progressing within 5 years.
- Carcinoma in situ is usually a high-grade lesion and patients have a 50–80% chance of progressing to invasive disease in 5 years.
- The staging system for bladder cancer is based on the depth of tumour invasion, which has a direct correlation with survival.

Clinical Presentation

Bladder cancer typically presents with painless macroscopic haematuria (80–90% cases). Of patients with macroscopic haematuria 15% have a bladder carcinoma, while approximately 6% of those with microscopic haematuria have a tumour. The presence of pain suggests an inflammatory component and should trigger the search for infection or calculus formation. The presence of irritative symptoms, such as frequency and dysuria, should not lull the clinician into assuming that bleeding is of a non-neoplastic origin, as this can be the first clear signal of a primary symptomatic *in situ* carcinoma or of advanced disease. Loin or back pain may herald a hydronephrotic kidney or an intra-abdominal lymphadenopathy.

Investigations

Haematuria may occur intermittently and therefore repeated urine samples should be performed to confirm the diagnosis. Gross painless haematuria should be referred promptly for urological opinion. The investigations that should be performed are summarized in *Table 16.3*. Asymptomatic haematuria occurs in 13% of the general

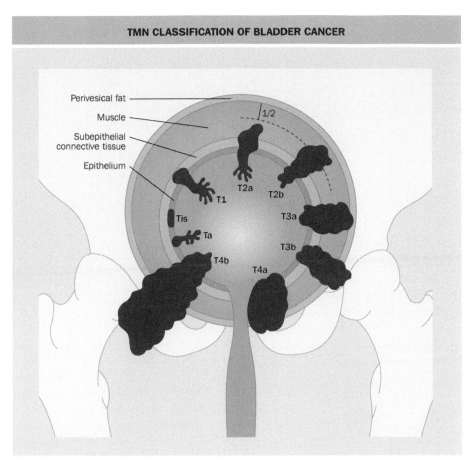

Figure 16.3. Tumour (T), node (N), and metastasis (M) stage of bladder cancer. This diagram is based on the pathological staging (pTMN).

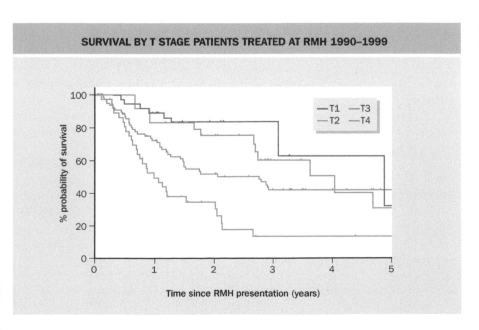

Figure 16.4. Survival by T stage: patients treated by radiotherapy at the Royal Marsden Hospital (RMH), 1990–1999.

Table 16.3. *Summary of investigations for bladder cancer*

Investigation by general practitioner	Investigation by urologist
Clinical examination, including rectal and vaginal examination	Clinical examination, including vaginal and rectal examination
Urine microscopy, culture, sensitivity, and cytology (repeated if haematuria is not confirmed)	Full blood count and biochemistry
	Chest radiography
Prompt referral to urologist if macroscopic or asymptomatic microscopic haematuria confirmed	Midstream urine sample microscopy and culture
	Cytology
Refer to urologist if persistent urinary tract infection in a woman or a single infection in a man	Intravenous urography and/or renal ultrasound
	Flexible cystoscopy and multiple biopsies

population. Of these, 14% have a significant cause for their bleeding and 6.5% have bladder cancer. The presence of asymptomatic haematuria without proteinuria should prompt urological referral. Ideally, the diagnosis of malignancy should be confirmed following a visit to a 'one-stop' haematuria clinic and removal of the tumour undertaken within 4 weeks of flexible cystoscopy. Proteinuria with microscopic haematuria most commonly results from urinary infection, particularly in women. However, if no infection is found, referral to a nephrologist is appropriate.

Screening

Screening of the general population increases the probability of diagnosis of the disease at an early stage, but has not been shown to have an impact on survival. However, high-risk patients with occupational exposure to carcinogens over a number of years are recommended to undergo regular urine cytological screening.

Superficial Bladder Cancer

Superficial bladder tumours are a heterogeneous group with different natural histories. Low grade Ta tumours run a benign course and are treated by excision alone, since they rarely recur. Papillary tumours of higher grade are associated with recurrence (57–85%), but seldom invade or metastasize. T1 tumours are characterized by more frequent recurrences and a greater propensity to progress to muscle invasive disease, especially if of high grade. For patients with Ta tumours 5-year survival is over 90% and it is 75% for those with T1 tumours.

Patients are particularly at risk when tumours recur within 6 months of the original resection or when high-grade disease is present (with or without CIS). In such cases intravesical installations with chemotherapeutic agents such as mitomycin C or immunological agents such as bacillus Calmette–Guérin (BCG) may reduce the risk of progression. A non-specific inflammatory reaction is thought to contribute to the cytotoxic effect, and toxicities are related to local effects and to the extent to which the agent is systemically absorbed. The latter depends on the size of the instilled molecule, the pH at time of instillation, and the timing of instillation relative to cystoscopy or biopsy. Vesical irritability results with dysuria, myelosuppression, and contact dermatitis. With BCG, a small proportion of patients develop systemic tuberculosis, requiring antituberculous treatment, and deaths have been reported.

Single installations of intravesical chemotherapy at the time of transurethral resection of bladder tumour (TURBT) reduce the risk of recurrence, as do more prolonged courses of weekly chemotherapy. However, there is little evidence that intravesical chemotherapy reduces the risk of progression in high-risk patients. Generally, BCG has been found to be more effective and may reduce the risk of progression, but because it is more toxic it is usually recommended for patients with a high risk of progression (e.g. CIS or high-grade T1 lesions) or following failure of intravesical chemotherapy.

CIS has an aggressive natural history, but combined endoscopic resection and subsequent instillation of BCG eradicates CIS for more than 1 year in 70% cases, and prevents subsequent disease for 5 years in 60% cases and 10 years in 40% cases. The role of maintenance therapy is unclear, and the timing of cystectomy in patients who have failed intravesical therapy remains controversial.

In conclusion, intravesical chemotherapy is effective at reducing tumour recurrence but has little effect on progression, while BCG reduces the rate of progression to muscle

Table 16.4. *Summary of intravesical treatment in bladder cancer*

Stage	Grade	Treatment
Ta/T1	1–2	Single, < 2 cm no indication
Ta/T1	1–2	Single > 2 cm treatment with mitomycin C post-transurethral resection of bladder tumour
Ta/T1	1–2	Single recurrences: single treatment with mitomycin C
		Multiple relapses or multiple tumours at relapse: a course of mitomycin C (40mg/40ml) weekly for 6 weeks or bacillus Calmette–Guerin (BCG) weekly for 6 weeks
Tis		Intravesical BCG (consider maintenance) or cystectomy
T1	3	Intravesical BCG or cystectomy

invasive disease and recurrence rates. Overall, only a third of patients need treatment, but all must be rigorously followed up to anticipate the development of recurrent disease. A summary is presented in *Table 16.4*.

Clinical presentation, key points

- 80–90% of cases present with painless macroscopic haematuria.
- Patients with gross painless haematuria and asymptomatic microscopic haematuria should be referred promptly to an urologist.
- The risk is greatest for those over 40 years of age with a history of exposure to a carcinogen.
- Screening of individuals does not affect survival, but does increase the probability of diagnosing disease at an early stage.

Invasive Bladder Cancer

The most effective curative treatment strategy for invasive bladder cancer remains uncertain, and practice varies considerably. Choices lie between radical cystectomy, initial radiotherapy with salvage cystectomy for recurrence, or a combination of treatments. For patients who are unfit for surgery or who have disease outside the bladder, radiotherapy is usually recommended. Surgery is preferred in patients with irritable bladder symptoms, extensive CIS, or bilateral renal obstruction or when radiotherapy is contraindicated because of concomitant medical conditions. In patients with squamous carcinoma or adenocarcinoma surgery is often preferred, but for the remainder who are suitable for either treatment, the choice is not simple.

In practice in the UK, in the absence of adequate randomized data to support either modality, the decision often depends on local expertise and patient preference.

Surgery

Radical cystectomy (involving resection of the bladder, prostate, seminal vesicles, female urethra, uterus, ovaries, and pelvic lymph nodes) followed by urinary diversion has been established as a curative treatment since the 1950s. Mortality was as high as 10–15%, but with modern techniques it has fallen to 1% in expert hands. Impotence was a frequent complication, but with the development of nerve-sparing techniques potency may be preserved. The use of continent urinary diversions has resulted in practical and psychological benefits to patients who previously would have had an ileal conduit, but such diversions are suitable for only a minority of patients in the UK. They are also associated with incontinence and infective complications. In carefully selected cases, a partial cystectomy may be performed, such as in patients with solitary tumours of the bladder dome and those with normal random biopsies from elsewhere in the bladder. Survival by stage following radical cystectomy is shown in *Table 16.2*. The pattern of failure in recurrence is usually with metastatic disease, which typically affects the lung, liver, or bone. About 10–20% patients develop pelvic recurrence of their disease after cystectomy.

Radiotherapy

In the UK, radical radiotherapy is the most common primary treatment for muscle invasive disease, with salvage surgery undertaken for treatment failures. Some series suggest that results with radiotherapy alone may be worse than those with cystectomy, but case selection and the availability of more detailed staging information following surgery influences these results. Patient preference is an important factor, and many patients prefer a bladder-sparing approach. The main criticism of radiotherapy is that complete responses are only seen in 50–60% of cases at their first 3-month cystoscopy, and local control is maintained in about half of these. The use of combined pre- or post-operative radiotherapy with surgery may be expected to improve results, but unfortunately this expected benefit has not been proved in randomized studies to date.

Radiotherapy to the bladder is usually well tolerated. Acute side effects include tiredness, urinary frequency, dysuria, and diarrhoea. These problems are usually controlled by simple medication and resolve within a few weeks of completion of therapy. Late complications include bladder shrinkage, urgency, and telangiectasia causing haematuria, and can be reduced with good radiotherapy techniques.

Chemotherapy

The usual pattern of failure after radical local treatment for bladder cancer is with systemic metastasis. Systemic therapy has therefore been investigated in an attempt to improve survival. Early single-arm studies were encouraging, and suggested response rates of 60–70% for localized tumours, with 30% of these being complete responses. However, a limited number of small randomized trials of adjuvant chemotherapy were completed with equivocal results, and failed to show a significant survival advantage. Research in this area continues. Recent larger-scale studies to investigate the use of neoadjuvant chemotherapy (given before radical local treatment) have suggested a small advantage. A metaanalysis to confirm results is awaited.

Palliative care

The aim of treatment is to both control symptoms and maintain quality of life. This should be carried out in a multidisci-plinary setting that involves the palliative care team within the hospital and in the community.

Chemotherapy

The use of chemotherapy in those fit enough to receive it is justified by reports of long-term survivors and the results of two randomized studies that indicated a survival benefit for more intensive regimens compared with less intensive or single-agent treatment. However, the most commonly used regimens have significant toxicity, which must be balanced against a modest survival advantage. The effect of chemotherapy on quality rather than duration of life remains unclear.

Radiotherapy

Radiotherapy provides effective palliation of symptoms from bone metastases and from uncontrolled pelvic disease. Short fractionation regimens with fewer hospital visits are preferable in the palliative setting.

Treatment, key points

- The most effective curative treatment for invasive bladder cancer is not known, and practice often reflects local expertise and patient preference.
- Adjuvant chemotherapy, despite initial promising results, has yet to be proved to improve survival.
- Judicious use of palliative radiotherapy and chemotherapy can improve symptom control and maintain quality of life in patients with incurable disease.

Future developments

Given our uncertainty about the optimal management of invasive bladder cancer it is perhaps unfortunate that there are no

Key points: bladder and/or urothelial cancers

95% of the cancers affect the bladder, 5% affect the upper tracts

90% of patients present with macroscopic haematuria

5–10% present with microscopic haematuria only

Both macroscopic and microscopic haematuria, when caused by a urothelial cancer, are intermittent; repeat urine testing can be negative for haematuria in the presence of a tumour

Reproduced from England Department of Health Cancer Referral Guidelines Consultation Document May 2000.

Referral proforma: urology cancer

Age:

Suspected cancer:

Prostate	☐	Kidney	☐
Bladder	☐	Testis	☐

Other..

Symptoms:	Yes	No	
Macroscopic haematuria			
Loin pain			
Testicular swelling			
Bone pain			
Lower urinary tract symptoms (e.g., hesitancy, poor stream, etc.)			

Other, please state.............................

Clinical examination:	Yes	No	
Renal mass			
Pyrexia			
Swelling in the body of the testis			
Prostate feels malignant on rectal examination			

Other, please state...................................

Investigations:	Yes	No	
Prostate-specific antigen.................ng/ml			
Haemoglobin................................g/dl			
Microscopic haematuria			
Mass detected on imaging			

Comments/other reasons for urgent referral

Reproduced from England Department of Health Cancer Referral Guidelines Consultation Document May 2000.

ongoing trials of the effectiveness of surgery against that of radio-therapy. However, we expect improvements in both modalities. The use of conformal radiotherapy techniques, with treatment of only part of the bladder for some of the treatment, may reduce morbidity and allow dose escalation. So far chemother-apy has made little impact in this disease, but it is hoped that the introduction of new agents such as gemcitabine and taxol will improve results. The application of molecular biological techniques may provide useful diagnostic and prognostic infor-mation and may also lead to novel treatments in the future.

Further Reading

Hall RR. *Clinical Management of Bladder Cancer*. London: Arnold, 1999.

Knowles MA. The genetics of transitional cell carcinoma: progress and potential clinical application. *BJU Int* 1999; **84**: 412–27.

Appendix

Guidelines for urgent referral: urological cancers

Macroscopic haematuria

Any swelling in the body of the testis in a man 15–55 years of age

Palpable renal masses

Incidental finding of a solid mass in the kidney on imaging

Bone pain accompanied by an abnormal prostate on rectal examination and/or a high prostate-specific antigen (PSA; >20ng/ml)

Clinically malignant prostate on rectal examination and a PSAlevel greater than 20 ng/ml

17 Renal Cell Cancer

Andy Webb and Martin Gore

Incidence

In the UK there are approximately 6000 new cases of renal cell carcinoma (RCC) per year. Men have a two to three times higher risk of developing RCC than women and the median age of diagnosis is 65 years, but the age range is wide and occasionally children are diagnosed. Various statistics relating to renal cell carcinoma are shown in *Figure 17.1*.

Aetiology

Several environmental factors, including chronic dialysis, obesity, and tobacco use, are associated with a higher risk of developing RCC (Linehan *et al.*, 1997). Families with Von Hippel–Lindau (VHL) disease have a very high risk of RCC, with 25–45% of individuals being affected (Choyke *et al.*, 1992). Studies of these families have identified the VHL tumour suppressor gene on 3p25. Both copies of this gene are inactivated in the tissue of all VHL-associated kidney cancers and in over 75% of sporadic clear cell kidney cancers (Latif *et al.*, 1993).

Clinical Presentation

Renal cancer can remain clinically occult for many years, and it is an incidental finding in a number of patients. Haematuria is the most common presentation (60%), followed by abdominal mass (45%) and pain (41%). The classic triad of all three clinical features occurs less frequently (19%). Approximately 75% of patients with metastatic RCC have metastases to the lung, with soft tissue, bone, liver, and the central nervous system being other common sites of disease. Patients may also complain of systemic symptoms such as lethargy caused by anaemia, pyrexia, fatigue, and weight loss (*Table 17.1*; Skinner *et al.*, 1971).

Investigations

Ultrasound, computed tomography (CT), and magnetic resonance imaging (MRI) together with excretory urography, arteriography, and venography can all add information as to the staging and operability of renal cancer. The first three techniques are the most frequently used because they are less invasive. Multiple imaging modalities may be necessary to define operability, particularly with large tumours.

Pathology

The most common histological type of kidney cancer is clear cell (75% of cases), and poor prognostic features include sarcomatoid changes and high nuclear grade.

Staging and Prognosis

The most commonly used staging classification is the Robson modification of the system described by Flocks and Kadesky (*Table 17.2*; Robson, 1982). The 5-year survival rates initially reported by Robson and colleagues were 66% for stage I, 64% for stage II, 42% for stage III, and 11% for stage IV patients. The survival rate for patients with stage IIIB RCC is much worse than for other stage III patients, with a 5-year survival of 18% (Skinner *et al.*, 1971) compared to 34–51% for the group as a whole. The survival of patients has remained the same since 1969, the date of Robson's classification system.

Table 17.1. *Incidence of presenting symptoms*

Symptom	Incidence (%)
Classic triad (haematuria, mass, pain)	19
Haematuria	59
Abdominal mass	45
Pain	41
Weight loss	28
Anaemia	21
Fever	7
Symptoms from metastases	10

RENAL CELL CARCINOMA STATISTICS

New renal cell carcinoma

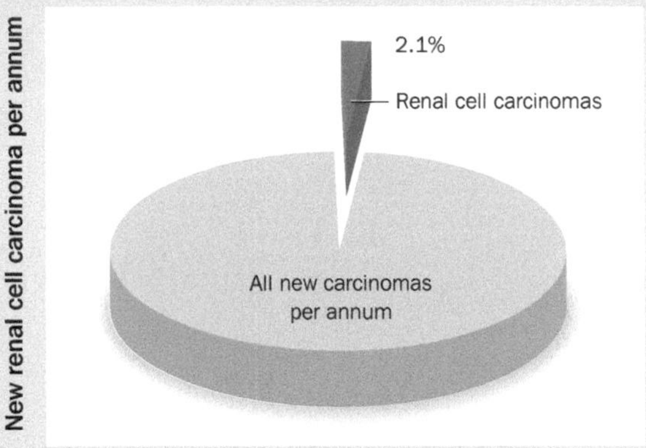

New cases per annum	5250
Males rank	10
Females rank	14
Deaths per annum	3033

Incidence

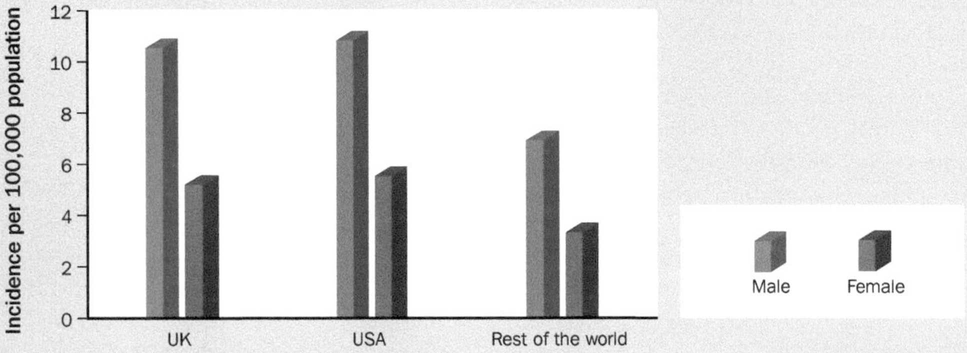

Survival rate

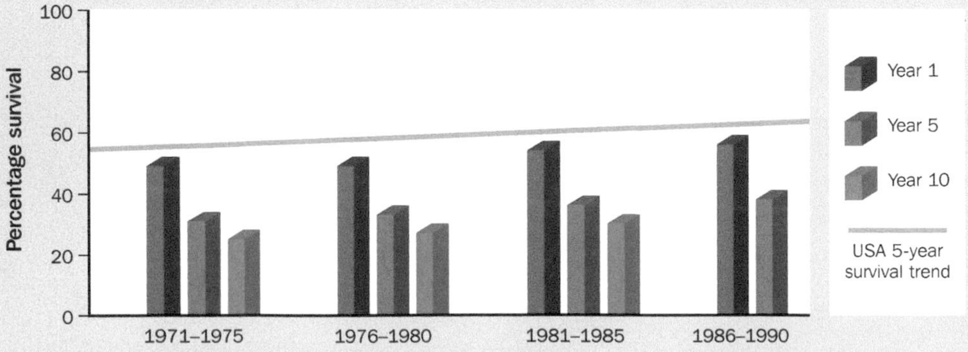

Figure 17.1. *Statistical data relating to renal cell carcinoma.*

Table 17.2. *Staging and 5-year survival*

Stage	Description	5-year survival (%)
I	Confined to kidney	56–100
II	Confined to Gerota's fascia	47–67
III	Involves renal vein/ inferior vena cava (IIIa) Involves local lymph nodes (IIIb)	34–51
IV	Through Gerota's fascia or extensive lymph node involvement or metastatic disease	0–18

A third of patients present with metastatic disease, and 40% of patients with localized disease relapse after nephrectomy. Although the prognosis for the majority of patients with metastatic disease is poor, the following features are associated with a relatively good prognosis (Elson *et al.*, 1988):

- long disease-free interval between initial nephrectomy and the development of metastases (>24 months);
- single site of metastatic disease;
- no symptoms.

Key points

- 6000 new cases in UK and 95,000 deaths per year worldwide.
- Families with Von Hippel–Lindau disease have a very high risk of renal cell carcinoma.
- Most patients present with at least one of the classic triad of symptoms – haematuria, pain, abdominal mass.
- 40% develop advanced disease after potentially curative nephrectomy.
- 33% present with advanced disease and prognosis is generally poor.

Treatment

Surgical management
Patients fit for surgery with stage I, II, or III RCC should have a standard radical nephrectomy. Patients with moderately enlarged abdominal lymph nodes (1–2cm) on CT scanning should also have a nephrectomy, because the enlarged nodes often result from reactive changes. Gross involvement of the renal vein or inferior vena cava requires careful staging. Minor extension into the vena cava can be removed through the renal vein or a vena cava incision. More extensive disease, such as tumour thrombus extending supradiaphragmatically, requires a thoracotomy and hypothermic circulatory arrest for successful removal. Although the operative mortality of such procedures is relatively high, the long-term outcomes are reasonably good.

In general, there is little indication for surgical resection if there is tumour extension beyond Gerota's fascia; extensive nodal involvement. Spontaneous remission of metastatic lesions following nephrectomy occurs in less than 1% of patients (Montie *et al.*, 1977), and thus nephrectomy is not indicated if the sole aim is to induce response in distant lesions. Recently, two randomized trials have shown a survival benefit for patients with metastatic disease who undergo nephrectomy. Other reasons for nephrectomy in this situation include:

- Large symptomatic primary tumour associated with metastatic disease of small–moderate volume. Nephrectomy palliates the symptoms of pain and haemorrhage, and also improves systemic constitutional symptoms. Nephrectomy has a lower morbidity than radiotherapy or embolization.
- Large asymptomatic primary tumour associated with small-volume metastatic disease. In this situation there is a high likelihood that local symptoms will occur before those from metastatic disease.
- Prior to entry into a clinical trial of immunotherapy. Improvements in the patient's immune response have been demonstrated following nephrectomy and thus there may be a better chance of responding following cytoreductive surgery.

Hormonal therapy
Medroxyprogesterone acetate (MPA) was the standard therapy for systemic treatment of metastatic RCC for many years. In 10 trials involving 173 patients, the cumulative response rate to MPA was 10% (Harris, 1983). The Medical Research Council (MRC) trial that compared MPA with interferon demonstrated a 7% response rate to MPA and a median survival of 6 months (Medical Research Council Renal Cancer Collaborators, 1999). Tamoxifen at low dose

(20 mg per day) showed very little activity, but some evidence indicates that at a higher dose (40 mg per day) activity may be increased. Despite low response rates to hormonal agents, they still perform an important part of the management of patients because they can provide good symptomatic improvement with little or no toxicity.

Chemotherapy

Studies using both single-agent and combination chemotherapy regimens report low response rates of short duration. In a review of 4093 treated patients in 83 phase II chemotherapy trials, the overall response rate was only 6.8%. The most active agent is 5-fluorouracil, with a response rate of 13.4% (Yagoda *et al.*, 1995). At present there is no role for chemotherapy alone in RCC.

Radiotherapy

Radiotherapy has clear symptomatic benefit in the treatment of bone metastases. It also has benefits in treating brain metastases, except where severe neurological deficits that cannot be reversed by corticosteroids are present. It can occasionally be used to treat specific sites of soft-tissue disease, but it is rarely of benefit in treating large primary renal tumours. No evidence from randomized trials indicates that radiotherapy has an adjuvant role post-nephrectomy (Linehan *et al.*, 1997).

Biological therapy

The importance of the immune system in metastatic RCC is evidenced by the observation that occasional spontaneous regressions occur and that there are host immune responses in patients who remain alive for years with metastatic disease. RCC is one of the few tumour types shown to respond to biological therapy and this remains the most promising area of research into future treatment options.

Interferons

Interferons have a wide range of actions, including immunomodulatory activity with enhancement of leukocyte-mediated cytotoxicity, antiproliferative effects on malignant cells, and antiviral activity. The majority of research has centred on the use of interferon alfa, because it has consistently shown the highest activity. Phase II studies show objective responses of 15–20%. An MRC study (Medical Research Council Renal Cancer Collaborators, 1999) randomized patients to 12 weeks of subcutaneous interferon alfa (10 megaunits subcutaneously three times a week) or MPA (300mg orally per day for 12 weeks). A total of 350 patients were randomized and evidence was obtained of a statistically significant response (14% versus 7%) and survival advantage (median 8.5

versus 6 months, $p = 0.017$) in favour of interferon alfa. Two other randomized trials have shown a statistically significant benefit in terms of survival for interferon alfa. A Cochrane meta-analysis also suggests an improvement in overall survival. The optimal duration of interferon alfa therapy has not been defined. Most patients who respond do so at 3–4 months, but later responses can occur. Our current practice is to continue treatment for patients who have responding or stable disease for as long as they are able to tolerate the side effects.

Fossa *et al.* (1995) compared interferon-treated patients with case controls obtained from the Eastern Cooperative Oncology Group database of patients who were in non-immunotherapy studies. Only patients with good prognosis disease had a significant survival benefit from interferon treatment. The prognostic categories were defined according to the factors set out in the section on prognosis: good, two or three favourable factors; moderate, one favourable factor; poor, no favourable factors.

A randomized double-blind trial of gamma interferon versus placebo in 196 patients with metastatic RCC showed similar response rates in both arms (4.4% versus 6.6%, respectively, $p = 0.54$) and no survival benefit (12.2 months with interferon versus 15.7 months with placebo, $p = 0.52$; Gleave *et al.*, 1995). The results show that not all interferons have activity in metastatic RCC and demonstrate the importance of randomised studies.

Interleukin-2

Interleukin-2 (IL-2) is a cytokine with no intrinsic anti-tumour activity, but it acts through immunological mechanisms, including activation of cytotoxic T-cells and the production of other cytokines. High-dose intravenous IL-2 is toxic and results in a vascular leak syndrome, hypotension, and renal, gastrointestinal, and haematological toxicities. Therefore, careful patient selection and inpatient monitoring are required. Fortunately, lower-dose subcutaneous outpatient regimens are also active with less toxicity. Cumulative data suggest overall response rates of 15–20%. A proportion of patients who achieve a complete remission appear to be long-term survivors (Bukowski, 1997). As with interferon alfa, the benefit of IL-2 appears to occur only in the good and moderate prognostic groups of patients when compared with case controls (Jones *et al.*, 1993).

Interferon alfa and interleukin-2 combination therapy

Interferon alfa may enhance IL-2 induced killing through cytotoxic lymphocyte activation by enhanced expression of the major histocompatibility complex (MHC) class 1 anti-

Key points: renal cancer

Macroscopic haematuria is the most common presenting symptom

Other presenting features:

loin pain

renal mass

microscopic haematuria

anaemia

pyrexia

May present as an incidental finding on abdominal imaging (e.g. computed tomography or ultrasound)

Reproduced from England Department of Health Cancer Referral Guidelines Consultation Document May 2000.

gens on tumour cells. This theoretical benefit has been investigated in a randomized three-arm trial. In this study, 425 patients were randomized to receive either interferon alfa (18mU subcutaneously three times a week for 10 weeks) or IL-2 (18mU/m^2 intravenously in 5-day cycles as two induction cycles and then four maintenance cycles), or a combination of the two with the same dose of IL-2 but only 6mU of interferon alfa. The IL-2 and interferon arm resulted in significantly higher response rate (18.6 versus 7.5% versus 6.5%, $p < 0.01$) and longer disease-free survival ($p = 0.01$). However, no overall survival benefit was found between any of the three groups (Negrier et al., 1998).

Interferon alfa, interleukin-2, and 5-fluorouracil

A major step in clinical research into new treatments occurred when Atzpodien et al. (1993) reported results of the addition of bolus 5-fluorouracil to subcutaneous interferon alfa and IL-2, with a response rate of 49% with acceptable toxicity. Subsequently, the same authors confirmed this activity in a randomized study to compare the combination of tamoxifen in 78 patients. There was a clear response advantage for the biochemotherapy group (39% versus 0%). In addition, progression-free and overall survival were significantly improved (median overall survival not reached after 42 months versus 14 months, $p < 0.04$; Atzpodien et al., 1997). At the Royal Marsden Hospital we have used continuous infusions of 5-fluorouracil via a Hickman line, together with subcutaneous interferon alfa and IL-2. In a group of patients with poor prognostic features, we have reported a response rate of 31% with activity being seen in all prognostic groups (Allen et al., 1999).

Adjuvant therapy

A significant number of patients (40%) relapse after nephrectomy for potentially curable disease. One randomized study of adjuvant interferon alfa versus observation after nephrectomy has been carried out, and resulted in no difference in the survival between the treatment arms (Pizzocaro et al., 1997).

Future directions

On the basis of randomized studies, interferon alfa has established itself as a standard treatment (Table 17.3).

Table 17.3. Systemic treatment option in metastatic renal cell carcinoma

Treatment	Response rate (%)	Median survival (months)
Hormone treatment	5–10	6
Chemotherapy	5–10	6–8
Interferon alfa	10–15	8–12
Interleukin-2	15–20	10–15
Interferon alfa + interleukin-2	20	10–15
Interferon alfa + interleukin-2 + 5-fluorouracil	20–40	10–40

Referral proforma: urology cancer

Age:

Suspected cancer:

Prostate	☐	Kidney	☐	
Bladder	☐	Testis	☐	

Other...

Symptoms:	Yes	No	
Macroscopic haematuria			
Loin pain			
Testicular swelling			
Bone pain			
Lower urinary tract symptoms (e.g., hesitancy, poor stream, etc.)			

Other, please state.............................

Clinical examination:	Yes	No	
Renal mass			
Pyrexia			
Swelling in the body of the testis			
Prostate feels malignant on rectal examination			

Other, please state...................................

Investigations:	Yes	No	
Prostate-specific antigen..................ng/ml			
Haemoglobin................................g/dl			
Microscopic haematuria			
Mass detected on imaging			

Comments/other reasons for urgent referral

Reproduced from England Department of Health Cancer Referral Guidelines Consultation Document May 2000.

Combinations of 5-fluorouracil, IL-2, and interferon alfa have increased response rates and studies are now accruing that compare interferon with this combination. New oral 5-fluorouracil compounds could replace intravenous 5-fluorouracil and may lead to improvements in toxicity as well as efficacy. Although 5-fluorouracil, IL-2, and interferon alfa combinations have improved the response rates, most patients still relapse and die. Therefore, maintenance strategies following this combination require investigation.

Similarly, because a significant number of patients relapse after potentially curative nephrectomy, the role of adjuvant therapy using the combination of 5-fluorouracil, IL-2, and interferon alfa is currently being investigated in a randomized trial against observation.

Other areas of active research include compounds that effect new blood-vessel formation (angiogenesis), vaccination, and other forms of immunotherapy.

Treatment, key points

- Nephrectomy should be attempted even in the face of metastatic spread in fit patients.
- Standard treatment for advanced disease is interferon alfa.
- Interferon alfa prolongs survival when compared to hormone therapy.
- High response rates have been achieved using combined biological and chemotherapies.

Further Reading

Allen M, Vaughan M, Johnston S, *et al.* Protracted venous infusion 5-fluorouracil in combination with subcutaneous interleukin-2 and alpha interferon in patients with metastatic renal cell carcinoma: A phase II study. *Br J Cancer.* 2000; **83**: 980–5.

Atzpodien J, Kirchner H, Hanninen EL, Deckert M, Fenner M, Pollwoda H. Interleukin-2 in combination with interferon-alpha and 5-fluorouracil for metastatic renal cell cancer. *Eur J Cancer.* 1993; **29A**: S6–8.

Atzpodien J, Kirchner H, Franzke A, *et al.* Results of a randomized clinical trial comparing SC interleukin-2, SC alpha-2a-interferon, and IV bolus 5-fluorouracil against oral tamoxifen in progressive metastatic renal cell carcinoma patients (Meeting abstract). *Proc Annu Meet Am Soc Clin Oncol.* 1997; **16**: 326.

Bukowski RM. Natural history and therapy of metastatic renal cell carcinoma: the role of interleukin-2. *Cancer.* 1997; **80**: 1198–220.

Choyke PL, Glenn GM, Walther MM, *et al.* The natural history of renal lesions in von Hippel–Lindau disease: a serial CT study in 28 patients. *AJR Am J Roentgenol.* 1992; **159**: 1229–34.

Elson PJ, Witte RS, Trump DL. Prognostic factors for survival in patients with recurrent or metastatic renal cell carcinoma. *Cancer Res.* 1988; 48: 7310–13.

Fossa S, Jones M, Johnson P, *et al.* Interferon-alpha and survival in renal cell cancer. *Br J Urol.* 1995; **76**: 286–90.

Gleave ME, Elhilali M, Fradet Y, *et al.* Interferon gamma-1b compared with placebo in metastatic renal-cell carcinoma. Canadian Urologic Oncology Group [see comments]. *N Engl J Med.* 1998; **338**: 1265–71.

Harris DT. Hormonal therapy and chemotherapy of renal-cell carcinoma. *Semin Oncol.* 1983; **10**: 422–30.

Jones M, Philip T, Palmer P, *et al.* The impact of interleukin-2 on survival in renal cancer: a multivariate analysis. *Cancer Biother.* 1993; **8**: 275–88.

Latif F, Duh FM, Gnarra J, *et al.* von Hippel–Lindau syndrome: cloning and identification of the plasma membrane Ca(++)-transporting ATPase isoform 2 gene that resides in the von Hippel–Lindau gene region. *Cancer Res.* 1993; **53**: 861–7.

Linehan W, Shipley W, Parkinson D. Cancer of the kidney and ureter. In: DeVita V, Hellman S, Rosenberg S, eds. *Cancer: Principles and Practice of Oncology,* Vol. 1. Philadelphia: Lippincott–Raven, 1997: 1271–1297.

Medical Research Council Renal Cancer Collaborators. Interferon-alpha and survival in metastatic renal carcinoma: early results of a randomised controlled trial. *Lancet.* 1999; **353**: 14–7.

Montie JE, Stewart BH, Straffon RA, Banowsky LH, Hewitt CB, Montague DK. The role of adjunctive nephrectomy in patients with metastatic renal cell carcinoma. *J Urol.* 1977; **117**: 272–5.

Negrier S, Escudier B, Lasset C, *et al.* Recombinant human interleukin-2, recombinant human interferon alfa-2a, or both in metastatic renal-cell carcinoma. Groupe Francais d'Immunotherapie [see comments]. *N Engl J Med.* 1998; **338**: 1272–8.

Pizzocaro G, Piva L, Costa A, Silvestrini R. Adjuvant interferon to radical nephrectomy in Robson's stages II and III renal cell carcinoma, A randomised study with biological evaluations. *Proc Am Soc Clin Oncol.* 1997; **16** :318.

Robson CJ. Staging of renal cell carcinoma. *Prog Clin Biol Res.* 1982; **100**: 439–45.

Skinner DG, Colvin RB, Vermillion CD, Pfister RC, Leadbetter WF. Diagnosis and management of renal cell carcinoma. A clinical and pathologic study of 309 cases. *Cancer.* 1971; **28**: 1165–77.

Yagoda A, Abi-Rached B, Petrylak D. Chemotherapy for advanced renal-cell carcinoma: 1983–1993. *Semin Oncol.* 1995; **22**: 42–60.

Appendix

Guidelines for urgent referral: urological cancers

Macroscopic haematuria

Any swelling in the body of the testis in a man 15–55 years of age

Palpable renal masses

Incidental finding of a solid mass in the kidney on imaging

Bone pain accompanied by an abnormal prostate on rectal examination and/or a high prostate-specific antigen (PSA; >20ng/ml)

Clinically malignant prostate on rectal examination and a PSA level greater than 20 mg/l

18 Germ Cell Tumours of Testis

Paula Wells and David Dearnaley

Germ cell tumours (GCTs) of the testis are the commonest malignancy in men aged 20–40 years. The incidence is rising and is increasing at a rate of 10–20% every 5 years. The increased understanding of the biology of these tumours and considerable therapeutic improvements in their management mean that 95% of these patients can now expect to be cured.

Incidence

Approximately 1600 cases are registered in England and Wales each year. A 15-year-old boy has a lifetime risk of developing a tumour of 1/500, but tumours are rare in those younger than 15 and older than 60 years of age. Of adult cases, 90% have a recognizable testicular primary, approximately 5% arise in the mediastinum and the remainder from the retroperitoneum or pineal body, or are of unknown primary site. Testicular GCTs are divided histologically into teratoma and seminoma, with a median age of presentation for teratoma of 25–30 years and for seminoma approximately a decade later. Various statistics relating to testicular tumours are presented in *Figure 18.1*.

Aetiology

GCTs are most common in Caucasians, with the highest incidence in Nordic countries, particularly Denmark and Norway. The main risk factor for tumour development is testicular maldescent, with a five-fold increase in incidence in those with unilateral descent, rising to a ten-fold risk with bilateral maldescent. Although the incidence of testicular maldescent is rising in the UK, only 10% of cases occur with this background. Prenatal influences are also thought to be important in tumour development. It is hypothesized that increased maternal weight that results in increased oestrogen exposure in utero may influence genital development. Furthermore, transplacental exposure to xenoestrogenic chemicals, such as dichlorodiphenyltrichloroethane (DDT), with anti-androgenic and immunosuppressive properties may contribute to the declining sperm count and rising inci-

Table 18.1. *Risk factors for testicular cancer*

Factor	Approximate increase in risk
Unilateral maldescent	×5
Bilateral maldescent	×10
Family history	×10
Contralateral testicular tumour	×10
Mumps orchitis/testicular atrophy	?
Childhood inguinal hernia	?
Carcinoma in situ	50% progression to invasive disease at 5 years

Life-time risk of testicular cancer in the UK: 1 in 450–500.

dence of GCT through more than one mechanism. The main risk factors are highlighted in *Table 18.1*.

Cytogenetics

Approximately 80% of GCTs are characterized by the presence of an isochromosome in the short arm of chromosome 12, but its precise role is as yet unknown. Genes that regulate the performance of cytochrome p450 enzymes or that are responsible for inactivating xenoestrogenic chemicals, and other unlinked genes that may influence the immunological response to the mumps virus, may also be important. Genetic studies continue in this area.

Pathology

The histopathology of these tumours is complex and the diagnosis must therefore be made by a pathologist skilled in tumour classification. The pathologist should assess malignant germ cell elements, note cord resection margins, and specifically comment on the presence of vascular invasion (the most important prognostic factor) in tumours. The

TESTIS TUMOURS STATISTICS

New testis tumours

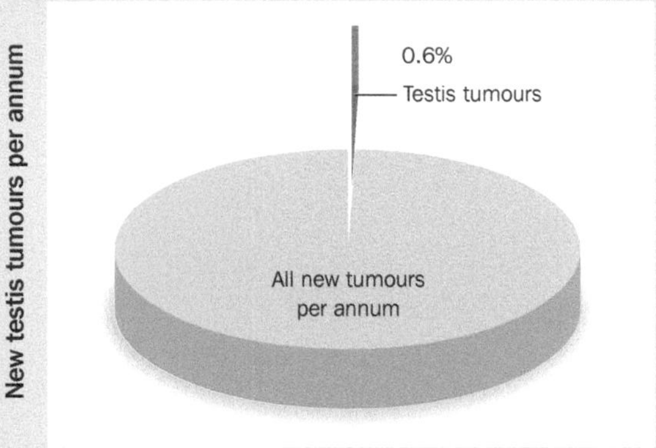

New testis tumours per annum

0.6%
— Testis tumours

All new tumours
per annum

New cases per annum	1380
Males rank	15
Females rank	—
Deaths per annum	77

Incidence

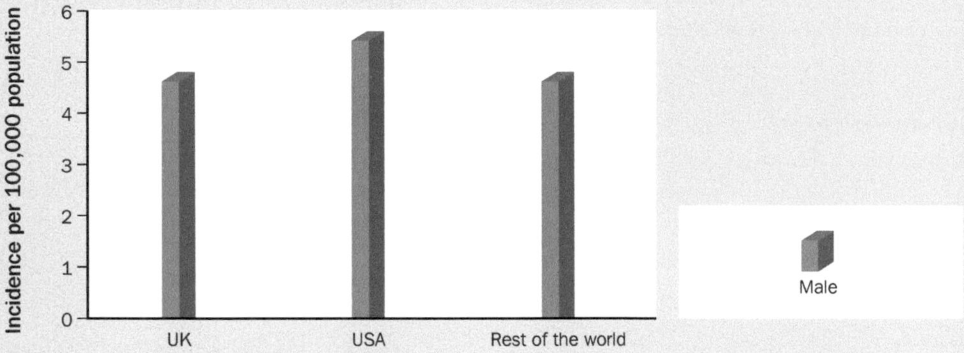

Incidence per 100,000 population

(bar chart, y-axis 0 to 6)

UK — approx 4.6
USA — approx 5.4
Rest of the world — approx 4.6

Male

Survival rate

Percentage survival

(bar chart, x-axis 1971–1975, 1976–1980, 1981–1985, 1986–1990)

Year 1
Year 5
Year 10
USA 5-year survival trend

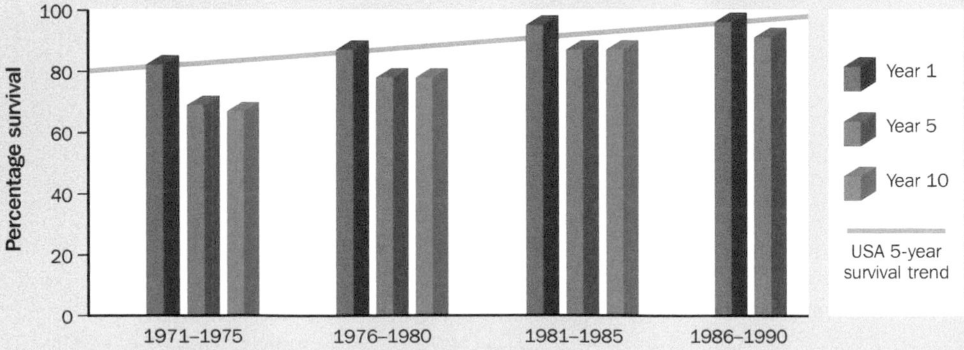

Figure 18.1. *Statistical data relating to testicular tumours.*

tumours are classified as seminomas or non-seminomatous, with 10% being mixed tumours. The pathological classification in *Table 18.2* represents that most commonly used in the UK.

Seminoma

There are some important variants of seminoma. Classic seminoma has a characteristic uniform solid-greyish appearance, and contain an admixture of tumour cells and lymphocytes microscopically. Anaplastic tumours appear more pleomorphic, but this is not of prognostic significance. Spermatocytic tumours occur in a more elderly population, metastasis is exceptional, and they are not associated with intratubular germ cell neoplasia or gonadal dysgenesis.

Non-seminomatous germ cell tumours

90% of cases contain mixed malignant elements. The most common histological subtypes are malignant teratoma undifferentiated (MTU) and malignant teratoma intermediate (MTI); both contain undifferentiated teratoma, although MTI also shows areas of differentiation and MTU has a higher propensity for metastasis. Teratoma differentiated (TD) pursues an indolent and usually benign course. Malignant teratoma trophoblastic (MTT) are composed of trophoblastic elements that produce human chorionic gonadotrophin (HCG) and are usually aggressive with widespread metastatic potential. Alpha-fetoprotein (AFP) is produced by yolk-sac elements, which are a common component of adult tumours. Pure yolk-sac tumours most usually arise in infancy and have low metastatic potential and good prognosis.

Staging

Careful clinical examination and routine biochemistry, haematology, and tests of tumour markers (HCG, AFP, lactate dehydrogenase) are required. Radiological investigations include chest radiography and computed tomography (CT) scans of the chest, abdomen, and pelvis in teratomas, which spread haematogenously and commonly involve the lung and liver, as well as in retroperitoneal or supradiaphragmatic lymph nodes. Seminomas metastasize in a predictable and contiguous fashion. Para-aortic lymph nodes are most commonly affected, and more distant nodal spread or bone involvement is most unusual in the absence of retroperitoneal disease. Prognostic factors are increasingly important in the management of metastatic GCTs. Conventional staging systems, such as the Royal Marsden

Table 18.2. *Pathology of male germ cell tumours*

Classical seminoma
Anaplastic seminoma
Spermatocytic seminoma
Malignant teratoma
Teratoma differentiated
Malignant teratoma undifferentiated
Malignant teratoma intermediate
Malignant teratoma trophoblastic
Yolk sac tumour
Combined tumour (seminoma and teratoma)

Table 18.3. *Royal Marsden Hospital Staging System*

Stage	Substage	Definitions
I		No evidence of metastasis
IM		Rising serum markers with no other evidence of metastasis
II		Abdominal node metastasis
	A	≤ 2cm in diameter
	B	2–5cm in diameter
	C	≥ 5cm in diameter
III		Supradiaphragmatic nodal metastasis
	M	Mediastinal
	N	Supraclavicular/cervical/axillary
	O	No abdominal node metastasis
	ABC	Node stage as defined as in stage II
IV		Extralymphatic metastasis
	L1	Three or fewer lung metastasis
	L2	Three or more lung metastasis all <2cm in diameter
	L3	Three or more lung metastasis one or more >2cm in diameter
	H+	Liver metastasis
	Br+	Brain metastasis
	Bo+	Bone metastasis

system (*Table 18.3*), describe disease extent and are supplemented by information from tumour markers to place patients into prognostic groups (*Table 18.4*). Individual prognostic factors are used to place patients into good, intermediate, or poor

157

Table 18.4. *Definition of the germ cell consensus classification: a prognostic factor-based staging system for metastatic germ cell cancers from the International Germ Cell Collaborative Group (1997)*

Prognosis	Parameter	Non-seminoma	Seminoma
Good	Tumour type	Testis/retroperitoneal primary and no non-pulmonary visceral metastases and good markers, all of:	Any primary site and no non-pulmonary visceral metastases and all of:
		Alpha-fetoprotein (AFP) <1000ng/ml	Normal
		Human chorionic gonadotrophin (HCG) <5000iu/l (1000ng/ml)	Any
		Lactate dehydrogenase (LDH) <1.5 times upper limit of normal	Any
	Proportion	56% of non-seminomas	90% of seminomas
	5-year progression-free survival	89%	82%
	5-year survival	92%	86%
Intermediate	Tumour type	Testis/retroperitoneal primary and no non-pulmonary visceral metastases and intermediate markers, any of:	Any primary site and non-pulmonary visceral metastases and:
		AFP >1000 and <10,000ng/ml	Normal
		HCG >5000 and <50,000iu/l	Any
		LDH >1.5 times upper limit of normal and <10 times normal	Any
	Proportion	28% of non-seminomas	10% of seminomas
	5-year PFS	75%	67%
	5-year-survival	80%	72%
Poor	Tumour type	Mediastinal primary or non-pulmonary visceral metastases or poor markers, any of:	No patients classified as poor prognosis
		AFP >10,000ng/ml	
		HCG >50,000iu/l	
		LDH >10 times upper limit of normal	
	Proportion	16% of non-seminomas	
	5-year PFS	41%	
	5-year survival	48%	

prognostic groups. Patients with a good prognosis may be considered for less intensive treatment regimens, while those in poor-risk groups may benefit from intensive therapy and should be entered into trials designed to test the utility of such schedules.

Serum markers

Increased levels of tumour markers are detected in the blood of many patients with GCTs and are vital for tumour diagnosis. They are also used to define the prognostic group into which a patient falls (which has implications for therapy), in the assessment of therapeutic response, on follow-up to confirm remission, and to follow patients who are on a surveillance programme following orchidectomy. Markers are measured pre- and post-orchidectomy and then weekly during treatment. AFP is an oncofetal antigen produced from foetal liver, yolk sac, and gastrointestinal tract, and it has a half life of 5–7 days. Increased AFP is found in 50–60% of malignant teratomas, levels are not elevated in pure seminomas. HCG is a glycopeptide secreted by the

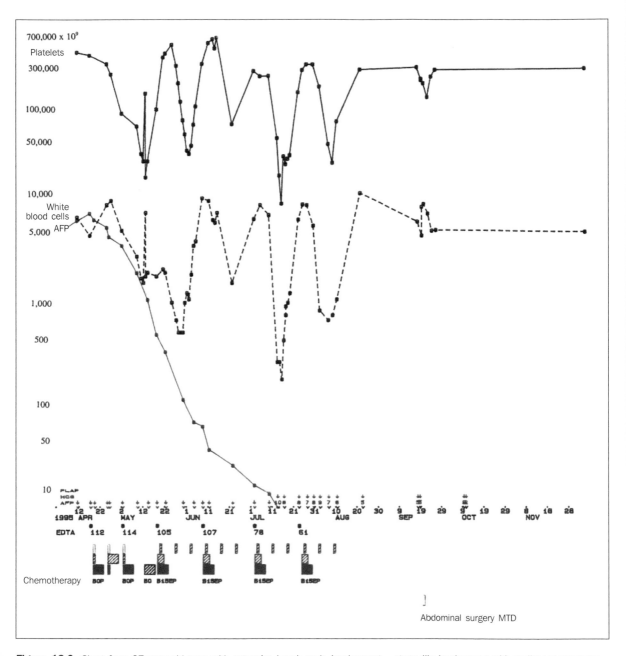

Figure 18.2. Chart from 27 year old man with extensive lymph node involvement – stage IIIc involvement with malignant teratoma intermediate. AFP level was markedly elevated before intensive weekly chemotherapy, but fell with the expected half-time of 5–7 days. After chemotherapy markers normalized but a residual abdominal mass was resected, which contained differentiated teratoma. The patient remains well 5 years after treatment.

placenta in pregnancy and the trophoblastic elements in testicular cancers. Its half-life is 24–36 hours. HCG levels are elevated in 10–25% patients with seminoma and 30–35% patients with malignant teratoma. The fall in serum markers in response to therapy is demonstrated in *Figure 18.2.*

Key points: testis

Scrotal swellings are seen relatively commonly in general practice

Solid swellings that affect the body of the testis have a high probability (>50%) of being caused by cancer, especially in men 15–55 years of age

Indeterminate swellings of the testicle have a low probability of being caused by cancer, especially in men over 55 years of age (1–4%)

Reproduced from England Department of Health Cancer Referral Guidelines Consultation Document May 2000.

Referral proforma: urology cancer

Age:

Suspected cancer:

Prostate	☐	Kidney	☐
Bladder	☐	Testis	☐

Other...

Symptoms:	Yes	No	
Macroscopic haematuria			
Loin pain			
Testicular swelling			
Bone pain			
Lower urinary tract symptoms			
(e.g., hesitancy, poor stream, etc.)			

Other, please state...............................

Clinical examination:	Yes	No	
Renal mass			
Pyrexia			
Swelling in the body of the testis			
Prostate feels malignant on rectal examination			

Other, please state....................................

Investigations:	Yes	No	
Prostate-specific antigen..................ng/ml			
Haemoglobin.................................g/dl			
Microscopic haematuria			
Mass detected on imaging			

Comments/other reasons for urgent referral

Reproduced from England Department of Health Cancer Referral Guidelines Consultation Document May 2000.

Key points

- Germ cell tumours occur most frequently in 20–40-year-olds and are increasing in incidence
- Intratubular germ cell neoplasia is a premalignant lesion associated with a 50% risk of tumour development within 5 years.
- Testicular tumours are more common in patients with a history of testicular maldescent.
- Serum alpha-fetoprotein and human chorionic gonadotrophin are helpful to diagnosis because either one or both are abnormal in 75% cases of malignant teratoma.
- Serum tumour markers are vital to diagnosis, assessment of prognosis, monitoring response to therapy, and on follow-up to confirm remission.
- Survival is related to stage at presentation, and therefore early diagnosis is vital; 95% patients are cured.

Management

Teratoma

The advent of effective cisplatin-based chemotherapy in the late 1970s dramatically changed treatment options for these patients.

Stage I

Stage I is defined by the absence of disease outside the testicle and the fall of serum markers to normal following orchidectomy. In the UK, a surveillance policy or entry of patients into trials that test adjuvant chemotherapy is the universal approach. A surveillance policy, if adopted, must be followed rigorously to ensure that relapse is detected at the earliest opportunity. At presentation 25–30% of cases have occult disease and will relapse, but the prompt initiation of chemotherapy should cure more than 90% of such patients to give an overall cure rate of 98%. Analysis of the pathological features of the primary tumour have identified vascular invasion as the most important prognostic factor. In these cases the risk of relapse is 50% and adjuvant chemotherapy may be considered.

Metastatic teratoma

Testicular teratoma is highly chemosensitive and modern chemotherapy regimes have resulted in a 80–90% cure rate. Standard therapy consists of bleomycin, etoposide, and cisplatin (BEP), which is given in three or four courses depending on the scheduling of the regime. Following chemotherapy, residual masses require careful evaluation and usually surgical resection. In view of the toxicity of treatment, notably the significant emetic effects, the renal and ototoxicity of cisplatin, and the potential life-threatening lung toxicity of bleomycin, dose modifications and drug substitutions have been investigated in patients with good prognosis. In the poor prognostic group and in relapsed patients, intensive regimens are being investigated, some with high-dose therapy and peripheral stem-cell rescue. Among patients with poor prognosis, cure can still be achieved in 60%. Following relapse, 20–25% patients become disease-free after salvage treatment. The choice of chemotherapy and management of side effects is best undertaken in specialized units and it is not surprising that experienced centres that see relatively large numbers of patients have better treatment results.

Seminoma
Stage I

Approximately two-thirds of cases fall into this group, with a 15% risk of subclinical abdominal nodal metastasis on presentation. The predictable pattern of spread and extreme radiosensitivity of the tumour has resulted in a policy of adjuvant nodal irradiation of abdominopelvic lymph nodes. This policy achieved cure rates of 98%, but the potential risk of secondary malignancy and chronic gastrointestinal disturbance led to studies aimed at reducing field size and dose, or at using patient surveillance.

The latter is more difficult than in teratoma in view of the lower incidence of marker positivity, difficulty in defining active disease on CT in some cases, and late relapses. Surveillance for these patients involves frequent radiological imaging with attendant radiation exposure, and thus this practice continues to be assessed in clinical studies. The policy that has resulted from recent Medical Research Council studies is that of para-aortic strip irradiation to a standard dose of 20Gy in 10 fractions, with suitable patients being entered into ongoing studies of chemotherapy.

Metastatic seminoma

Patients with stage II nodal metastases that can safely be encompassed by a radiation field are treated with radiotherapy. In practice, this usually means that masses <5 cm are irradiated and those >5 cm are treated with chemotherapy as for stages III and IV disease. The combination chemotherapy schedules used are the same as those used in teratoma; cisplatin-based combinations achieve long-term survival rates of 90%. Residual masses following chemotherapy are usually kept under surveillance as resection is hazardous because of their high fibrous tissue content and proximity to blood vessels. Sometimes consolidation radiotherapy may be required if signs of activity remain.

Fertility and psychological aspects of the disease

GCTs often occur at the start of the patient's family and professional life, at a time when good health is often taken for granted. In addition to the toxicity of treatment, considerable psychological stress may arise from lack of confidence regarding the patient's health and, occasionally, a change in personal and professional relationships. In some patients psychological help may be required.

Another important issue is that of fertility. About 25% of men with GCTs have impaired fertility at diagnosis, which may be further affected by their treatment. However, with modern radiotherapy techniques long-term fertility should not be impaired and although chemotherapy regimes reduce sperm counts initially, these usually recover to normal within 2–3 years. The teratogenic risk is of concern, but studies of children born to men previously treated for this disease have not revealed evidence of developmental abnormalities. In view of these uncertainties sperm banking is offered to all patients.

Conclusion

GCTs have an importance in oncology that far outweighs their incidence; they provide a model of curable cancer in which the use of tumour markers, aggressive combination chemotherapy, and combined modality treatment can be investigated. The high cure rates also permit evaluation of the long-term sequelae of both the diagnosis of life-threatening disease and its treatment.

Management, key points

- In stage I teratoma, prospective studies have shown close surveillance to be as safe as adjuvant treatment, without the toxic effects. Relapse occurs in approximately 50% of cases with pathological lymphovascular invasion and chemotherapy may be offered in these cases.
- Metastatic non-seminoma is treated with combination chemotherapy; approximately one-third of patients subsequently require surgical excision of residual masses.
- Prognosis following chemotherapy is related to stage. Of patients with small-volume disease 95% are cured, but large-volume disease with poor prognostic features has survival probabilities of 50–70%.
- Seminoma is extremely radiosensitive and radiotherapy to para-aortic nodes is indicated in stage I and small-volume stage II disease.
- Advanced stages of seminoma are very sensitive to platinum-based chemotherapy regimes and cure rates are very high.

Further Reading

Clinical Oncology Information Network (COIN). Guidelines on the management of adult testicular germ cell tumours. *Clin Oncol.* 2000; **12(suppl)**: S173–210.

Dearnaley DP, Huddart RA, Horwich A. Managing testicular cancer. Clinical review. *BMJ.* 2001; **322**: 1583–8.

International Germ Cell Cancer Collaborative Group. International germ cell consensus classification: a prognostic factor-based staging system for metastatic germ cell cancers. *J Clin Oncol.* 1997; **15**: 594–603.

Sandberg AA, Meloni AM, Suijkerbuijk RF. Review of chromosome studies in urological tumours: III. Cytogenetics and genes in testicular tumors. *J Urol.* 1996; **155**: 1531–56.

Appendix

Guidelines for urgent referral: urological cancers

Macroscopic haematuria in adults

Microscopic haematuria in adults over 50 years

Swellings in the body of the testis

Palpable renal masses

Solid renal masses found on imaging

Elevated age-specific prostate specific antigen (PSA) in men with a 10 year life expectancy

A high PSA (>20 ng/ml) in men with a clinically malignant prostate or bone pain

Any suspected penile cancer

Reproduced from National Institute for Clinical Excellence. *Guidelines on Cancer Services. Improving Outcomes in Urological Cancers*, London: NICE, 2002.

19 Cancer of the Endometrium, Cervix, Vulva, and Vagina

Khalil Razvi and Peter Blake

Endometrial Cancer

Incidence
Endometrial cancer is the fifth most common cancer in women in England and Wales, with an estimated incidence of 13.8 per 100,000 women in 1997. It has a preponderance towards the white populations in western Europe and North America, while the incidence is much lower in Asian women. It is a disease that predominates in post-menopausal women, with 92% of cases in women over 50 years of age. The overall mortality rate of 30% at 5 years reflects the tendency for this tumour to be diagnosed early. Various statistics relating to endometrial cancer are shown in *Figure 19.1*.

Pathology
Invasive cancers
Approximately 60% are adenocarcinomas, while a further 20% are adenoacanthomas (adenocarcinomas with a benign squamous component) and 10% are adenosquamous carcinomas (in which the squamous component is also malignant). The other subtypes are rare and include clear-cell carcinoma, papillary serous carcinoma, squamous cell carcinoma, and metastatic carcinoma.

Endometrial hyperplasia
Although not a malignancy, endometrial hyperplasia is associated with an increased predisposition to endometrial cancer. It can be divided into simple or complex without atypia and simple or complex with atypia. The risk of progression to malignancy in a simple hyperplasia without atypia is only 1%,

but it approaches 30% for complex hyperplasia with atypia (*Table 19.1*).

Aetiology
Unopposed oestrogenic stimulation of the endometrium forms the basic aetiology of many of the risk factors for this disease (*Table 19.2*). It is also commonly found in association with diabetes mellitus and hypertension, which probably reflects the common predisposing factor of obesity in all of these clinical states. Obese women have higher blood oestrogen concentrations because of peripheral conversion of androgens into oestrogens in fat tissue. There is also a familial association in the Lynch type II syndrome, in which it is associated with colorectal and ovarian cancer in some families.

Clinical features
The cardinal symptom is that of post-menopausal bleeding. Although there are many causes of post-menopausal bleeding, up to 20% of such women ultimately have a genital tract malignancy. It can also manifest with other abnormal vaginal bleeding, including intermenstrual bleeding, post-coital bleeding, and menorrhagia. Women on hormone replacement therapy (HRT) with breakthrough bleeding for which no obvious cause is found should also be investigated.

In the perimenopausal period, abnormal uterine bleeding is usually ascribed to menopausal changes and may not be investigated. This is reasonable if the menstrual periods become progressively lighter and further apart, but any other pattern should be evaluated. Most young patients who

Table 19.1. *Endometrial hyperplasia: classification and risk of progression and/or regression*

Histological diagnosis	Cytological atypia	Regression (%)	Persistent (%)	Progressed to carcinoma
Simple	Absent	80	19	1
Complex	Absent	80	17	3
Simple atypical	Present	9	23	8
Complex atypical	Present	57	14	29

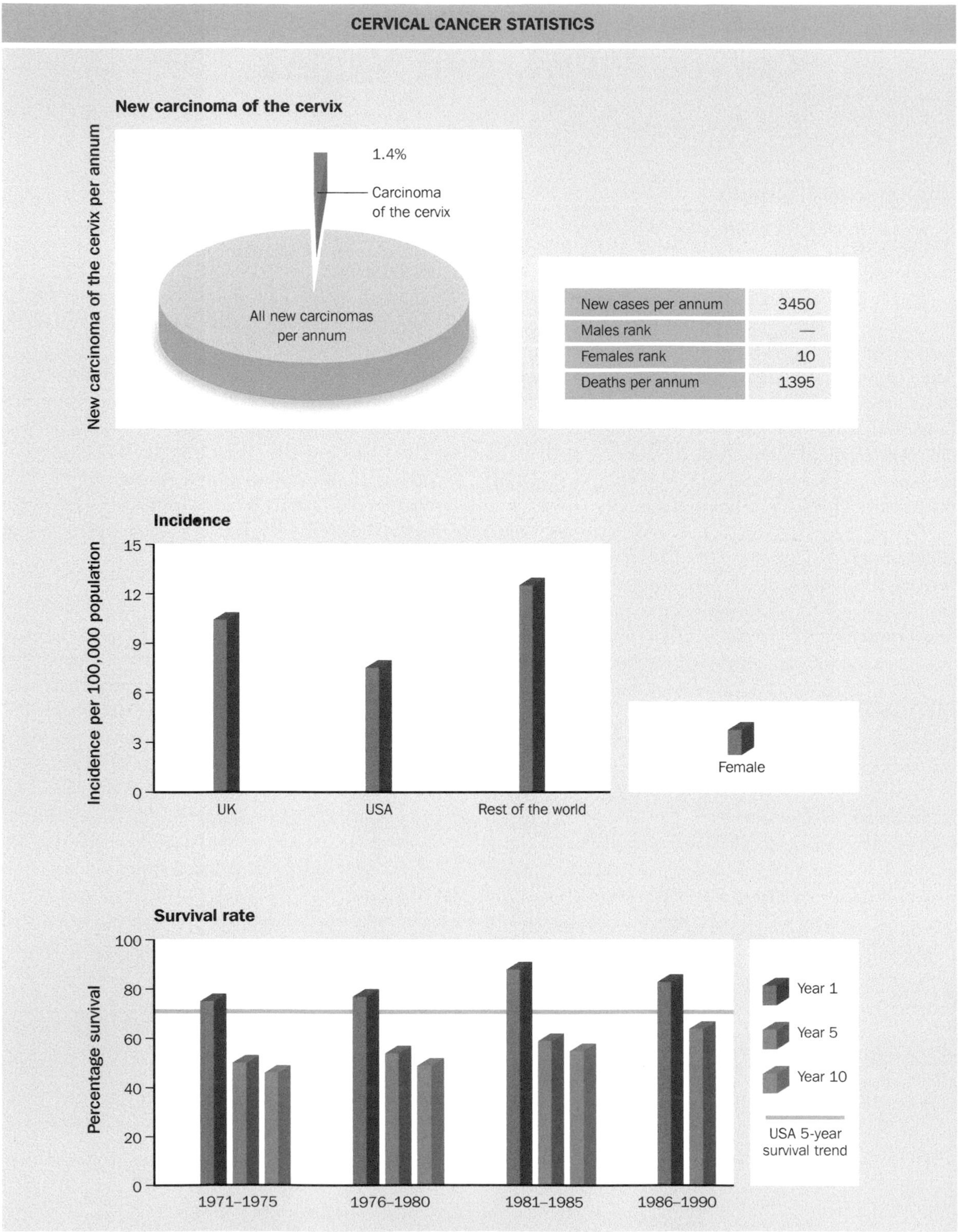

CERVICAL CANCER STATISTICS

New carcinoma of the cervix

New carcinoma of the cervix per annum

1.4%

Carcinoma
of the cervix

All new carcinomas
per annum

New cases per annum	3450
Males rank	—
Females rank	10
Deaths per annum	1395

Incidence

Incidence per 100,000 population

UK USA Rest of the world

Female

Survival rate

Percentage survival

1971–1975 1976–1980 1981–1985 1986–1990

Year 1

Year 5

Year 10

USA 5-year
survival trend

Figure 19.1. Statistical data relating to cervical cancer.

Table 19.2. *Risk factors for endometrial cancer*

Early menarche (<12 years of age)

Late menopause (after 52 years of age)

Nulliparity

Obesity

Chronic anovulation (e.g. polycystic ovarian disease)

Granulosa – theca cell tumour of the ovary

Tamoxifen therapy

Lynch type II syndrome

develop endometrial cancer are obese and are often associated with anovulatory menstrual cycles (and, hence, polycystic ovarian disease and infertility). Occasionally, a woman may present with vaginal discharge which may be due to an associated pyometra.

Screening is currently not cost-effective for the detection of either hyperplasia or cancer of the endometrium, and clinical examination may often be unremarkable except for the evidence of bleeding and uterine enlargement. Therefore, it is important that appropriate referral of symptomatic patients is made so that the benefit of early presentation of this disease is not lost.

Guidelines for urgent referral

- Visible tumour on the cervix on speculum examination.
- Visible tumour on the vulva.
- Palpable pelvic mass or suspicious mass on pelvic ultrasound.
- More than one episode or a single heavy episode of post-menopausal bleeding.
- Post-coital bleeding that persists for more than 4 weeks.

Investigations
General practice
It is important that a thorough history and physical examination, including pelvic examination, be carried out. Patients with abnormal bleeding because of poor compliance on the contraceptive pill or HRT can be excluded easily. A cervical smear is taken if indicated; about one-third to half of the patients have a positive smear because of shedding of abnormal endometrial cells. However, a negative smear does not rule out endometrial cancer. A full blood count is performed if the bleeding is significant.

Hospital
A transvaginal ultrasound scan is a useful initial investigation, as it is simple and allows measurement of endometrial thickness as well as visualization of the ovaries. A meta-analysis of 35 studies found that transvaginal ultrasound scanning is accurate and that women with post-menopausal bleeding, who are not on HRT, have an incidence of 10% endometrial cancer with an abnormal scan, but only 1% if the scan is normal. An endometrial thickness of more than 5 mm in the post-menopause and more than 15 mm in the pre-menopause is abnormal.

The most important test for assessment is that of an endometrial biopsy. Traditionally, this would entail a formal dilatation and curettage (D and C) under anaesthesia, but it is now possible to perform an outpatient endometrial biopsy with an accuracy approaching 90%. However, if the ultrasound suggests a thickened endometrium or if insufficient material is obtained on outpatient biopsy, then a hysteroscopy with D and C is carried out. This has the advantage of visualizing any abnormal areas in the uterine cavity and assessing the endocervical canal. It can be performed as a day case, avoiding hospitalization.

If cancer is diagnosed, the optimum treatment is dependent on the stage and grade of the disease and the nodal status. Blood investigations include renal and liver function tests with a full blood count. A chest radiograph is obtained and further assessment of the tumour using magnetic resonance imaging (MRI) allows pre-operative estimation of the depth of myometrial invasion and nodal status, although a transvaginal ultrasound is also quite accurate in estimating the depth of myometrial involvement. Computed tomography (CT) scanning is less accurate in determining myometrial invasion. An audit performed in southern England examining clinical management and outcome revealed that only about one-third of women received proper staging investigations and treatment according to local guidelines, and those who were not treated appropriately had a significant reduction in survival.

Staging and 5-year survival
The staging of endometrial cancer is performed according to the Fédération Internationale de Gynécologie et d'Obstétrique (FIGO) classification (*Table 19.3*). This requires a surgicopathological staging, although in many cases a lymphadenectomy is not performed and nodes cannot be assessed. The tumour is graded histologically into grade

Table 19.3. *Stage and survival in endometrial cancer (modified FIGO staging)*

Stage		Percentage of total	5-year survival
I	Tumour confined to the uterus	75	72
Ia	Tumour confined to the endometrium		
Ib	Myometrial invasion <50%		
Ic	Myometrial invasion >50%		
II	Involvement of cervix	11	56
IIa	Endocervical gland involvement only		
IIb	Cervical stromal invasion		
III		11	31.5
IIIa	Tumour invades uterine serosa or adnexae or positive ascites and/or peritoneal washings		
IIIb	Vaginal involvement		
IIIc	Para-aortic or pelvic lymph node metastases		
IV		3	10.5
IVa	Carcinoma involving mucosa of the bladder or rectum		
IVb	Distant metastases including intra-abdominal and/or inguinal lymph nodes		

1 (well differentiated), grade 2 (moderately differentiated), and grade 3 (poorly differentiated). In addition, the depth of myometrial invasion is measured. There are other prognostic factors identified in endometrial cancer, but stage of disease, depth of myometrial invasion, and tumour grade correlate well with nodal metastasis and survival (*Table 19.4*).

Treatment
Surgery
Around 90% of women with endometrial cancer are treated with primary surgery. This is a total abdominal hysterectomy with bilateral salpingo-oophorectomy (TAHBSO). Pelvic and para-aortic lymphadenectomy are not routinely performed in the UK (although FIGO staging requires these nodes to be assessed). This is partly because a significant proportion of the surgery is undertaken by the general gynaecologist and the patient's medical condition sometimes precludes extensive surgery. Also, whether lymphadenectomy improves survival is still unclear and is the subject of current trials. Certainly, it has been shown that 10% of apparent stage I disease and 20% of stage II disease have positive lymph nodes at lymphadenectomy (thus making them stage IIIc). If cervical involvement is diagnosed pre-operatively, then a radical hysterectomy (or radiotherapy) is performed, as in cancer of the cervix. Patients diagnosed as having stage III and IV disease at the initial assessment are usually referred

Table 19.4. *Prognostic factors associated with adverse outcomes in endometrial cancer*

Stage of disease
Tumour grade
Myometrial involvement
Older age and obesity
Lymph node and lymphovascular space involvement
Histological subtype (e.g. clear cell, squamous, papillary serous types)
Positive peritoneal cytology
Negative steroid-receptor status
Tumour aneuploidy

for radiotherapy, although palliative surgery is sometime carried out.

Radiotherapy
Radiotherapy can prolong survival in women with advanced or recurrent disease, or when surgery is not appropriate. It can be given as an adjuvant to surgery, and historical data suggest that it reduces the rate of pelvic and vault recurrence in high-risk stage I and in stage II disease, for which algorithms have been devised (*Table 19.5*). Currently clinical trials are under way to assess the efficacy and side-effects of adjuvant radiotherapy in high-risk stage I disease after surgery, as the combi-

Table 19.5. *An example of an algorithm for the use of adjuvant radiotherapy to the pelvis[a] and vaginal vault[b] post-operatively in early stage disease*

Tumour grade	FIGO Ia	FIGO Ib	FIGO Ic
1	No adjuvant radiotherapy	No adjuvant radiotherapy	Pelvic and vault radiotherapy
2	Vault radiotherapy alone	Vault radiotherapy alone	Pelvic and vault radiotherapy
3	Pelvic and vault radiotherapy	Pelvic and vault radiotherapy	Pelvic and vault radiotherapy

[a]Pelvic radiotherapy is usually delivered in 20–25 fractions over 4–5 weeks on a daily basis using a linear accelerator.
[b]Vault radiotherapy is usually delivered as brachytherapy using a remote afterloading system.

nation of radiotherapy and surgery increases the morbidity to the patient over that of surgery alone.

Radical radiotherapy (up to a dose of 80Gy to the endometrium) is sometimes employed in the patient who has early stage endometrial cancer and who is medically unfit for surgery. This is usually by a combination of external and intracavitary radiotherapy. Palliative radiotherapy is mainly aimed at advanced endometrial cancer that is not amenable to surgery or for metastatic and recurrent disease. It is quite useful for the control of vaginal bleeding and bone pain.

Chemotherapy and hormonal therapy

At present there is no definite evidence of the efficacy of chemotherapy or hormonal therapy in the treatment of endometrial cancer. Progestogens are most frequently prescribed, especially in treating recurrent disease, although a meta-analysis of six randomized controlled trials that compared progestogens with no hormone treatment showed no significant reduction in death rates. Similarly, there is no strong evidence for the use of tamoxifen or gonadotrophin-releasing hormone analogues.

The use of chemotherapy is limited to fit patients with systemic disease. Response rates to combination chemotherapy of 20–35% have been reported, but the response is usually partial and of short duration. The drugs commonly used are the platinum compounds, doxorubicin, and epirubicin.

Conclusion

Carcinoma of the endometrium predominates in postmenopausal women. As bleeding is an early symptom, the vast majority are diagnosed as stage I and II. The primary treatment is TAHBSO, which is usually followed with radiotherapy to the pelvis and/or the vaginal vault in patients who are considered to be at increased risk of recurrence. There is at present an increasing interest in the role of lymphadenectomy, which may obviate the need for post-oper-

ative radiotherapy. Chemotherapy has a limited role and is sometimes used in systemic disease. The use of hormonal agents, although common, remains to be proved effective. Follow-up in the first 2 years is every 3–4 months (as the highest risk of recurrence is at this time) and then usually every 6 months for 5 years.

Cancer of the Cervix

Incidence

With the National Cervical Screening Programme, the rate of cervical cancer in the UK dropped from 15.4 to 8.9 cases per 100,000 population between 1990 and 1996. It is now the ninth most common cancer among females, with a lifetime risk of 1 in 126. While the incidence of invasive cancer is falling, it is associated with a concomitant rise in screening-detected preinvasive lesions [cervical intraepithelial neoplasia (CIN)]. The disease predominates in women over 45 years of age, with a peak incidence in the age group 45–50 years. There has recently also been an increase of cases in women aged between 25 and 34 years. Various statistics relating to cancer of the cervix are shown in *Figure 19.2*.

Pathology

The majority of cases (85%) are squamous cell carcinomas, while the most common of the remainder are adenocarcinoma and adenosquamous carcinoma (*Table 19.6*). Precursor lesions are well established for squamous cancers (CIN), but less so for adenocarcinomas [cervical glandular intraepithelial neoplasia (CGIN)].

Cervical intraepithelial neoplasia

The transformation zone of the cervix denotes the area in which the endocervical columnar epithelium undergoes metaplasia into squamous epithelium; this zone is usually

CANCER OF THE UTERINE BODY STATISTICS

New cancer of the uterus body

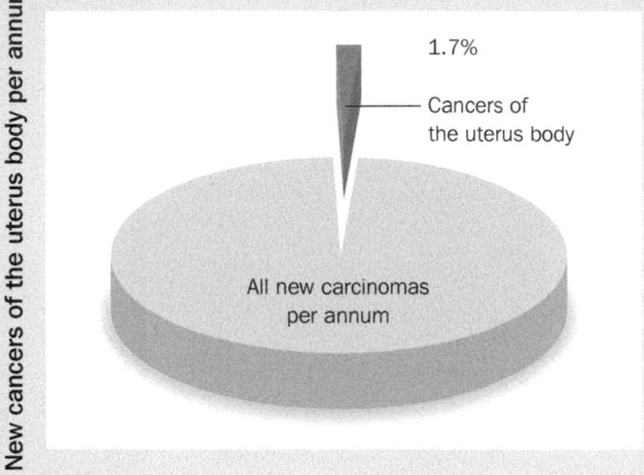

New cases per annum	4090
Males rank	—
Females rank	5
Deaths per annum	871

Incidence

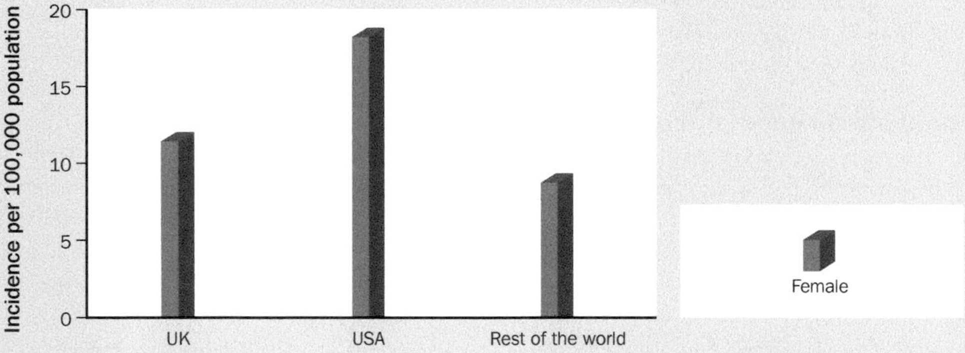

Survival rate

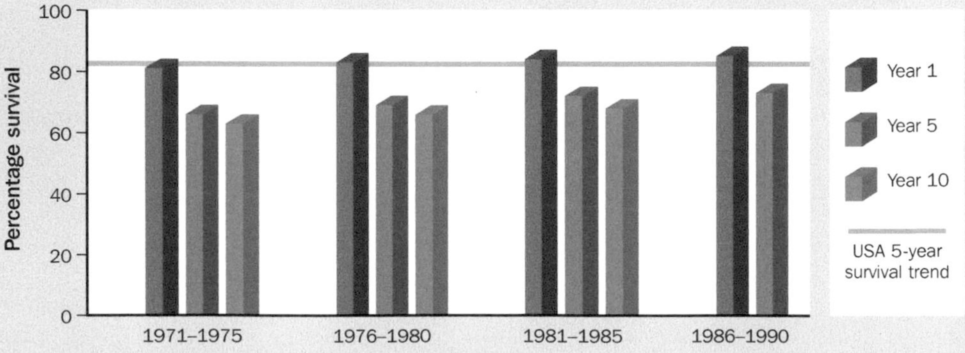

Figure 19.2. *Statistical data relating to cancer of the uterine body.*

Table 19.6. Pathology of cervical cancer

Histological type	Frequency (%)
Squamous cell carcinoma large cell non-keratinizing large cell keratinizing small cell	80–90
Adenocarcinoma endocervical endometrioid clear cell adenosquamous adenoid cystic	10–15
Rare tumours adenosarcoma leiomyosarcoma malignant melanoma metastatic tumours	<5

situated just inside the endocervical canal. At puberty and in pregnancy, the columnar epithelium of the cervix comes out onto the ectocervix as a result of the influence of oestrogens. As it becomes exposed to the vaginal milieu, it undergoes metaplasia to produce a larger transformation zone than is normally the case. Occasionally, this process becomes disrupted and dysplastic transformation occurs, which is precancerous. CIN refers to this dysplastic change in squamous cells and is graded according to severity. Cells from the transformation zone can be obtained at cervical smear and assessed using the Papanicolaou (Pap) stain. It is postulated that the exposure of the cervix to certain agents, such as the human papilloma virus (HPV), results in an increased risk of developing CIN or of CIN progressing to higher grades or invasive disease.

The natural history of CIN shows that the development of invasive cancer is a slow process, which may take up to 20 years to develop. In patients with CIN I, about one-third regress back to normal and careful follow-up is all that is necessary. With CIN II and CIN III, the risk of progression to malignancy is higher and treatment is necessary. Studies have shown that for inpatients with CIN III, 30–70% will develop invasive carcinoma over a period of 10–12 years, but in 10% this occurs within a year. Treatment is either ablative or excisional. Ablative therapies include cryosurgery and laser ablation of the cervix. Excisional treatments include knife conization, laser conization, and the now popular large-loop excision of the transformation zone, which can be an outpatient procedure. One advantage of excisional treatments is that histological verification is obtained and may be crucial if occult invasive cancer is not to be missed.

Cervical glandular intraepithelial neoplasia

The precursor of adenocarcinoma of the cervix is CGIN, which may only occasionally reveal itself on a cervical smear showing abnormal glandular cells. Unlike CIN, in which the basement membrane between the epithelium and the stroma is clearly defined, allowing accurate grading, the basement membrane around intracervical glands is harder to define and grading is not possible. In addition, the natural history of progression of this lesion is not so well established. Also, it is not possible to assess this lesion adequately with colposcopy, as it is usually in the endocervical canal. The only reliable way to assess this further is via a cone biopsy. As abnormal glandular cells can also arise further up the gynaecological tract (e.g. in the endometrium, fallopian tube, and ovary), it is important to obtain an endometrial biopsy and to assess the adnexae for any abnormalities.

Squamous cell carcinoma

Microinvasive cancer

Microinvasive cancer refers to invasion that is not visible to the naked eye, but microscopically has a depth of invasion up to 5mm and a width of no more than 7mm. In the FIGO classification, it is further subdivided into Ia1 (depth <3mm) and Ia2 (depth <5mm), with the maximum width remaining the same. This subdivision has come about more recently because Ia1 disease has a negligible risk of nodal disease compared with Ia2, in which the risk approaches 10%.

Invasive cancer

These tumours are usually easily visible on the ectocervix with speculum examination, may be exophytic or endophytic in type, and may infiltrate the surrounding areas, including the vagina and the parametrium. They are divided into three grades of differentiation, from well differentiated (GI) to poorly differentiated (G3). The majority of squamous tumours are of the large cell type (well and moderately differentiated), while the small cell type (poorly differentiated) includes variants with a very poor prognosis, such as neuroendocrine tumours, and a high propensity to undergo bloodborne spread.

Adenocarcinoma

Although previously reported as an uncommon type of cervical cancer, accounting for about 5% of cases, over the past

Table 19.7. Aetiology of cervical cancer

Sexual behaviours	Early onset of sexual intercourse
	Multiple sexual partners
Viral infections	Human papilloma virus (subtypes
	16, 18, 31, 33)
	Human immunodeficiency virus
	?Herpes simplex virus 2 infection
Oral contraceptive pill	?Due to regular screening
Smoking	
Immunosuppression	Renal transplant
	Systemic lupus erythematosus

Table 19.8. Causes of an abnormal Papanicolaou smear

Cervical cancer
Cervical intraepithelial neoplasia
Other genital tract cancer (e.g. vaginal, vulval, endometrium,
    fallopian tube, ovary)
Atrophic changes
Infection (e.g. cervicitis, trichomoniasis)
Previous radiation treatment
Regeneration from injury

few years the incidence has increased to about 15%. These tumours arise from the glandular epithelium of the endocervical canal and glands. The preinvasive lesion is difficult to identify because many of the glands and crypts lie deep within the cervical stroma and may give a false histological impression of invasive disease. Adenocarcinomas and adenosquamous carcinomas are considered to have a worse prognosis than squamous cancers, although this may result from the greater tumour bulk, stage for stage.

Aetiology

A number of aetiological factors have been identified, as shown in *Table 19.7*. It has been shown that earlier onset of sexual activity in the teens is associated with a higher incidence of both CIN and invasive cancer. This implies that the adolescent cervix, in which the transformation zone is large, is prone to oncogenic agents. The relationship between HPV, CIN, and cervical cancer has been well studied. Between 90–100% of invasive squamous cancers have an underlying HPV 16 infection, while HPV 18 is associated with adenocarcinoma of the cervix. Although the type 2 herpes simplex virus (HSV) was previously implicated, its role is more likely secondary, as a co-factor. The evidence linking oral contraceptive usage with cervical cancer is more tenuous, but it may be that such women are probably more frequently screened and hence have better detection rates.

It is now accepted that a woman with human immunodeficiency virus (HIV) infection who develops carcinoma of the cervix has clinical acquired immunodeficiency syndrome (AIDS). Women on long-term immunosuppressive therapy (e.g. because of renal transplant or systemic lupus erythematosus) are more prone to develop CIN and, hence, cervical cancer. Smoking is also thought to have an immunosuppressive effect on the cervix, as well as a direct tumourogenic effect on the cervical epithelium.

Screening

Cervical screening is now well established in the UK, after large-scale screening programmes in Iceland, Finland, and British Columbia showed a significant reduction in the overall incidence and mortality from cancer of the cervix. In Iceland between 1986 and 1995, screening resulted in a 76% reduction in mortality and a 67% reduction of incidence of cervical cancer. The rates for adenocarcinoma and adenosquamous carcinomas are, however, unaffected by screening. Women between the ages of 20 and 60 years are offered screening every 3–5 years on the National Health Service cervical screening programme. However, only 83% availed themselves of it between 1992 and 1994. Despite this, in England and Wales there has been a 42% drop in new cases between 1990 and 1996. It must be remembered that the Pap smear is a screening tool and that most abnormal smears are not the result of cancer (*Table 19.8*).

Clinical features

Cancer of the cervix usually presents with abnormal vaginal bleeding (post-coital, intermenstrual, or post-menopausal) or an offensive vaginal discharge, pelvic pain, or leg pain (indicative of nerve involvement and advanced disease). Occasionally, an early lesion may present with an abnormal PAP smear (*Table 19.9*).

The main clinical finding is an obvious growth or ulceration on the surface of the cervix or an enlarged cervix (when the lesion is in the endocervical canal). Tumour may have extended into the vagina, and parametrial involvement may be apparent on rectal examination. Evidence of nodal spread,

Table 19.9. *Symptoms and signs of cervical cancer*

Symptoms	Signs
Abnormal vaginal bleeding (post-coital, intermenstrua, lpost-menopausal)	Cervical tumour (extension into parametrium, uterosacral
Vaginal discharge	ligaments, extension onto vagina)
Pain (pelvic, backache, referred leg pain (nerve involved)	Nodal disease (supraclavicular nodes, inguinal nodes,
Bladder symptoms (advanced disease), haematuria, frequency	pelvic side wall nodes on rectal examination)
Rectal symptoms (advanced disease), tenesmus, rectal bleeding	Lymphoedema of the leg
Asymptomatic – abnormal Papanicolaou smear	Obstructive uropathy (uraemia, palpable kidneys)

lymphoedema, obstructive uropathy, and deep vein thrombosis may be apparent.

Colposcopy

Colposcopy is the examination of the cervix using a low-power binocular microscope and is a diagnostic tool used in women with an abnormal cervical smear. Using acetic acid and iodine to stain the cervix and upper vagina, abnormal areas indicative of CIN or even cancer can be detected and biopsies can be taken. This allows accurate diagnosis and management of preinvasive and early invasive lesions that are not visible to the naked eye.

Guidelines for urgent referral

- Visible tumour on cervix with speculum examination.
- Visible tumour on the vulva.
- Palpable pelvic mass or suspicious mass on pelvic ultrasound.
- More than one episode or a single heavy episode of post-menopausal bleeding.
- Post-coital bleeding that persists for more than 4 weeks.

Investigations
General practice

A pelvic examination is an important initial assessment in any woman with symptoms in the gynaecological tract and the cervix should be inspected and a smear taken if necessary. Women with an obvious tumour should be urgently referred to the nearest cancer centre. Those with normal findings but an abnormal Pap smear, indicative of premalignancy or cancer, should be referred for a colposcopic evaluation.

Hospital

The most important investigation is an examination under anaesthesia (EUA), which should ideally be performed jointly by the gynaecologist and the clinical oncologist (radiotherapist). This allows the disease to be staged and the appropriate treatment chosen. EUA entails a detailed abdominal and pelvic examination plus cystoscopy and sigmoidoscopy to rule out local spread of disease. Biopsies of the tumour can also be taken if a histological diagnosis has not been made. Endocervical and endometrial biopsies can also be taken as necessary. Patients with occult lesions should have colposcopically directed biopsies of suspicious areas or a cone biopsy for diagnosis.

Other investigations include an intravenous urogram (IVU) to look for evidence of ureteric obstruction (which indicates Stage IIb disease). A CT scan or MRI of the abdomen and pelvis is also commonly performed to assess the liver, nodal status, and evidence of local spread. Meta-analytical studies do not show any difference between CT scans and MRI in terms of accuracy of lymph-node evaluation, but MRI seems better at evaluating early disease, whereas CT is better for late disease. A chest radiograph is also obtained to look for lung metastases.

Staging and survival

Staging of cervical cancer is based on the system devised by FIGO (1997) (*Table 19.10*). This is a clinical staging system (except for Stage Ia, which requires histology) based on the findings at EUA plus results of the IVU and chest radiography, although further imaging is usually performed in the UK as described above. As the FIGO staging is a basic clinical system the results of imaging investigations and measurements must be stated separately. In patients with early Stage I disease and negative nodes, the 5-year survival is over 90%. More advanced stages have worse prognoses and it is unusual for Stage IV disease to be cured.

Table 19.10. FIGO staging and 5-year survival of carcinoma of the cervix

Stage	Features	5-year survival (%)
0	Preinvasive (cervical intraepithelial neoplasia III)	
I	Invasive cancer confined to the cervix	76
Ia	Invasive cancer identified only microscopically and not wider than 7mm in diameter	
Ia1	Stromal invasion up to 3mm in depth	
Ia2	Stromal invasion greater than 3mm and up to 5mm in depth	
Ib	Lesions greater than Ia2, whether seen clinically or not	
Ib1	Lesions up to 4cm in size	
Ib2	Lesions greater than 4cm in size	
II	Extension into the vagina, but not the lower third, or infiltration of the parametria, but not to the side wall	55
IIa	Involvement of the upper two-thirds of vagina	
IIb	Infiltration of the parametria, but not to the side wall	
III	Extension of the cancer to the pelvic side wall or lower third of the vagina	30
IIIa	Involvement of the lower third of the vagina, but not the pelvic side wall	
IIIB	Extension to the pelvic side wall, hydronephrosis, or non-functioning kidney	
IV	Extension outside the reproductive tract	7
IVa	Involvement of the mucosa of the bladder or rectum	
IVb	Distant metastasis or disease outside the true pelvis	

Treatment
Surgery

The definitive treatment for cervical cancer is either surgery or radiotherapy. The standard surgical treatment for invasive cervical cancer is a radical hysterectomy and pelvic lymphadenectomy. This entails the removal of the uterus, upper vagina, and parametria with the pelvic lymph nodes. The ovaries can be conserved in pre-menopausal women. Surgery is applicable in patients with up to Stage IIa disease and is inappropriate when the tumour has spread into the parametrium (Stage IIb and above).

Women who have early Stage Ia1 disease can be cured by a cone biopsy if they wish to retain their fertility, or by a simple hysterectomy otherwise. A radical trachelectomy (removal of the cervix with the parametrium) with pelvic lymphadenectomy is a surgical technique that is sometimes offered to young women with early stage disease (usually Ia2 and Ib1) and who strongly wish to retain their uterus for fertility.

The advantages of surgery compared with radiotherapy are that the vagina remains pliable and ovarian function can be preserved. The small risk of a second malignancy with radiotherapy is also avoided and surgical findings can give valuable information that can guide further management.

Radiotherapy

Radiotherapy can be used as primary treatment at all stages of the disease, although surgery is preferable in the early stages if the patient is surgically fit. It is also used as primary treatment in women with a high risk of nodal involvement, which include large-volume tumours, poor tumour differentiation, and lymphovascular space involvement.

Treatment usually involves external beam radiotherapy to the whole pelvis followed by intracavitary brachytherapy, in which the radiation source is placed into the uterine cavity and upper vagina. Radiotherapy invariably results in ovarian ablation and HRT may be needed.

Adjuvant radiotherapy is widely prescribed after radical surgery for patients found to have histological indicators of a poor prognosis (node positivity, lymphovascular space involvement, and narrow margins of excision). Although there is evidence that adjuvant radiotherapy can improve pelvic control, no firm evidence indicates that long-term survival is improved. Moreover, the complication rates in women who have undergone both modalities of treatment are much higher than those in women who have undergone either treatment alone.

Chemotherapy
Concurrent chemoradiotherapy
Data accrued from randomized controlled trials show that women with high-risk cervical cancer have a significantly improved survival rate when chemoradiation is used compared with radiotherapy alone. Radiotherapy is combined with platinum-based chemotherapy (usually cisplatin as a single agent) and a 10–20% increase in survival at 3 years has been reported. However, acute toxicity is significant with this regime and the late side effects are still to be assessed.

Other chemotherapy
The use of neoadjuvant chemotherapy before radiotherapy has been largely disappointing. There is no standard protocol, and most studies have shown little or no survival benefit. However, neoadjuvant chemotherapy before radiotherapy is now being studied.

Recurrent disease
Women with recurrent cervical cancer confined to the central pelvis after previous surgery or radiotherapy can occasionally be treated by pelvic exenteration and 5-year survival rates of up to 50% can be achieved. Cases for exenteration are carefully selected, so the majority of women referred are eventually found to be unsuitable for the procedure.

Occasionally, radical radiotherapy can be used for recurrences after surgery and, again, long-term survival rates of up to 40% can be achieved in patients who are carefully re-staged and treated. Chemoradiotherapy may prove to be particularly beneficial in this group of patients. Chemotherapy in recurrent disease may provide some palliation with response rates of up to 40%, albeit of a short duration. Newer chemotherapeutic agents, such as taxanes and topoisomerase-I inhibitors, are also being studied.

Cancer of the Vulva

Incidence
Vulval cancer is uncommon and accounts for approximately 4% of all female genital tumours. Approximately 800 new cases are registered in the UK each year (registration data up until 1992), and the most recent mortality figures recorded 340 deaths in 1996, producing a mortality rate from this disease of just under 50%. The number of women who develop vulval cancer is expected to rise.

Pathology
Vulval intraepithelial neoplasia and Paget's disease
Vulval intraepithelial neoplasia (VIN) and Paget's disease are thought to be possible precursor lesions, with the patholog-

Table 19.11. Vulval intraepithelial neoplasia (VIN) terminology

Squamous vulval intraepithelial neoplasia	
VIN I	Mild dysplasia
VIN II	Moderate dysplasia
VIN III	Severe dysplasia or carcinoma in situ
Non-squamous vulval intraepithelial neoplasia	
Paget's disease	

ical features of VIN similar to those of CIN. Approximately 40% of VIN occurs in women under 40 years of age, with the incidence increasing thereafter. Its malignant potential is thought to be less than 5% with a latent period of progression of 2–8 years. Paget's disease is rare and unlike Paget's disease of the breast, which has a high incidence of underlying adenocarcinoma, no more than one-third of cases of Paget's disease of the vulva are associated with an adenocarcinoma (*Table 19.11*).

Microinvasive disease
Microinvasive disease invades less than 1 mm, but it is important to distinguish this from deeply invasive disease because there is no associated nodal disease and inguinofemoral node dissection is not required.

Invasive disease
Squamous cell carcinoma of the vulva accounts for 85% of all invasive vulval cancers. Less than 5% are melanomas and the remainder are carcinomas of Bartholin's gland, other adenocarcinomas, basal cell carcinomas, verrucous carcinomas, rhabdomyosarcomas, and leiomyosarcomas.

Aetiology
The aetiology of vulval cancer is still not very clearly defined. However, precursor lesions include squamous vulval intraepithelial neoplasia (VIN), Paget's disease, melanoma in situ, and the non-neoplastic epithelial disorders of the vulva.

HPV and type 2 HSV have also been implicated as co-factors and tumours occur more frequently in women who are immunosuppressed.

Clinical presentation
The most common symptom is that of vulval itching, which occurs in about two-thirds of patients (*Table 19.12*). Up to half

Table 19.12. Symptoms and signs of vulval cancer

Symptoms	Signs
Itching	Lump, polyp or swelling
Mass or ulcer	Ulcer
Pain, burning, or soreness	Colour change (whitening, pigment, deposition)
Warts in post-menopausal women	A clinical 'wart'
Bleeding and/or discharge	Irregular fungating mass
	An ulcer with raised, rolled edges
	Enlarged groin nodes

of the patients also present with a vulval mass or ulcer, which may be associated with discharge or bleeding. Unfortunately, usually a delay of months occurs between the onset of symptoms and the seeking of medical advice by many patients, which is often compounded by delays in appropriate referral.

In women with VIN, 20–45% of cases are asymptomatic and are most frequently found after previous treatment for CIN or cancer of the cervix or anus. Note that only a minority of suspicious vulval lesions ultimately reveal a malignancy. At present, there is no method of screening for this disease.

Guidelines for urgent referral

- Visible tumour on the cervix with speculum examination.
- Visible tumour on the vulva.
- Palpable pelvic mass or suspicious mass on pelvic ultrasound.
- More than one episode or a single heavy episode of post-menopausal bleeding.
- Post-coital bleeding that persists for more than 4 weeks.

Investigations
General practice
In patients with symptoms and signs of vulval cancer, a pelvic examination is an important initial assessment, but may not be possible if discomfort and pain is associated with a vulval lesion. A cervical smear, if applicable, should be performed. The patient is then referred to a local gynaecologist with experience in gynaecological oncology or to the nearest gynaecological cancer centre. As many of these patients are elderly, it is expedient if co-existing medical conditions are controlled while referral is made.

Hospital
The diagnosis of vulval cancer is usually confirmed by biopsy prior to definitive treatment. Colposcopy is sometime undertaken in addition if preinvasive disease is suspected in the lower genital tract. If inguinal nodes are palpable or enlarged on imaging, an ultrasound-guided fine needle aspiration is performed for cytological assessment.

An EUA and a full-thickness biopsy of the lesion plus any other suspicious areas is undertaken. This is a very important step because it helps to confirm the diagnosis as well as delineate the extent of the lesion. If the lesion is small, an excision biopsy is undertaken.

Other investigations include a full blood count, urea and electrolytes, and chest radiography. Appropriate imaging of the pelvis by either CT or MRI is performed to identify the full extent of the disease, especially in advanced disease.

Staging and 5-year survival
The staging of vulval cancer as described by FIGO (2002) is given in *Table 19.13* and is a surgicopathological staging system. Note that the clinical assessment of lymph-node status is usually inaccurate and, even when clinically not evident, about 30% of groins have metastatic disease. The importance of this cannot be understated, since survival is dependent on the extent and amount of groin node disease, as indicated in *Table 19.14*. As a consequence, groin nodes should be surgically assessed in all but Stage Ia squamous cell carcinoma, verrucous tumours and basal cell carcinomas.

Treatment
Surgery
Early stage disease
In small tumours it is important to excise radically as much of the primary tumour as possible, with surgical margins of at least 1cm, while avoiding extensive surgical and psycho-

Table 19.13. *Stage and survival in vulval cancer*

Stage	Features	5-year survival (%)
0	Preinvasive carcinoma	
I	Tumour confined to vulva or perineum with no lymph node metastases	69
Ia	Lesion 2cm or less on vulva and/or perineum with stromal invasion up to 1mm	
Ib	As in Ia except stromal invasion is >1mm	
II	Tumour confined to vulva and/or perineum and more than 2cm in greatest dimension; no lymph node metastases	49
III	Tumour of any size arising on the vulva and/or perineum with adjacent spread to lower urethra or anus and/or Unilateral regional (inguinal and/or femoral) lymph node metastases	32
IVa	Tumour invading any of the following: upper urethra, bladder mucosa, rectal mucosa, pelvic bone and/or Bilateral regional lymph node metastases	13
IVb	Any distant metastases including pelvic lymph nodes	

Table 19.14. *Survival in groin node positive squamous carcinoma of the vulva*

Groin node status	5-year survival (%)
Negative	92
Positive	
ipsilateral	75
bilateral	30
contralateral	27
>2 nodes	25
>6 nodes	0

logical morbidity. The traditional radical vulvectomy is now used in only selected cases. Groin node dissection is also undertaken except in the instances described above.

Advanced disease

Treatment is more individualized in advanced disease, with multimodality treatment gaining prominence. The size and location of the tumour influences surgical management and a wide radical local excision is still the aim, with groin node dissection. A radical vulvectomy is employed in some cases in which clear margins cannot be obtained with more limited surgery. If sphincter damage is a distinct possibility, then consideration is

given to radiotherapy as a primary or neoadjuvant role. Otherwise, stomas and reconstructive pelvic surgery are needed.

Radiotherapy

When surgery is not possible, then primary radical radiotherapy to a maximum dose of 75–70 Gy is usually given by a combination of external radiotherapy and brachytherapy. However, this may vary depending on the clinical context. When the surgical resection margin is less than 8 mm, if two or more lymph nodes are involved or if there is extracapsular spread in a node, then adjuvant radiotherapy is given usually at a dose of 45–50 Gy in 5–6 weeks.

Chemotherapy

Chemotherapy has a small role to play as most patients are elderly and who may have co-existent medical problems. No randomized data show that chemotherapy is superior to radiotherapy alone, although two studies suggest that preoperative chemoradiation in advanced vulval cancer reduces the need to perform de-functioning stomas.

Morbidity of treatment

The morbidity of treatment of this condition has been well studied and can be broadly divided into those related to relapsed disease and those related to primary treatment, either surgery (*Table 19.15*) or radiotherapy. In relapsed disease, it is sometimes not possible to conserve sphincter function of

Key points: gynaecological cancer

Ovarian cancer

Uncommon below 40 years of age

Symptoms – often vague and/or non-specific abdominal symptoms

90% of patients have a palpable palvic mass

Usually diagnosed late

Endometrial cancer

Most patients (95%) present with post-menopausal bleeding

Uncommon in pre-menopausal women

Cervical cancer

Incidence is similar across all adult age groups

Screening programme aims to identify precursor lesions

Typical symptoms are post-menopausal, post-coital, and persistent inter-menstrual bleeding

Usually (80%) diagnosed on speculum examination

Up to 40% are screen detected

Any clinical suspicion is an indication for referral and not for a cervical smear

Vulval cancer

Most cases occur in women over 65 years of age

Patients usually present with bleeding, discomfort, itch, or a burning sensation

90% of patients have a visible tumour on clinical examination

Reproduced from England Department of Health Draft Cancer referral Guidelines Consultation Document 2001.

Guidelines for urgent referral: gynaecological cancer

Urgent referral

Visible tumour on cervix on speculum examination

Visible tumour on vulva on clinical examination

Palpable pelvic mass

Suspicious pelvic mass on pelvic ultrasound

More than one or a single heavy episode of post-menopausal bleeding (PMB)

Post-coital bleeding (PCB) that persists for more than 4 weeks

Hormone replacement therapy (HRT); unexpected or prolonged bleeding persisting for more than 4 weeks after stopping HRT

Early referral

Indications for 'early' referral (i.e. within 4–6 weeks), but not 'urgent' referral:

single episode of PMB

single episode of PCB

Referral proforma: gynaecological cancer

Age:

Cancer type:

Ovary	☐	Endometrium	☐
Cervix	☐	Vagina/vulva	☐

Menopausal status

Pre-menopausal	☐
Post-menopausal (>1 year since last menopause	☐
Hysterectomy	☐
On HRT	☐

Symptoms:

Bleeding	☐
Post-coital	☐
Post-menopausal	☐
Single episode	☐
More than 1 episode	☐

Duration of PB bleeding .... weeks

Abdominal symptoms

	Yes	No
Examination		
Abdominal mass		
Pelvic mass		
Visible cervical lesion		
Visible vulval lesion		

Pelvic ultrasound   Noter done ☐   Negative ☐   Positive ☐

Comments/other reasons for urgent referral

Table 19.15. Surgical morbidity

Wound breakdown

Deep vein thrombosis and/or pulmonary embolism

Sexual dysfunction: stenosis, psychosexual

Lymphocysts

Wound infection

Incontinence

Pressure sores

Lymphoedema

the bladder or anus and reconstructive procedures may be needed. Relapse in the skin bridge between the vulva and the groin poses a difficult problem and survival is poor.

Follow-up and care

As local relapse is not uncommon, follow-up of patients should be in the oncology clinic. Long-term follow-up is advised, as the risk of developing other genital tract cancer is not insignificant. Patients are usually seen every 3–6 months in the first 3 years and yearly thereafter.

Cancer of the Vagina

Incidence, pathology, and aetiology

Cancer of the vagina is a very rare tumour of mainly elderly women, with an annual incidence of about 1 per 100,000 women and a lifetime risk of less than 1%. The most common site is the upper third of the vagina. The aetiology is unknown, although chronic irritation (e.g. procidentia or the use of a pessary) may be an underlying cause. Women exposed as foetuses to diethylstilboestrol are at risk of developing clear-cell adenocarcinoma of the vagina, but this risk is very low. HPV has also been implicated.

Although vaginal intraepithelial neoplasia (VAIN) is considered to have a malignant potential, the relationship is not as well proved as that in CIN. More than 90% are squamous in type, with 5% being adenocarcinomas, and, rarer still, are melanomas and sarcomas.

Clinical presentation and investigations

Most cases of vaginal cancer are picked up at an advanced stage after the development of post-menopausal bleeding. Other symptoms include vaginal discharge, urinary symptoms, and pelvic pain. Some cases are asymptomatic and are picked up via routine cervical screening or the colposcopic assessment of abnormal smears.

Once vaginal cancer is suspected, the patient should be referred immediately to a gynaecological oncologist. The most important investigation is an EUA with assessment of the bladder and rectum. Biopsies are taken for histological confirmation. Other investigations include renal and liver function tests, radiology of the renal tract, and CT or MRI scans of the abdomen and pelvis.

Staging and prognosis

Staging is clinical, based on the above-mentioned investigations. At presentation, cases are equally divided between stage I, II, or advanced stage (one-third each). The prognosis of this condition correlates very closely with the stage and degree of differentiation (*Table 19.16*).

Management

Radiotherapy is the main treatment modality of vaginal cancer. It is usually given either as a combination of external radiation and brachytherapy or as brachytherapy alone. Combined therapy is useful to treat tumours of the upper two-thirds of the vagina. Tumours in the middle and lower two-thirds of the vagina and stage I and IIa disease are usually treated with brachytherapy alone. External beam radiotherapy is used as sole treatment in cases with advanced disease for which palliation is desired. Radiotherapy can lead to complications such as vaginal stenosis and delayed vaginal healing.

Surgery is mainly carried out for small, stage I lesions in which local excision is possible. Surgical extirpation of upper vaginal tumours requires a radical hysterectomy and pelvic lymphadenectomy, with a partial or complete vaginectomy with or without vaginal reconstruction. Pelvic exenteration is rarely performed for central disease. Experience of chemotherapy is quite limited in squamous lesions, although it is the mainstay of treatment in the very rare vaginal rhabdomyosarcomas (sarcoma botryoides) in young girls.

Further Reading

Union Internale Contre le Cancer. FIGO staging. *TNM Classification of Malignant Tumours*, 6th edition. Sobin LH and Witterkind CL (eds). New York: Wiley-Liss, 2002.

20 Ovarian Cancer

Ian Jacobs and Martin Gore

Incidence

Ovarian cancer is the commonest gynaecological malignancy being responsible for nearly 7,000 cases a year in the UK and 4,500 deaths. Twice as many women die of ovarian cancer than cervical and uterine combined. This makes it the fourth commonest malignancy in women and the fourth commonest cause of cancer death (*Table 20.1*). The median age of onset is 65 and it is rare under the age of 30 (*Table 20.2*). Various statistics relating to ovarian cancer are shown in *Figure 20.1*.

Pathology

The majority of malignancies of the ovary are epithelial cancers (*Fig. 20.2*). An important group of ovarian malignan-cies are however, metastases, commonly from the breast or GI tract; these tumours often have a signet ring appearance and are called Krukenberg tumours.

There are also several uncommon primary tumours of the ovary including granulosa cell tumour, Sertoli-Leydig tumour and arrhenoblastoma where surgery is the main-stay of their treatment and germ cell tumours (teratoma, dysgerminoma) which are mainly treated with chemother-apy. These rare malignancies are important as they occur in young women usually between the ages of 15 and 35, and can be managed by fertility-sparing surgery followed up by combination platinum-based chemotherapy.

Approximately 10% of epithelial ovarian malignancies are so called borderline and are characterized by features of malignancy (nuclear atypia, cellular multilayering, increased mitotic activity) but unlike invasive cancers there is no invasion of the stromal tissue. Borderline tumours are typically stage I (see *Table 20.6*) but they can be associated with invasive metastatic disease. The treatment of these tumours is primarily surgical and the impact of chemother-apy for those presenting with stage III disease (see *Table 20.6*) is unclear. The prognosis for borderline tumours is extremely good partly because the majority of patients have stage I disease: 5 year-survival rates for stage I disease are over 95% and as high as 75% for stage III disease.

Aetiology

A number of risk factors and protective factors have been identified for epithelial ovarian cancer (*Table 20.3*). A

Table 20.1. *Cancer in women. UK – 1999–2001 ( ) rank*

	Incidence	Mortality
Breast	39290 (1)	12990 (2)
Lung	14830 (3)	13040 (1)
Colon	16810 (2)	7360 (1)
Ovary	6890 (4)	4660 (4)
Cervix	3240 (4)	1170 (12)
Uterus	4880 (8)	1050 (17)
Total	133790	74420

Table 20.2. *Epithelial ovarian cancer. Age distribution*

Age (years)	No. of cases
<45	532 (10%)
45–54	794 (15%)
55–64	1,263 (25%)
>65	2,583 (50%)

Table 20.3. *Risk/protective factors for ovarian cancer*

Risk	Protective
Age	Parity
Family history	Pill
BRCA1/2 mutations	Oophorectomy
?Ovarian stimulation	Hysterectomy
	Sterilisation

OVARIAN CANCER STATISTICS

New ovarian cancer

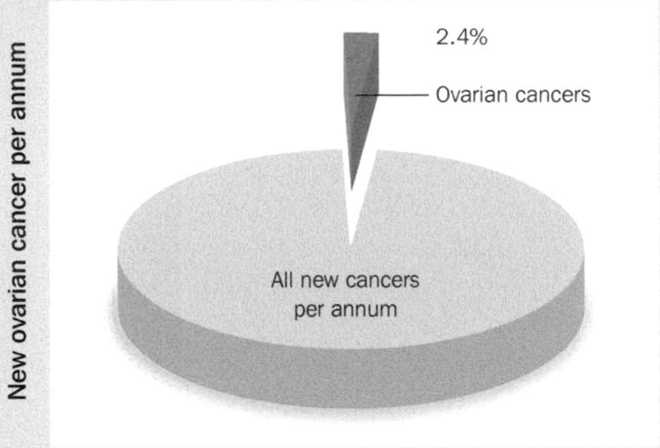

New cases per annum	5910
Males rank	—
Females rank	4
Deaths per annum	4491

Incidence

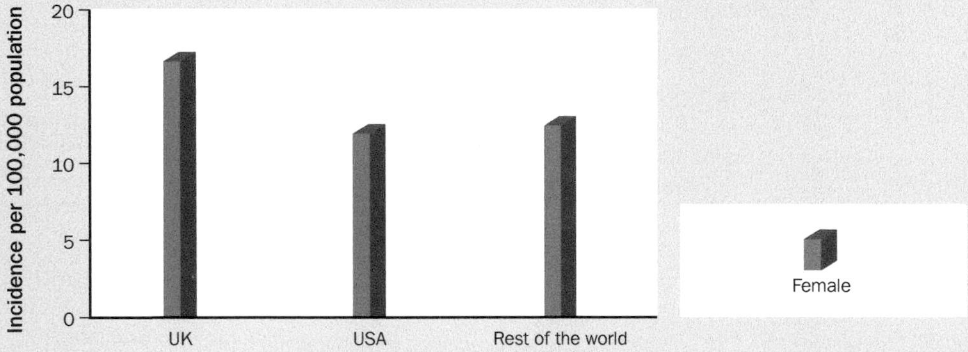

Survival rate

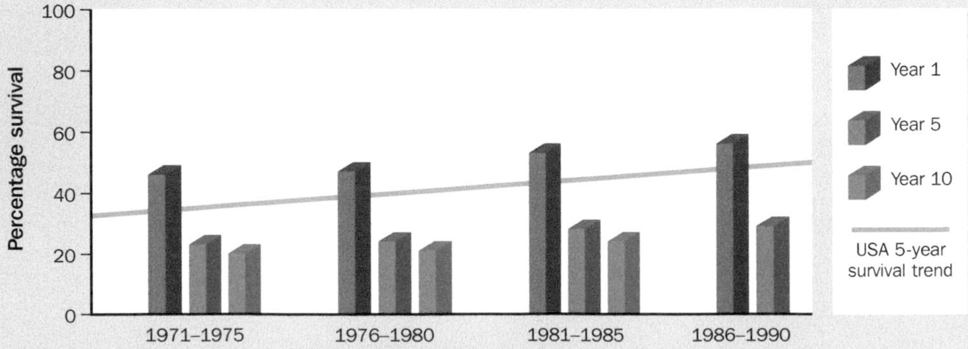

Figure 20.1. *Statistical data relating to ovarian cancer.*

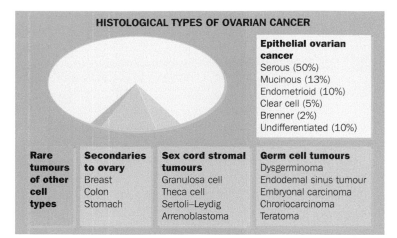

Figure 20.2. *Histological types of ovarian cancer.*

Key points

- Patients with suspected ovarian cancer should be referred to a specialist in a cancer unit/centre.
- Risk factors for ovarian cancer related to family history, parity, pill usage.
- The majority of patients present with advanced disease and have a 5-year survival of 30%.
- Most important prognostic factor in ovarian cancer is the amount of residual disease left behind after initial surgery.

Table 20.4. *Hereditary ovarian cancer syndromes. Suggestive family histories*

Site-special ovarian cancer	2 ovarian cancers in family members linked by 1st degree relationships
Breasts/ovarian cancer	1 ovarian cancer *PLUS* 1 breast cancer (occurring <50 years of age) in family members linked by 1st degree relationships OR
	1 ovarian cancer *PLUS* 2 breast cancers (occurring <60 years of age) in family members linked by 1st degree relationships
Lynch type II	Colorectal cancer *PLUS* Endometrial cancer *PLUS* Ovarian cancer in family members linked by 1st degree relationships
1st degree relationships = parent/child/sibling	

small but important group of families have a high frequency of specific cancers suggestive of a hereditary syndrome and such syndromes can include ovarian cancer. The hereditary cancer syndromes that involve ovarian cancer account for approximately 10% of ovarian cancers and are summarised in *Table 20.4*. The risk of ovarian cancer for various groups of the population is shown in *Fig. 20.3*.

Hereditary Ovarian Cancer

It is important that female members of families with a history suggestive of a hereditary ovarian cancer syndrome are

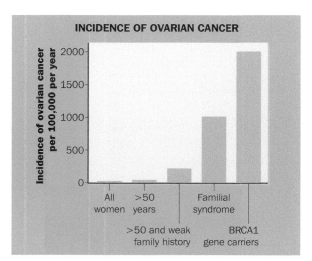

Figure 20.3. *Incidence of ovarian cancer amongst different groups of women.*

Key points

- Majority of malignancies of the ovary are epithelial cancers.
- Symptoms of ovarian cancer are notoriously nonspecific.
- Routine population-based screening is NOT currently recommended.
- A careful family history should be taken.
- Current treatment involves primary surgery and platinum-based chemotherapy.

counselled by an oncologist or a cancer geneticist with expertise in this area.

It is now possible to test for ovarian cancer causing mutations within 2 specific genes (BRCA1 and 2). These genes normally function as tumour suppressors and when mutated are responsible for the majority of cases of familial ovarian cancer. In order to find a mutation it is usually necessary to have a blood DNA sample from at least one affected individual in the family.

The risk of developing ovarian cancer in a woman who has a mutation in the BRCA 1 gene is about 40% by the time she is 80 but the risk appears to vary between families and with different mutations of these genes. The risk of developing ovarian cancer in women who have a mutation in the BRCA 2 gene is lower, approximately 20% by the age of 80.

It seems likely that BRCA1 and 2 mutations account for most but not all cases of hereditary ovarian cancer and that there are additional as yet undiscovered genes resulting in predispositions to ovarian cancer.

Patients who have been identified as having a genetic predisposition to ovarian cancer can be offered prophylactic bilateral oophorectomy followed by HRT when they have completed their family. The risks of HRT in patients who have a hereditary predisposition to breast cancer are not yet clear. Although prophylactic oophorectomy protects against ovarian cancer these patients may still be at a small risk of developing intra-abdominal carcinomatosis thought to arise from the peritoneum which contains cells which share an embryological origin with the ovaries.

Clinical Presentation

The symptoms of ovarian cancer are notoriously nonspecific and the practitioner needs to be constantly aware of the pos-

sibility of this diagnosis. Frequently, patients complain of nonspecific abdominal discomfort or pain for several months before a diagnosis of advanced disease is made. These gastrointestinal symptoms often mimic irritable bowel syndrome and typically include the complaint of abdominal bloating. Often, the diagnosis is only suspected once ascites develops.

Women may also present with a palpable abdominal mass, clinically evident ascites or a pelvic mass palpable on biannual examination. More specific gynaecologic symptoms such as vaginal bleeding and pelvic discomfort are only occasionally seen. Patients with very advanced (stage IV, see *Table 20.6*) disease may present with shortness of breath due to the presence of pleural effusions.

Screening

Routine population-based screening is not currently recommended because there is as yet no definitive evidence about the overall implications of population screening. Current methods of detection do not have 100% sensitivity for the early stages of ovarian cancer and there are well documented disadvantages such as anxiety which are created by false positive results and their subsequent investigation (*Table 20.5*). Randomized trials of screening the general population are underway involving women over 50 years of age and will report in the next few years. Encouraging preliminary results suggest that screening may improve survival.

Screening should currently be limited to women who are members of families with a hereditary predisposition as described above. Screening of this group of women should be organised after counselling in a cancer genetics clinic and usually consists of annual transvaginal ultrasound and serum

Table 20.5. Advantages and disadvantages of ovarian cancer screening

Advantages	Disadvantages
Early detection may improve survival	The economic cost of screening
Early detection may allow for less radical treatment	Anxiety associated with false positive results
Possible cost saving associated with less treatment and palliative care	Morbidity associated with surgical investigation of false positive results
Reassurance of women with negative results	False reassurance of some women

CA 125 measurement. A national Familial Ovarian Cancer Screening Study has recently been commenced to document the results of screening this high risk group.

Arrangements for cancer genetics counselling vary from area to area. The quickest way to access information on local facilities for women at risk is via the specialists in gynaecological cancer at the local regional cancer centre.

Women with only one relative with ovarian cancer are at slightly higher risk of developing ovarian cancer than the general population (4% versus 1% lifetime risk, respectively). Routine provision of screening is not recommended for these women.

Investigations

a) In general practice

In patients with symptoms or signs suggestive of ovarian cancer the initial investigation is a pelvic examination. Ultrasound scan of the pelvis or abdomen is very important if available. If the scan reveals an adnexal mass the assessment may establish the differential diagnosis between physiological, benign and malignant changes. Features suggestive of ovarian cancer include solid areas (*Fig. 20.4*), multiple cysts, thick septae dividing cysts (*Fig. 20.5*) and increased blood flow on colour flow doppler assessment. Transvaginal ultrasound scans are particularly accurate in assessing the ovaries.

b) In hospital

If the ultrasound scan reveals a significant volume of ascites this can easily be tapped and may help in establishing a diagnosis of malignancy. Serum tumour markers may be helpful in the differential diagnosis as CA 125 is elevated (>30 U/ml) in over 80% of patients presenting clinically with ovarian cancer. It should however be noted that moderate CA 125 elevation (up to 100 U/ml) can occur in a spectrum of physiological situations (pregnancy, menstruation) as well as benign conditions (benign tumours, fibroids, endometriosis). Higher levels can be seen from any cause of peritoneal irritation and in congestive cardiac failure. Very high values can occur in the advanced stages of many other cancers (eg. breast, lung colon) particularly when associated with ascites. CEA is a useful serum marker to differentiate ovarian cancer from gastro-intestinal malignancy. In younger patients measurement of AFP and hCG should be considered as these markers are elevated in many germ cell tumours.

Scoring systems have been described incorporating ultrasound findings, CA 125 level and menopausal status which have > 90% accuracy in differentiating benign from malig-

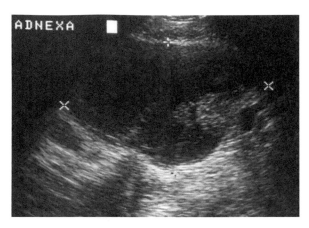

Figure 20.4. *Transvaginal ultrasound demonstrating a left-sided malignant ovarian cyst containing solid areas.*

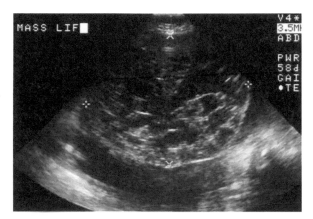

Figure 20.5. *Transvaginal ultrasound demonstrating a large multilobulated cystic ovarian cancer with thick septae.*

nant ovarian tumours. If the findings on cytological examination of tapped ascites suggest that malignancy is present or the ultrasound/CA 125 results are suspicious referral to a gynaecological oncologist should be organised. Sometimes further investigation to establish a primary site (eg. with CT/MRI) is required but in patients with a complex adnexal mass and elevated CA 125 it may be reasonable to proceed directly to surgery (*Fig. 20.6*).

The algorithm for investigating patients with adnexal masses is set out in *Fig. 20.7*.

Stage and 5-Year Survival

The features of the individual stages of ovarian cancer as defined by FIGO and the 5-year survival rates for each stage

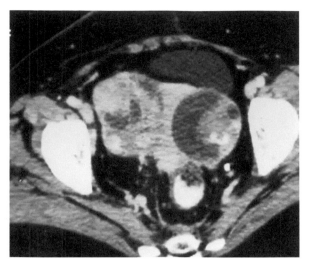

Figure 20.6. CT scan demonstrating bilateral cystic ovarian cancer.

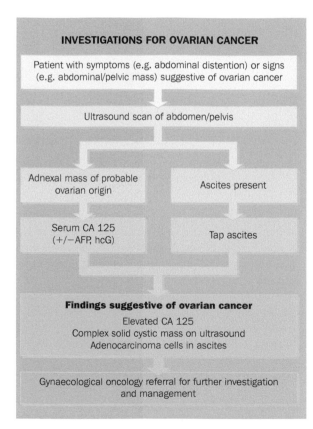

INVESTIGATIONS FOR OVARIAN CANCER

Patient with symptoms (e.g. abdominal distention) or signs (e.g. abdominal/pelvic mass) suggestive of ovarian cancer

Ultrasound scan of abdomen/pelvis

Adnexal mass of probable ovarian origin

Ascites present

Serum CA 125 (+/−AFP, hcG)

Tap ascites

Findings suggestive of ovarian cancer
Elevated CA 125
Complex solid cystic mass on ultrasound
Adenocarcinoma cells in ascites

Gynaecological oncology referral for further investigation and management

Figure 20.7. Algorithm for investigation of patient with symptoms and/or signs of ovarian cancer.

are shown in Table 6. The term advanced disease refers to stages III-IV, although some include stage II in this definition. Stage Ia or b disease with a tumour which is well or moderately differentiated is categorized as early epithelial ovarian cancer of good prognosis whereas patients with stage Ic, II, poorly differentiated tumours or clear cell histology are described as having early epithelial ovarian cancer of poor prognosis. The distinction is important as patients with good prognosis early disease have survival rates of approximately 90% and do not need adjuvant chemotherapy after surgery. Randomised trials are ongoing defining the role of chemotherapy in poor prognosis early disease. Surgery and chemotherapy for ovarian cancer should be delivered at a cancer centre.

Surgery

Surgery for ovarian cancer has 2 objectives: thorough staging and maximum tumour debulking (cytoreduction). A mid line incision is required, a total abdominal hysterectomy, bilateral salpingo-oophorectomy and omentectomy should usually be performed and as much tumour as possible resected. If stage I disease is suspected then thorough exploration of the abdominal cavity, peritoneal washings, multiple peritoneal biopsies of suspicious areas, omentectomy and sampling of para-aortic and pelvic lymph nodes is essential to exclude occult advanced disease. It is extremely important that stage I disease is accurately defined at surgery because otherwise patients with apparent stage I but actual stage III disease may not receive the chemotherapy they require.

One of the most important prognostic factors in ovarian cancer is the amount of residual disease left behind after initial surgery (*Table 20.7*). The intention of surgery for advanced ovarian cancer is not to leave any residual tumour or at the most, 1–2 cm nodules, this is known as optimal debulking. The rationale is to reduce the number of potentially chemoresistant clones. The prognosis of patients with a residual single mass of 5 cm is substantially worse than for patients who have a hundred intra-peritoneal nodules of less than 0.5 cm. Unfortunately, despite maximum surgical effort optimal debulking is only achieved in approximately 50% of patients with stage III disease.

A randomized trial in Europe demonstrated that for patients in whom optimal debulking at presentation was not possible, debulking half way through their chemotherapy (after 3 cycles) confered a significant survival benefit. This approach is currently being further evaluated.

Women who wish to retain their fertility and who have early disease of good prognosis may be considered for con-

Table 20.6. *Staging of ovarian cancer according to the International Federation of Gynaecological Oncology (FIGO)*

		5-yr survival
Stage I	Growth confined to the ovary	75%
a	One ovary, capsule intact, no surface tumour, no ascites*	
b	Both ovaries, capsule intact, no surface tumour, no ascites	
c	Capsule breached by tumour, washings/ascites with malignant cells	
Stage II	Growth with pelvic extension	45%
a	Uterine or tubal extensions/metastases	
b	Extension to other pelvic tissues	
c	a or b, capsule(s) ruptured, surface tumour, malignant ascites or positive peritoneal washings	
Stage III	Growth with intraabdominal extension (including retroperitoneal or inguinal nodes, omentum, surface of small bowel and liver surface)	20%
a	Microscopic intraabdominal extension	
b	<2 cm diameter nodules	
c	>2 cm diameter nodules and retroperitoneal or inguinal lymph node involvement	
Stage IV	Distant metastases	8%
a	Cytologically positive pleural effusion, liver parenchymal, lung etc.	

*These patients have 5 years survival rate of 90% in some series

Table 20.7. *Prognosis related to extent of disease after cytoreductive surgery.*

Residual tumour after primary surgery for stage III ovarian tumour	5 year survival
0	65%
<1 cm	50%
1–2 cm	30%
2–5 cm	20%
>5 cm	10%

servative surgery i.e. unilateral salpingo-oophorectomy. These patients must have thorough surgical staging including pelvic/para-aortic lymph node sampling and be carefully counselled. Women who have had conservative surgery for early stage ovarian cancer are often advised to have their remaining ovary removed once they have completed their family. The follow up of these patients requires careful planning with regular serum CA 125 estimations and transvaginal ultrasound examinations to follow the remaining ovary.

Women who develop menopausal symptoms following surgery for ovarian cancer or young women who have had both ovaries removed either therapeutically or prophylactically, should be considered for hormone replacement therapy.

Chemotherapy

Patients with stage Ic, II, III and IV disease require chemotherapy. Platinum-based treatment (cisplatin, carboplatin) is essential and in the UK, single agent carboplatin was until recently considered standard therapy. However, two randomised trials established that the combination of platinum plus paclitaxel (Taxol) as the gold standard treatment for ovarian cancer. A recent trial has called this into question but internationally platinum-paclitaxel remains standard of care. NICE guidance requires this to be discussed and patients given a choice.

Randomized trials strongly suggest that carboplatin and cisplatin are equally effective. Carboplatin has a much more favourable toxicity profile than cisplatin causing less nausea and vomiting and almost no oto-, neuro- or nephrotoxicity at standard doses. Carboplatin is prescribed according to the patientís glomerular filtration rate because it is largely excreted unchanged through the kidneys. Several different formulae are used in this context.

The aggressiveness of chemotherapy depends on the clinical circumstances so that a woman of 50 with optimally debulked disease who has a chance of prolonged disease-free interval or even cure should be treated with platinum–paclitaxel combinations whereas an elderly patient with bulky disease and a poor performance status in whom palliation is the main aim can be reasonably given single agent carboplatin. Patients usually receive 6 cycles of chemotherapy unless there is evidence of disease progression. Each cycle is given intravenously via a bag and giving set. Regimens vary but usually the administration of each cycle takes about 4 hours with antiemetics being given orally and/or intravenously at the time of treatment. Most regimens can be given in the outpatient setting and cycles are given every 21–28 days.

The progress of treatment is followed by physical examination and serial measurement of the serum CA 125 usually taken prior to each cycle of therapy. Calculations can be made to define response or progression according to the CA 125 measurements. The definitions need to be applied bearing in mind that sometimes the CA 125 may rise or fall due to circumstances other than progression or response, eg. abdominal paracentesis. There is now debate whether routine serial imaging procedures such as US or CT are of value.

The majority of patients who relapse following first-line chemotherapy do so within 18 months of completing therapy and all are incurable. Response rates to further chemotherapy in these patients depend on the interval between the relapse and previous treatment. Patients who have been in partial or complete remission for one year or more have a higher chance of responding again to treatment (*Table 20.8*). The chemotherapy agents commonly used for treating relapsed disease are shown in Table 20.8, for the patients who relapse within 12 months the response rate is usually 15–20%. Second remissions tend to be shorter than the first, lasting about 6 months.

Table 20.8. Response rates to chemotherapy at relapse

| | Treatment-free interval (months) | | |
	<12	12–24	>24
Single agents (paclitaxel, topotecan, etoposide , docetaxel, liposomal, doxorubicin)	15–30%	–	–
Platinum rechallenge	15–30%	30%	60–80%
Platinum-based combinations	45–65%	–	–

Palliative Care

One of the major problems in patients with recurrent/progressive disease is bowel obstruction. This may involve the large or small bowel and is often at multiple sites. It may respond to conservative management and only occasionally will patients benefit from surgery involving stoma formation or a bypass procedure.

Conservative management for intestinal obstruction includes no oral intake, nasogastric tube, iv hydration, iv anti-emetics and sometimes steroids. For terminally ill patients nasogastric tubes are often not used and patients are allowed to eat and drink. In this situation they vomit once or twice a day but are able to at least in part satisfy some of their hunger.

Increasing gastrostomy tubes are used in order to relieve the abdominal distension and vomiting associated with obstruction.

Further Reading

Harries M, Gore M. Part I. Chemotherapt for epithelial ovarian cancer: treatment at first diagnosis. *Lancet Oncol* 2002; **3**(9): 529–36.

Harries M, Gore M. Part II. Chemotherapt for epithelial ovarian cancer: treatment at first diagnosis. *Lancet Oncol* 2002; **3**(9): 537–45.

21 Leukaemia and Myeloma

Bhawna Sirohi and Ray Powles

Leukaemias

Leukaemia is a malignant disease of the bone marrow and blood characterized by abnormal clonal proliferation and accumulation of mature and immature blood precursors. Before 1975 almost all patients with leukaemia died within a year. Now approximately 50% under the age of 50 years are cured. The common types of leukaemia are divided into four categories: myelogenous or lymphocytic, both of which can be acute or chronic.

Acute Leukaemias

Acute leukaemia is a rapidly progressing disease that results in the accumulation of immature functionless cells in the marrow and blood, such that the marrow often can no longer produce enough normal red blood cells, white blood cells (WBCs), and platelets. Depending on the cell lineage involved, acute leukaemia is classified as acute myelogenous leukaemia (AML) or acute lymphoblastic leukaemia (ALL).

Incidence

The incidence of acute leukaemia in the UK is 9 per 100,000 population. Both subtypes can occur in all age groups, but ALL also occurs as the usual variety in children. Both types are slightly more common in males, and the incidence of AML increases with age. Various statistics relating to leukaemia are shown in *Figure 21.1.*

Aetiology

While the exact cause is not known, a number of predisposing factors implicated are ionizing radiation, aromatic hydrocarbons (such as benzene), cigarette smoking, electrics-related occupations, certain anticancer drugs (such as alkylating agents and plant alkaloids), and radiotherapy for other primary malignancies. Acute leukaemia occurs with increased frequency in congenital diseases such as Down's, Fanconi, Kline–Felter, Wiskott–Aldrich, and Bloom syndromes.

Classification

It is important to distinguish between ALL and AML because the natural history, prognosis, and therapy of the two are different. The most widely used classification of acute leukaemia is that proposed by the French–American–

Table 21.1. *French–American–British (FAB) classification of acute myeloid leukaemia (AML)*

FAB type	Morphology	Frequency (%)
M0	Acute leukaemia with minimal evidence of myeloid differentiation	2
M1	AML without maturation	19
M2	AML with maturation	24
M3	Acute promyelocytic leukaemia	10
M3V	Variant form of promyelocytic leukaemia	
M4	Acute myelomonocytic leukaemia	30
M5a	Acute monoblastic leukaemia	5
M5b	Acute monocytic leukaemia	5
M6	Acute erythroleukaemia	4
M7	Acute megakaryocytic leukaemia	1

Table 21.2. *French–American–British (FAB) classification of acute lymphocytic leukaemia (ALL)*

FAB type	Morphology	Frequency
L1	Small, uniform cells with high nuclear:cytoplasm ratio	75% of childhood ALL
L2	Large, heterogeneous cells with low nuclear:cytoplasm ratio	70% of adult ALL
L3	Burkitt's type of B-cell origin, large, uniform cells with vacuolated cytoplasm	Rare

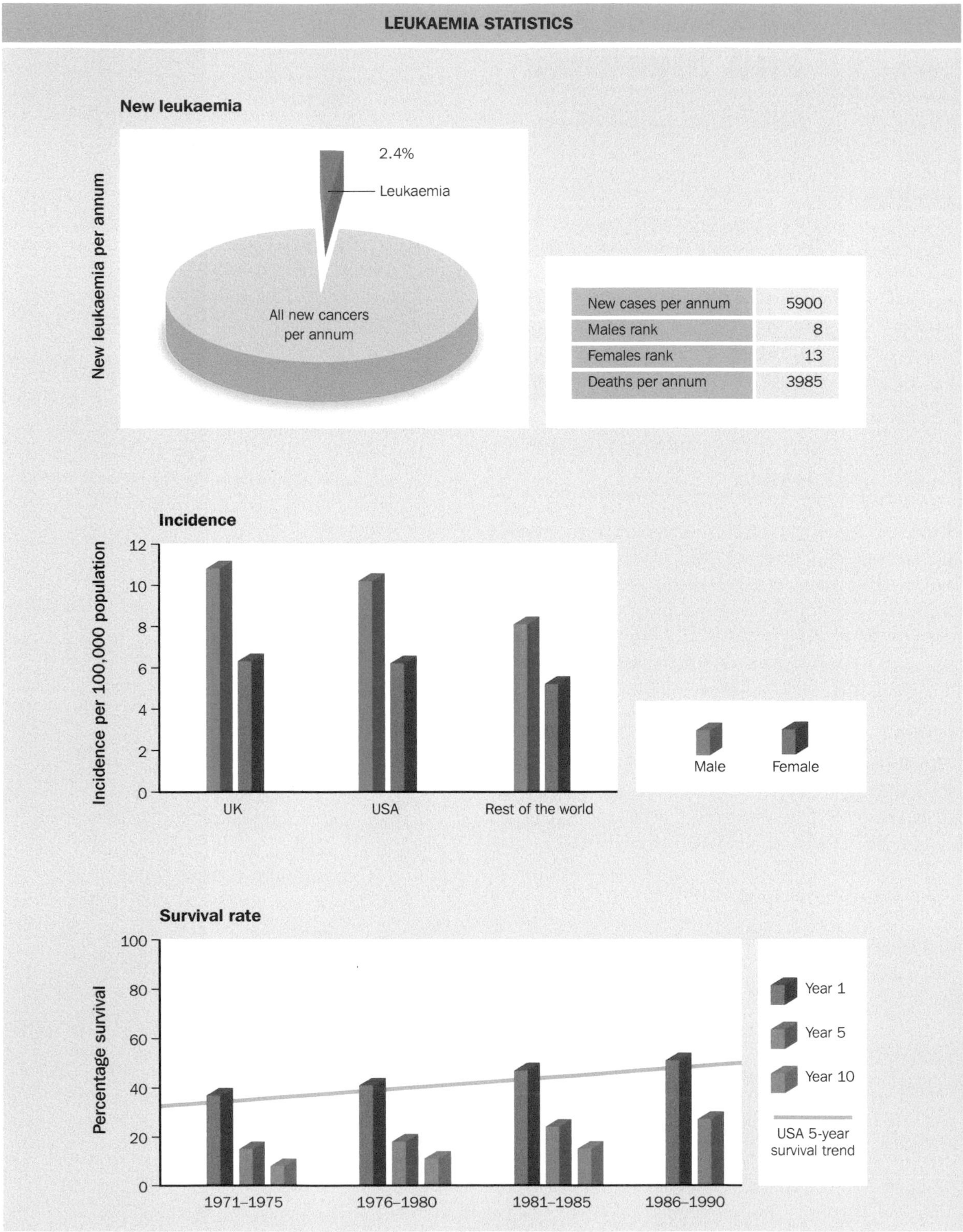

LEUKAEMIA STATISTICS

New leukaemia

New cases per annum	5900
Males rank	8
Females rank	13
Deaths per annum	3985

Incidence

Survival rate

Figure 21.4. *Statistical data relating to leukaemia.*

190

Table 21.3. *Chromosomal abnormalities associated with acute leukaemia*

FAB subtype	Karyotype	Relative prognosis
Acute myeloid leukaemia		
M1	−5, −7, +8	Poor
M2	t(8;21)	Good
M3	t(15;17)	Good
M4	inv 16, −16	Good
Acute lymphocytic leukaemia		
L1 or L2	Hyperdiploidy	Good
L1 or L2	6q−	Good
L3	t(8;14)	Poor
L1 or L2	Philadelphia +ve t(9;22)	Poor
L1 or L2	TEL AML1	Good
Biphenotypic		
L2 or M4	t(4;11)	Poor

British (FAB) cooperative group, which is based on morphology and chemistry (*Tables 21.1* and *21.2*). Chromosomal abnormalities associated with acute leukaemia are given in *Table 21.3*.

Using heteroantisera and monoclonal antibodies, ALL cells can be divided into various types as shown in *Table 21.4*. All types of ALL, except B-cell, have elevated terminal deoxynucleotidyl transferase (TdT) expression. This elevation is extremely useful in diagnosis; if concentrations of the enzyme are not elevated the diagnosis is suspect. However, 20% of cases of AML may also express TdT.

Investigations

Investigations required for diagnosis are given in *Table 21.5* and those used to guide therapy in *Table 21.6*.

Clinical features

Most of the clinical features result from bone marrow failure secondary to the leukaemia (i.e. anaemia, infections, and bleeding). One-third of patients with AML are acutely ill at presentation because of significant skin, soft-tissue, or respiratory infection. Petechiae with or without bleeding may be present. Patients with M3 AML may have severe haemorrhaging and secondary disseminated intravascular coagulation. Mild hepatosplenomegaly may be present. Leukaemias with monocytic component M4 and M5 may be associated with gingival hypertrophy and skin lesions from leukaemic infiltration. Chloromas (solid masses consisting of leukaemia cells) are present in about 5% of patients and commonly

Table 21.4. *Acute lymphocytic leukaemia cell types*

Cell	Characteristic feature(s)	Prognosis
T-ALL	Propensity for mediastinal mass and central nervous system involvement	Poor
Common ALL (CALLA)	CD10 antigen, B-cell antigens, immunoglobulin gene rearrangement	Good
Null ALL	Lacks CD10 or B-cell markers	Poor
Pre-B-ALL	Similar to CALLA but expresses cytoplasmic immunoglobulin	Good
B-ALL	Rare, expresses monoclonal surface membrane immunoglobulin	Poor

Table 21.5. *Investigations for diagnosis*

Peripheral blood	Full blood count, differential count (leukaemic blasts), cytochemistry, karyotype, immunophenotype, serum lysozyme, serum lactate dehydrogenase
Bone marrow	Differential count, cytochemistry, karyotype, immunophenotype, immunofluorescence studies for terminal deoxynucleotidyl transferase, trephine biopsy to assess cellularity and fibrosis
Cerebrospinal fluid examination	All patients of ALL (because ALL often involves the central nervous system) and in patients of AML who have neurological symptoms
Urine lysozyme	Elevated in M4 and M5

Table 21.6. Investigations used to guide therapy

Blood grouping	Patient and family
Human leucocyte antigen typing	Patient and family
Cytomegalovirus serology	
Coagulation profile	
Surveillance cultures	Blood, urine, stool, throat, perineum
Chest radiograph	
Serum chemistry	Electrolytes, uric acid, renal, and liver function
Urine examination	

nosis is made. The most common presentation is one of patients who see their general practitioner (GP) because they feel they have flu-like symptoms, perhaps with some bruising, and they look pale. The GP rightly diagnoses intercurrent infection and often sends them home to bed with antibiotics. After 24–40 hours the patient is less well and the GP becomes alerted to the deteriorating situation, but might not immediately suspect leukaemia. However, a blood count and film at the local hospital that is seen by a laboratory technician and the district general hospital haematologist results in the diagnosis being made. The haematologist contacts the GP by telephone, says there is a suspicion of leukaemia and requests an immediate bone marrow examination. At this point the patient may be critically ill with septicaemia. Life-saving supportive therapy (see below) should be undertaken within hours.

associated with M4 and M5. Massive mediastinal lymphadenopathy is a particular feature of T-ALL. Increased intracranial pressure secondary to meningeal leukaemia is rare but is most commonly seen in B-ALL and M4 patients, who are usually young.

Presentation of new patients to their general practitioner
Leukaemia patients in general should be seen by the specialist unit that is going to treat them on the same day as the diag-

Prognostic factors
The prognostic factors for AML and ALL are given in *Table 21.7*.

Definition of complete remission
Complete remission is defined as restoration of normal peripheral blood counts, maturation of all haemopoietic cell lines, and <5% blasts forms in a normocellular bone marrow

Table 21.7. Prognostic factors for acute myeloid leukaemia (AML) and acute lymphocytic leukaemia (ALL)

Type	Favourable	Unfavourable
AML	Young age Reactivity with cell surface marker CD2 (T1) FAB types M2, M3, M4, t(8;21), t(15;17), inv 16	Older age FAB types M6, M7 Hyperleucocytosis Prior treatment with radiation or cytotoxic drug therapy (secondary leukaemia) Low labelling index/aneuploidy Trisomy 8 Deletion of all or parts of chromosome 5 and/or 7 Abnormalities of chromosome 11 and band q23
ALL	Achievement of complete remission in less than 4 weeks TEL-AML1 gene rearrangement Hyperdiploidy ACALLA+, early B-cell, L1	Male sex Age <2 years or >10 years White blood cell count >20 ∞ 10^9/l B-cell phenotype (L3) T-cell Presence of Philadelphia chromosome Meningeal involvement Presence of myeloid markers on surface (biphenotypic disease)

for at least 4 weeks. Achievement of complete remission has been associated with a reduction in the leukaemic burden from 10^{12} cells (1 trillion) to 10^9 cells. This occurs 4–6 weeks into treatment (see below), at which point the patient is probably completely well (with alopecia), and ordinary hospital tests do not indicate any illness. Despite this enormous destruction of tumour cells the remaining clinically unidentifiable 10^9 cells represent the minimal residual disease and must be eliminated if relapse is to avoided. This is the rationale for post-remission therapy in AML and reinduction and/or consolidation therapy in ALL.

Management

Patients with acute leukaemia are treated with a curative intent. Treatment also depends on patient's age, risk, course of illness (relapse or diagnosis), and performance status.

General

The first 24 hours are critical to a successful outcome. Particularly important is the immediate treatment of infection, which is usually systemic, often with septicaemia, and requires combinations of several broad-spectrum intravenous antibiotics. These antibiotics sometimes need to be given even before the patient has reached the ward.

Supportive therapy with packed cells should be given for severe anaemia, but needs to be undertaken carefully in very ill patients, who may be in heart failure because of their very high WBC counts. Blood-cell separators can be used to reduce the white cell numbers if the count is extremely high. Patients need additional support with fluids. Platelet transfusions, with or without heparin and/or fresh frozen plasma and other clotting factors, may be required for bleeding problems that need careful and exact diagnosis.

Definitive treatment strategies

In acute leukaemias the blast cell morphology, immunophenotype, and genotype are important factors in selection of treatment. For example, ALL and AML require different drug programmes, B-cell and T-cell leukaemias need to be treated differently from precursor ALL to achieve equivalent cure rates, and AML M3 uniquely responds to all-trans-retinoic acid (ATRA). With regard to genotype, children with hyperdiploid ALL or ALL expressing the TEL AML1 fusion gene are usually cured by antimetabolite-based therapy, while those with *bcr-abl*-positive ALL are not.

Acute myeloid leukaemia

The first month of treatment should ideally be undertaken in a specialist leukaemia centre. During this period intensive cytotoxic drug treatment is given, during which time there is no effective normal bone marrow function. The chemotherapy can therefore be delivered only within an environment that is capable of giving the very best state-of-the-art supportive therapy. Approximately 10% of patients die from bone marrow failure at this stage.

Remission-induction therapy consists of 1–2 courses of intensive drug treatment to achieve a complete remission. The two treatments are given 1 month apart and each requires an inpatient stay of 1 month. Usually, three intravenous drugs are given simultaneously for 7–10 days and then bone marrow recovery is awaited during the next 3 weeks. The main combination is anthracycline (daunorubicin or idarubicin) and cytosine arabinoside (ara-C), which results in complete remission rates of approximately 65%. A third drug, etoposide or 6-thioguanine, is often added, as an Australian study suggested that the addition of etoposide to the two-drug regimen yielded statistically significantly better disease-free survival (Bishop *et al.*, 1990). Some evidence suggest that idarubicin is superior to daunorubicin and that high-dose ara-C has a favourable impact on duration of remission. Post-remission therapy includes one or two courses of the same drugs to further reduce the subclinical tumour burden.

ATRA is standard treatment, together with cytotoxic chemotherapy, for patients with acute promyelocytic leukaemia.

Principles of bone marrow transplantation

In the late 1960s the Nobel Prize Laureate, Don Thomas, proposed and was successful in transplanting bone marrow from a sibling and curing the patient. Prior to bone marrow transplantation (BMT) patients should be in remission, at which time they are clinically well. They are then given very intensive treatment to destroy the few remaining leukaemia cells still present. Unfortunately, this destroys all their normal marrow, but they can be rescued with human leucocyte antigen (HLA)-matched sibling marrow. This marrow is accepted easily because the chemotherapy received by the patient also destroys any remaining immunity. The problems are that the intensive treatment is toxic and the donor marrow, which is in effect a new immune system, may attack the patient [graft-versus-host disease (GVHD)]. Enormous work has been undertaken over 20 years to optimize this form of transplant (allogeneic) and up to 70% of patients are now cured by this treatment (*Table 21.8*). Our longest survivor at the Royal Marsden Hospital (the first such transplant in Europe) has now been off all treatment for 28 years.

More recently, patients have had transplants using their own marrow (autologous BMT; *Table 21.9*). Patients in

Table 21.8. Success rates with allogeneic bone marrow transplantation in acute myeloid leukaemia

Patient type	Estimated cure rate (%)
Failed induction therapy	15–20
In second remission	30
In untreated first relapse	35
In first remission	40–70

Table 21.9. Overview of studies of autologous bone marrow transplantation in acute myeloid leukaemia

Therapy	Survival rate (%)
Chemotherapy	30–35
Autologous bone marrow transplantation	40–60

complete remission have 2% of their marrow removed and stored. All the remaining marrow cells are destroyed using intensive chemotherapy and the patients are then 'rescued' with the stored 2% marrow being reinfused after the chemotherapy. The principle of this treatment is that in the 2% of bone marrow that is harvested and reinfused, there are very few leukaemia cells and these may not survive the process of harvest, storage, and reinfusion, while the normal cells do.

Current situation with bone marrow transplantation
Many cancer centres in North America and Europe now offer autologous BMT to younger patients with AML who are in their first complete remission.

The situation concerning allogeneic BMT for AML is clear-cut. All patients under 55 years of age who have an HLA-matched sibling (one patient in three) should be offered an allogeneic BMT if they are in the first complete remission, and this should be optimally undertaken about 5 months after diagnosis.

Patients who do not have an HLA-matched sibling may receive allogeneic cells if a donor can be found from the matched, unrelated Anthony Nolan Panel.

Newer methods for bone marrow transplantation
Traditionally, bone marrow is harvested from the pelvis using multiple needle punctures while the donor is under general anaesthesia. During the past 5 years an alternative

source of cells, from the peripheral blood using a blood–cell separator, has been used. The bone marrow cells are made to pass into the peripheral circulation after stimulation using granulocyte colony stimulating factor (GCSF) given subcutaneously to the donor for a few days prior to collection. This source of cells produces faster recovery of the blood counts in the patient and is therefore cheaper, easier, and safer. It also probably produces a greater immunotherapy effect than bone marrow cells, which helps prevent leukaemic relapse (graft-versus-leukaemia effect).

Acute lymphoblastic leukaemia
It is commonly perceived that ALL is the leukaemia of childhood, but it occurs in even larger total numbers in adults. The childhood variety was the first success story of a cure in cancer, and even now most children are cured with chemotherapy alone (up to 75%). However, unlike in AML, these children need up to 2 years of maintenance chemotherapy after the initial period in hospital. For adults the treatment is more like that for AML, as all patients require several periods of treatment in hospital for intensive chemotherapy and/or BMT.

Induction of remission
Treatment usually consists of a regimen that includes a combination of vincristine, prednisolone, and anthracycline, with or without asparaginase, which results in a complete remission rate of up to 80%. Once complete remission has been achieved, additional courses of chemotherapy are given as consolidation (ara-C, etoposide, teniposide, and cyclophosphamide).

Central nervous system prophylaxis
Central nervous system (CNS) prophylaxis is an important part of the treatment of patients with ALL. Combined cranial radiotherapy and intrathecal administration of methotrexate (MTX) reduces the risk of CNS relapse to approximately 5%. Leucoencephalopathy is a rare but serious complication that results from white matter degeneration and necrosis associated with intrathecal MTX therapy and cranial radiotherapy. In view of complications of radiotherapy, some centres use high-dose intravenous MTX $(1–3g/m^2)$ with leucovorin rescue together with intrathecal MTX as a substitute for radiation. Combination triple intrathecal chemotherapy with MTX, ara-C and hydrocortisone is employed to treat meningeal disease.

Maintenance therapy
Even after several months of relatively intensive treatment some leukaemia cells remain, and the strategy to eradicate

these is long-term administration of continuous low-dose oral chemotherapy for a period of 2–3 years (daily 6-mercaptopurine and weekly MTX, both given orally). Periodic intensification with vincristine and prednisolone is used by some centres.

Transplantation
The main aspects are:

- The role of allogeneic BMT in patients who have ALL is in the treatment of patients with unfavourable cytogenetics – Philadelphia chromosome-positive (Ph +ve), L3 morphology, and very high presenting WBC count.
- Increasingly, a role for autologous BMT for adult patients with ALL appears to be as a form of intensive chemotherapy that can delivered safely.
- Patients with adult ALL autografted in first complete remission have a long-term leukaemia-free survival (LFS) of 30–40%, which when followed by maintenance chemotherapy for 2 years results in a LFS of 56% at 5 years.

Chronic Leukaemias

In contrast to the acute leukaemias, chronic leukaemias exhibit an accumulation of morphologically mature rather than immature cells in the lymphoid or myeloid cell lines. Since maturing cells have less capacity for division, lower growth fractions are presumed to be a reason for their resistance to cure by chemotherapy aimed at dividing cells.

Chronic myeloid leukaemia
Chronic myeloid leukaemia (CML) is a relatively rare form of leukaemia characterized by presentation with a very large spleen and a high WBC count. Until recently it was incurable and had a chronic progressive course.

Incidence
The incidence is 1.3 per 100,000 people per year and the age-related incidence is higher in men than in women.

Aetiology
No clear correlation with exposure to cytotoxic drugs has been found, but there is an effect of radiation. Cigarette smoking accelerates the progression to blast crises and therefore has an adverse effect on survival.

Clinical presentation
Quite a few patients are diagnosed while still asymptomatic during health screening tests. Presenting features include fatigue, malaise, weight loss, or symptoms relating to splenic enlargement, which is sometimes massive and results in abdominal enlargement and pain. Occasionally, the presenting feature is severe abdominal pain from a splenic infarct. Patients often have high WBC counts, which may sometimes be so raised as to produce leucostatic manifestations with impaired cerebral optic coronary and splenic blood flow. Over a matter or hours such patients can become critically ill with cerebral infarcts, cardiac arrhythmia, and sudden death. Priapism is an unusual but extremely distressing problem that can produce long-term difficulties in the patient who survives. The white cells are mature and continue to function, so that patients have more than enough neutrophils to fight infection. Thus, infectious problems are not a feature of CML. The same applies to platelet production; platelets are found in abundance and function well, so bleeding is not a problem.

Occasionally, CML presents in a form that has 'evolved' into an acute leukaemia (see below).

Haematological findings
Increased WBC counts with various degrees of immaturity of the granulocytic series are found, and usually circulating blasts are <5%. Platelet counts are almost always elevated at diagnosis and a mild degree of normocytic, normochromic anaemia is present. Leucocyte alkaline phosphatase is characteristically low in CML. Serum levels of vitamin B_{12} and vitamin B_{12}-binding proteins are increased. Increased histamine production secondary to basophilia may occur in later stages and cause diarrhoea and flushing.

At diagnosis bone marrow cellularity may be increased, primarily of the myeloid and megakaryocytic lineages, with an altered myeloid to erythroid ratio.

Over a period of time, usually approximately 3 years, the disease evolves into a form of acute leukaemia that produces bone marrow failure and is very difficult to treat. Average survival, even with supportive therapy and drugs, is <6 weeks when this occurs. This evolution is called blast crises and is diagnosed when there are >30% blasts in the peripheral blood or bone marrow.

Chromosomal findings
The cytogenetic hallmark of CML found in 90–95% of cases is a translocation of the short arm of chromosome 9 to the long arm of chromosome 22, the t(9;22) (q34;q11). The product of the fusion gene resulting from t(9;22) is believed to play a central role in the initial development of CML.

Table 21.10. Response criteria in chronic myeloid leukaemia

	Response	Criteria
Haematological	Complete response	White blood cells $<10 \times 10^9/l$, normal morphology
		Normal haemoglobin and platelet counts
	Incomplete response	White blood cells $\geq 10 \times 10^9/l$
Cytogenetic		[percentage of marrow metaphases with t(9;22)]
	Complete response	0
	Partial response	≥ 35
	Minor response	36–85
	No response	85–100
Molecular		Presence of bcr-abl transcript by reverse-transcriptase
		polymerase chain reaction
	Complete response	None
	Partial response	Any

Prognostic factors

Median survival is about 4 years. The Sokal index identifies percentages of circulating blasts, spleen size, platelet count, cytogenetic clonal evolution, and age as the most important prognostic indicators (Sokal *et al.*, 1984).

Management

The goal of treatment is firstly to obtain immediate control of symptoms caused by the high WBC count and large spleen. This usually takes 3–4 weeks, and over the next 6 months additional methods may be used to attain molecular remission and cure, particularly for patients under 55 years of age. The response criteria are shown in *Table 21.10.*

Immediate treatment

New patients with very high WBC counts ($>150 \times 10^9/l$), with or without problems associated with leucostasis, should have emergency leukapheresis using a blood–cell separator, which can be life-saving. Under no circumstances should these patients be given red cells before leukapheresis, regardless of how anaemic they are, because this leads to further haemoconcentration and may precipitate a catastrophic cerebral event. If a patient has leucostasis and is very ill, it may be life-saving simply to bleed the patient into a bag and replace the blood with saline.

Chemotherapy

For patients with high WBC counts at presentation allopurinol should be given for 24 hours, after which hydroxyurea should be started at an initial dose of 1–4g/day, and the dose reduced by half with each 50% reduction of the leucocyte count. Cytological remissions with hydroxyurea are uncommon. Intensive combination chemotherapy has also been used in chronic-phase CML; 30–50% of patients achieve complete cytogenetic responses, and this can be used as a stepping stone to an autologous transplant (see below).

Allogeneic bone marrow transplantation

BMT is the only curative therapy for CML and, when feasible, is the treatment of choice. It has become clear that patients should be relatively young (less than 65 years) and have a healthy and histocompatible donor. Survival following BMT in the accelerated and blastic phases of the disease is significantly worse and associated with a very high rate of relapse. The Seattle data demonstrate that transplantation early in the chronic phase (1–2 years from diagnosis) is superior to later transplant.

Autologous bone marrow transplantation

The problem with the an autologous transplant in CML depends is the ability to obtain a complete cytogenetic remission (i.e. Ph −ve), so that suitable cells can be collected for rescue.

A retrospective analysis of over 200 autografts performed for CML at eight centres worldwide suggests that autografts prolong survival in both the chronic or accelerated phases of the disease, when compared retrospectively with conventional therapy. The median duration of cytogenetic remission was 14 months (range, 2–68 months).

Approaches to the treatment of minimal residual disease following autografting, such as immune modulation, are currently being investigated.

Leukapheresis and splenectomy

Intensive leukapheresis may control blood counts in chronic-phase CML and should be reserved for emergencies in which leucostasis-related complications such as pulmonary failure or cerebrovascular accidents are likely. It may also help pregnant, women in whom it is important to avoid potentially teratogenic drugs. Splenectomy is now reserved for symptomatic relief of painful splenomegaly unresponsive to chemotherapy or for signs of hypersplenism. Splenic radiation is used on rare occasions to reduce the size of the spleen.

Treatment of blast crisis

Treatment depends on the phenotype of the blast cells, myeloid or lymphoid, and therefore AML or ALL regimens are used, respectively. Erythroid blast crisis is also treated as for AML.

Post-transplantation treatment

Evidence of an immunologically mediated graft-versus-leukaemia effect is provided by the observation that donor leucocyte infusions without prior chemotherapy or GVHD prophylaxis can induce haematological and cytogenetic remissions in CML patients who have relapsed after allogeneic BMT.

Interferon

When allogeneic BMT is not feasible, interferon alfa therapy is the treatment of choice. Haematological remissions are generally achieved within 1–2 months of starting interferon alfa. Cytogenetic response generally start at 3–12 months and complete cytogenetic responses, which occur in up to 26% of patients, may require 6 months to 4 years of treatment.

STI-571

An experimental drug (signal transduction inhibitor STI-571), specifically designed to inhibit the excessive tyrosine kinase activity in CML cells, has been found to be very effective in producing complete molecular remissions. It is now licensed for use in patients with CML refractory or intolerant to interferon. 60% of the patients attain major cytogenic response, which is complete in about 40% of patients.

Chronic lymphocytic leukaemia

Chronic lymphocytic leukaemia (CLL) is a disease that only really becomes common after 70 years of age, and for the majority of patients who are elderly it is a relatively benign disease.

Incidence

The most common chronic leukaemia is B-cell CLL, which presents with an asymptomatic lymphocytosis in patients with a median age of 60 years.

Diagnosis

Diagnosis is often made incidentally from a persistent lymphocytosis ($>5 \times 10^9$/l). CLL cells are generally clonal populations of mature B-lymphocytes that exhibit monoclonal surface immunoglobulin. An unusual feature is expression of the CD5 membrane antigen seen on mature T-lymphocytes.

Clinical course

Cells accumulate slowly in the bone marrow, spleen, liver, and lymph nodes. Approximately half of all CLL patients exhibit decreased immunoglobulin production and show an increased susceptibility to infection.

The disease course is dependent on the leukaemia burden, which can be assessed by clinical staging systems such as that proposed by Rai *et al.*, 1975 and Binet *et al.*, 1981 (*Table 21.11*).

Occasionally, CLL transforms into a clinically and morphologically more aggressive phase that resembles prolymphocytic leukaemia, and 5% of CLL patients subsequently develop a large-cell lymphoma (Richter's syndrome).

Treatment

A proportion of patients remain asymptomatic and do not need any treatment, eventually dying from an unrelated cause. In the rest of the patients, the disease can usually be kept under control for 9–10 years, infection being the predominant cause of death.

For patients over 55 years of age no advantage is gained from starting treatment unless there is a clinical indication such as anaemia, recurrent infection, bleeding, bulky lymphadenopathy, or increasing splenomegaly.

Choices for initial therapy are many, but generally involve alkylating agents given daily or in a pulsed fashion with or without prednisone. The most commonly used drug is chlorambucil, which results in complete response rates of 25%, response duration of 2 years, and median survival of 4 years.

The nucleoside analogues fludarabine, pentostatin, and cladribine are very active in CLL. In previously treated patients the response rate to fludarabine is around 50% (15% complete remission, 40% partial response). In previously untreated patients, complete remission rates are over 30% with 45% partial responses. Intravenous immunoglobulin has been given to patients who are hypogammaglobu-

Table 21.11. *Staging of B-cell chronic lymphocytic leukaemia and relation to survival*

Classification	Stage	Clinical features	Median survival (years)
Rai	0	Lymphocytosis	12
	I	Lymphocytosis + adenopathy	9
	II	Lymphocytosis + splenomegaly	7
	III	Anaemia	1–2
	IV	Thrombocytopenia	1–2
Binet	A	No anaemia or thrombocytopenia, <3 nodes involved	>10
	B	No anaemia or thrombocytopenia, >3 nodes involved	5
	C	Anaemia and/or thrombocytopenia,	2

linaemic. In these studies a significant decrease in serious infections occurred, but the treatment is very costly. Early results with autologous and allogeneic BMT in CLL are encouraging, but a longer follow-up is necessary.

Multiple myeloma

Multiple myeloma represents a malignant proliferation of plasma cells derived from a single clone.

Aetiology

The cause of myeloma is not known, though it has been associated with radiation and exposure to petroleum products.

Incidence

Myeloma increases in incidence with age. The median age at diagnosis is 68 years and it is rare under 40 years of age. The yearly incidence is around four per 100,000, and males are slightly more commonly affected than females.

Diagnosis and staging

Myeloma can be a very insidious disease, presenting with vague symptoms of back pain and recurrent infections. Osteoporosis, vertebral collapse, and hypercalcaemia can occur and some patients present with renal failure (*Table 21.12*). Occasionally, hyperviscosity occurs with consequent CNS signs – this is most often encountered when the M component is IgM.

The classic triad of myeloma is marrow plasmacytosis (more than 10%), lytic bone lesions, and a serum and/or urine M component on electrophoresis (IgG, A, M, D, E). Diagnosis may be made in the absence of bone lesions if the plasmacytosis is associated with a high or progressive increase in M component over time, or if extramedullary mass lesions develop.

The staging system for patients with myeloma is a functional system for predicting survival and is based on a variety of clinical and laboratory tests (*Table 21.13*).

Variants of myeloma

Solitary bone plasmacytoma and extramedullary plasmacytoma are associated with an M component in fewer than 30% of cases, affect younger individuals, and are associated with median survivals of 10 years or more. Both tumours are highly responsive to local radiation therapy and if an M component is present it should disappear after treatment. Solitary bone plasmacytomas may recur in other bony sites or evolve into myeloma. Extramedullary plasmacytomas rarely recur or progress.

Monoclonal gammopathy of uncertain significance

The most difficult differential diagnosis in patients with myeloma involves the separation from individuals with benign monoclonal gammopathy of uncertain significance (MGUS), previously known as benign paraproteinaemias. MGUS occurs in 1% of the population over 50 years of age, and in up to 10% over 75 years of age. Patients with MGUS usually have <10% plasma cells in the bone marrow, less than 30g/l of M component, no urinary Bence Jones protein, and no anaemia, renal failure, lytic bone lesions, or hypercalcaemia. Patients with MGUS require no treatment and their survival is about 2 years shorter than age-matched controls in the general population who do not have MGUS.

Investigations

A full blood count with differential is obtained, as is the erythrocyte sedimentation rate (ESR). The ESR is often elevated, and in the differential count plasma cells can be seen.

Table 21.12. *Pathogenesis and clinical manifestations of multiple myeloma*

Clinical finding	Underlying cause	Pathogenic mechanism
Hypercalcaemia, pathologic fractures, cord compression, lytic bone lesions, osteoporosis, bone pain	Skeletal destruction	Tumour expansion; production of osteoclast activating factors (OAF) by tumour cells
Renal failure	Light chain proteinuria, hypercalcaemia, urate nephropathy, amyloid glomerulopathy (rare) Pyelonephritis	Toxic effects of tumour products, light chains, OAF, DNA breakdown products Hypogammaglobulinaemia
Anaemia	Myelophthisis, decreased production, increased destruction	Tumour expansion; production of inhibitory factors and autoantibodies by tumour cells
Infection	Hypogammaglobulinemia, decreased neutrophil migration	Decreased production due to tumour-induced suppression; increased IgG catabolism
Neurological symptoms	Hyperviscosity, cryoglobulins, amyloid deposits Hypercalcaemia, cord compression	Products of tumour; properties of M component; light chains OAF
Bleeding	Interference with clotting factors, amyloid damage of endothelium, platelet dysfunction	Products of tumour; antibodies to clotting factors; light chains; antibody coating of platelets
Mass lesions		Tumour expansion

A diagnosis of plasma cell leukaemia is made if there are >2000 plasma cells/μl. This may be seen in disproportionate frequency in IgD and IgE myeloma.

Serum calcium, urea, nitrogen, creatinine, and uric acid levels may be increased. Protein electrophoresis followed by immunofixation is carried out to detect paraprotein and measure serum immunoglobulins. Urine electrophoreses is required for Bence Jones proteinuria. Serum alkaline phosphatase is usually normal, even with extensive bone involvement, because of absence of osteoblastic activity. β_2-microglobulin is an important prognostic marker, but is elevated in patients with renal failure and those on interferon maintenance therapy.

A skeletal survey is carried out, and a bone marrow aspirate obtained to show plasma cell infiltration. A marrow biopsy is required for cellularity, light chain restriction studies, and amyloid staining.

If AL amyloidosis is suspected a serum amyloid protein scan is obtained. The serum M component will be IgG in 53%, IgA in 25%, IgD in 1%; 20% of patients have only light chains in serum or urine.

A small proportion of patients may have non-secretory multiple myeloma with no M component or light chains in the urine. They usually have extensive bone marrow involvement and often lytic lesions in the bones.

Treatment

Of patients with myeloma, 10% have an indolent course and demonstrate only very slow progression of the disease over many years. Such patients require anti-tumour treatment only when the serum M component rises above 50g/l or progressive bone lesions develop.

All patients with stage II or III disease, and stage I patients who exhibit Bence Jones proteinuria, progressive lytic bone lesions, vertebral compression fractures, recurrent infections, or a rising serum M component, should be treated with systemic combination chemotherapy.

Early initial supportive care
When patients first present to their GPs with myeloma it is usually with back pain, pain in other bony areas, and/or intercurrent infections. The presentation can often be indo-

Table 21.13. Myeloma staging system

Stage	Criteria	Estimated tumour burden ($\propto 10^{12}$ cells/m²)
I	All the following: Haemoglobin >100g/l (>10g/dl)	<0.6 (low)
	Serum calcium <3 mmol/L (<12 mg/dL)	
	Normal bone radiograph or solitary lesion	
	Low M-component production:	
	IgG level <50g/l (<5g/dl)	
	IgA level <30g/l (<3g/dl)	
	Urine light chain <4g/24h	
II	Fitting neither I nor III	0.6–1.20 (intermediate)
III	One or more of the following:	
	Haemoglobin <85g/l (<8.5g/dl)	
	Serum calcium >3mmol/l (>12mg/dl)	
	Advanced lytic bone lesions	
	High M-component production: IgG level >70g/l (>7g/dl)	
	IgA level >50g/l (>5g/dl)	
	Urine light chain >12g/24h	>1.20 (high)

Subclassification based on serum creatinine levels

Level	Stage	Median survival (months)	
A <177μmol/l	IA	61	
B >177μmol/l	IIA,B	55	
	IIIA	30	
	IIIB	61	15

Staging based on serum β₂-microglobulin levels

Level	Stage	Median survival (months)
<0.004g/l	I	43
>0.004g/l	II	12

lent and then suddenly cascade into a desperate situation of a patient who is very ill with hypercalcaemia, uraemia, dehydration, and infection. Survival at this time will be 1–2 days with no acute medical support. Hypercalcaemia generally responds to corticosteroid therapy, hydration, and bisphosphonates.

In the event of acute renal failure, plasmapheresis is approximately 10 times more effective at clearing light chains than peritoneal dialysis, and acutely reducing the protein load results in functional improvement. Plasmapheresis may also be the treatment of choice for hyperviscosity syndromes.

Infections need aggressive treatment with broad-spectrum intravenous antibiotics. Patients can develop cord compression which may require urgent radiotherapy or surgery.

The role of surgery for the prophylactic nailing and pinning of lesions that occupy more than 50% of the circumference of the long bones is important and can be undertaken, like radiotherapy, at the same time as chemotherapy.

Key points: leukaemia and myeloma

Leukaemia

75% occur in patients over 60 years of age, but patients of any age can be affected

Risk factors include previous chemotherapy and/or radiotherapy and exposure to radiation

Most cases are diagnosed following a blood count undertaken because of symptoms and/or signs of bone marrow failure (fatigue, pallor, bruising, bleeding, infections, etc.)

Some leukaemias may present with lymphadenopathy and/or hepatosplenomegaly

Myeloma

99% of patients are over 40 years of age and 95% are over 50 years of age

Clinical features include:

   bone pain with or without bone fractures

   symptoms of anaemia

Renal impairment

Erythrocyte sedimentation rate or plasma viscosity may be grossly elevated

Reproduced from England Department of Health Cancer Referral Guidelines Consultation Document May 2000.

Guidelines for urgent referral: haematological malignancies

Blood count and/or film suggestive of leukaemia: anaemia ± abnormal white blood cell counts (high or low) ± low platelet count

Lymphadenopathy (>1cm) persisting for 6 weeks

Hepatosplenomegaly

Bone pain associated with anaemia and raised erythrocyte sedimentation rate (or plasma viscosity)

Bone radiographs reported as being suggestive of myeloma

Constellation of three or more of the following symptoms: fatigue, night sweats, weight loss, itching, pain on drinking alcohol, breathlessness, bruising, recurrent infections, bone pain

Definitive treatment

The standard treatment previously consisted of intermittent pulses of melphalan and prednisolone, but it did not result in complete remissions although the overall response rate was 40–60%.

Most centres in Europe and the USA now use infusional combination chemotherapy via a Hickman line with vincristine, doxorubicin, and methylprednisolone given over about 5 months followed by one or two courses of high dose melphalan 200mg/m^2 and an autologous transplant. The patient requires 1 month in hospital for each course of high-dose therapy. Complete remissions are obtained with this programme in 50–75% of patients. These complete remissions are associated with symptomatic responses, such as reduction in bone pain and sometimes also healing of bone lesions.

A French randomized study showed that when conventional chemotherapy is compared with high-dose treatment, the median disease-free and overall survival is significantly better in the high-dose therapy patients. It is possible to give high-dose chemotherapy to patients who are more than 65 years of age

Preliminary results from the French randomized study to compare the single versus double transplants post-infusional chemotherapy have shown benefit with double transplants.

Maintenance therapy

Maintenance therapy with interferon may prolong the duration of response, and a recent analysis by the Oxford group demonstrated that it also significantly prolongs overall survival by 6–7 months.

Referral proforma: haematological malignancies

Age:

Malignancy suspected

Leukaemia	☐
Lymphoma (Hodgkin's disease or non-Hodgkin's lymphoma)	☐
Myeloma	☐

Symptoms	Yes	No	
Fatigue			
Night sweats			
Weight loss			
Itching			
Pain on drinking alcohol			
Breathlessness			
Bruising			
Recurrent infections			
Bone pain			

Clinical examination	Yes	No	
Pallor			
Lymph nodes:			
neck			
axilla			
groin			
other			
Hepatomegaly			
Splenomegaly			
Bruising and/or petechia			
Stomatitis and/or mouth ulcers			

Investigations

Haemoglobin..

White cell count...

Platelets...

Erythrocyte sedimentation rate..

Chest radiography..

Comments/other reasons for referral:

Reproduced from England Department of Health Cancer Referral Guidelines Consultation Document May 2000.

With sequential therapy (i.e. infusional chemotherapy followed by consolidation with high-dose melphalan with autologous stem cell rescue and interferon maintenance), the median overall survival ranges from 5 to 6 years and the median event-free survival is 3–4 years. Patients who attain complete remission do significantly better than those who do not.

Bisphosphonates
Compelling evidence now indicates that bisphosphonates (clodronate, pamidronate) given at all stages during the management of myeloma reduce bone damage and symptoms, and in the remission phase may even be associated with bone healing. Patients benefit symptomatically in terms of pain control, and there is early evidence that bisphosphonates, by making bones more normal, prevent myeloma cells proliferating and so help to treat the underlying disease.

Allogeneic bone marrow transplantation
Patients under 55 years of age who have a histocompatible sibling may be given the opportunity of an allogeneic BMT early in the management of their disease. Approximately 50% of patients given this treatment are cured by the procedure, but only if their disease is not far advanced and they have not had extensive previous treatment.

Conclusions

Enormous advances have been made in the management of leukaemias and myeloma over the past two decades, with responses to treatment now being not only curative but also giving to patients a quality of life that is normal in terms of activities, occupations, and family life.

Further Reading

Binet JL, Auquier A, Dighiero G, *et al.* A new prognostic classification of chronic lymphocytic leukemia derived from a multivariate survival analysis. *Cancer.* 1981; **48**: 198–206.

Bishop JF, Lowenthal RM, Joshua D, *et al.* Etoposide in acute nonlymphocytic leukemia. Australian Leukemia Study Group. *Blood.* 1990; **75**: 27–32.

Mehta J, Singhal S (eds). *Myeloma.* London: Martin Dunitz, 2002.

Rai KR, Sawitsky A, Cronkite EP, *et al.* Clinical staging of chronic lymphocytic leukemia. *Blood.* 1975; **46**: 219–34.

Sokal JE, Cox EB, Baccarani M, *et al.* Prognostic discrimination in 'good-risk' chronic granulocytic leukemia. *Blood.* 1984; **63**: 789–99.

22 Lymphoma

Nick Maisey and David Cunningham

Overview, key points

- Lymphomas are rare malignancies
- The majority are idiopathic
- Biopsy samples are necessary for diagnosis
- A large proportion of patients are curable

Incidence

Incidence, key points

- Lymphoma is more common in males
- Hodgkin's disease has a bimodal age distribution
- Non-Hodgkin's disease is more frequent in older patients

Non-Hodgkin's lymphomas (NHL) represent approximately 3–5% of malignant deaths in developed countries, with an annual UK incidence of 8240 and a mortality of 4317. The incidence and mortality of Hodgkin's disease is approximately one-third to one-half of that of NHL. The majority of cases are male in both Hodgkin's disease and NHL. Hodgkin's disease has a characteristic bimodal distribution, with incidence peaks in young adults and a later peak in older adults. The age distribution of NHLs varies between different histological subgroups and countries, with a higher incidence of high-grade lymphomas in the younger population and lower-grade lymphomas being more common in the elderly. Various statistics relating to NHL and Hodgkin's disease are shown in *Figures 22.1* and *22.2*.

Pathology

Pathology, key points

- The WHO adaptation of the Revised European and American Lymphoma (REAL) classification covers both Hodgkin's disease and NHL (*Table 22.1*)
- Lymphomas are subdivided according to cell type and morphology
- Several causes of lymph node enlargement may mimic lymphoma (*Table 22.2*)

Hodgkin's lymphoma
The malignant cells (mononuclear Hodgkin and multinucleate Reed–Sternberg cells) form the minority of the tumour mass, the rest of which is composed of inflammatory and fibrotic tissue. The Reed–Sternberg cell is not pathognomonic for Hodgkin's disease and may be seen in other conditions. The WHO classification describes classical Hodgkin's lymphoma (consisting of Nodular sclerosis Hodgkin's lymphoma, Lymphocyte-rich classical Hodgkin's lymphoma, Mixed cellularity Hodgkin's lymphoma and Lymphocyte depletion Hodgkin's lymphoma) as well as Nodular lymphocyte predominance Hodgkin's lymphoma.

Non-Hodgkin's lymphoma
Classification is based on the morphological appearances, and for practical purposes can be divided into low-grade and high-grade lymphomas. The low-grade lymphomas (small lymphocytic and follicular lymphoma) tend to be indolent in behaviour and responsive to chemotherapy, but are rarely curable. High-grade lymphomas (the majority being diffuse large B-cell lymphomas) are generally more aggressive, and a large proportion are curable. Rarer subtypes include mantle-zone lymphoma, mucosal-associated lymphoid tissue (MALT) lymphoma, lymphoblastic lymphoma, Burkitt's lymphoma, and T-cell lymphomas.

Aetiology

Aetiology, key points

- Viruses may play a role in the development of lymphoma (e.g. Epstein–Barr virus, human immunodeficiency virus, human T-cell leukaemia/lymphoma virus 1 and/or 2)
- Some genetic factors have been identified
- Several conditions (congenital and acquired) predispose to the development of non-Hodgkin's disease

NON-HODGKIN'S LYMPHOMA STATISTICS

New Non-Hodgkin's lymphoma

New Non-Hodgkin's lymphoma per annum

3.4%

Non-Hodgkin's lymphoma

All new cancers per annum

New cases per annum	8240
Males rank	6
Females rank	8
Deaths per annum	4470

Incidence

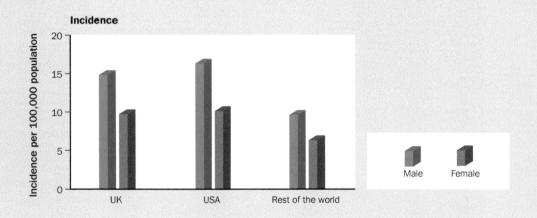

Incidence per 100,000 population

UK   USA   Rest of the world

Male   Female

Survival rate

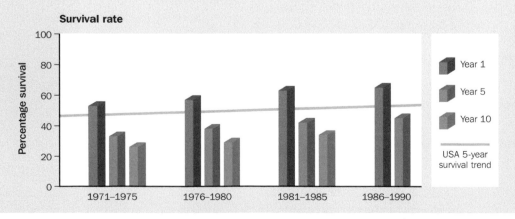

Percentage survival

1971–1975   1976–1980   1981–1985   1986–1990

Year 1

Year 5

Year 10

USA 5-year survival trend

Figure 22.1. *Statistical data relating to non-Hodgkin's lymphoma.*

HODGKIN'S DISEASE STATISTICS

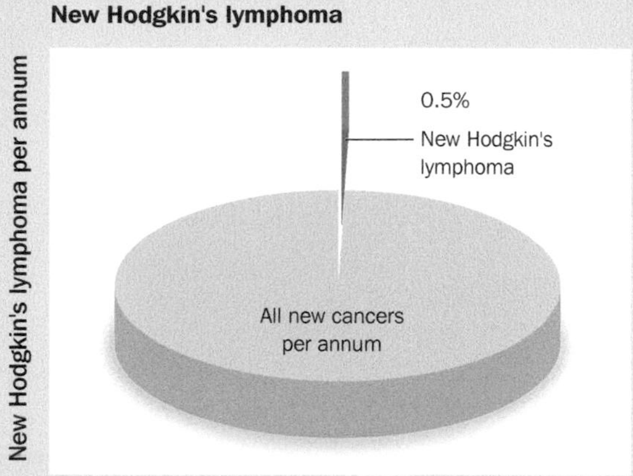

New cases per annum	1140
Males rank	16
Females rank	19
Deaths per annum	306

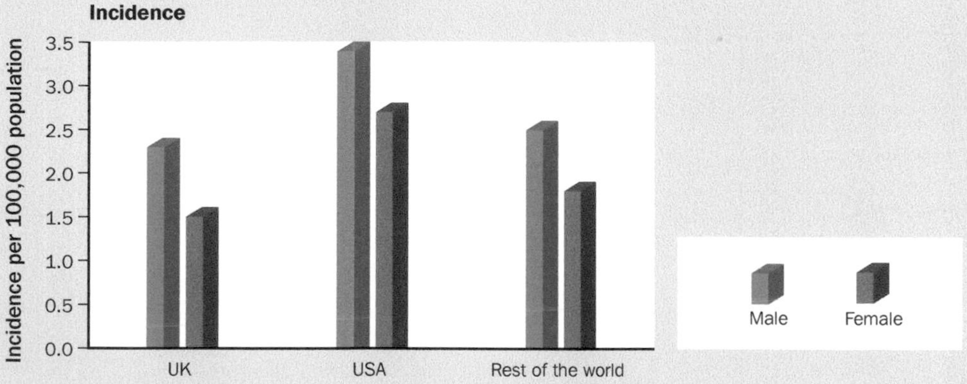

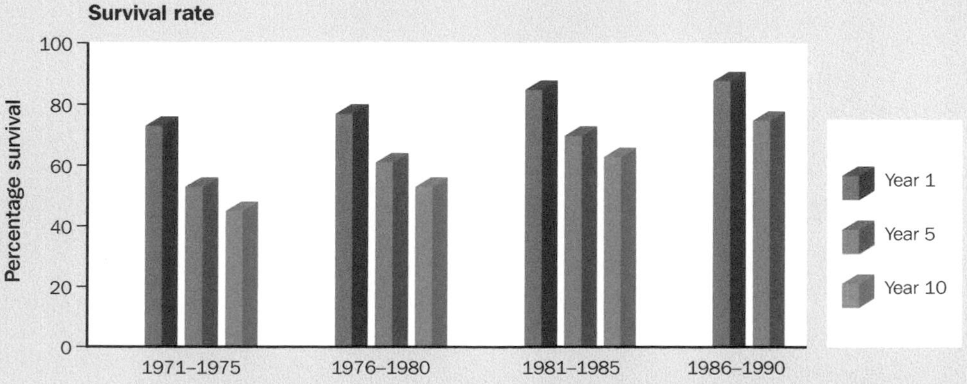

Figure 22.2. *Statistical data relating to Hodgkin's disease.*

Table 22.1 *The WHO adaptation of the Revised European and American Lymphoma classification of lymphomas*

B-cell neoplasms

Precursor B-cell neoplasm
    Precursor B-lymphoblastic leukemia/lymphoma
Mature (peripheral) B-cell neoplasms
    B-cell chronic lymphocytic leukemia / small lymphocytic lymphoma
    B-cell prolymphocytic leukemia
    Lymphoplasmacytic lymphoma
    Splenic marginal zone B-cell lymphoma (+/- villous lymphocytes)
    Hairy cell leuekmia
    Plasma cell myeloma/plasmacytoma
    Extranodal marginal zone B-cell lymphoma of mucosa-associated lymphoid tissue type
    Nodal marginal zone lymphoma (+/- monocytoid B-cells)
    Follicle center lymphoma, follicular,
    Mantle cell lymphoma
    Diffuse large cell B-cell lymphoma
    • Medlastinal large B-cell lymphoma
    • Primary effusion lymphoma
    Burkitt's lymphoma/Burkitt's cell leukemia

T-cell and natural killer cell neoplasms

Precursor T cell neoplasm
    Precursor T-lymphoblastic lymphoma/leukemia
Mature (peripheral) T cell and NK-cell neoplasms
    T cell prolymphocytic leukemia
    T-cell granular lymphocytic leukemia
    Aggressive NK-Cell leukemia
    Adult T cell lymphoma/leukemia (HTLV1+)
    Extranodal NK/T-cell lymphoma, nasal type
    Enteropathy-type T-cell lymphoma
    Hepatosplenic gamma-delta T-cell lymphoma
    Subcutaneous panniculitis-like T-cell lymphoma
    Mycosis fungoides/Sézary's syndrome
    Anaplastic large cell lymphoma, T/null cell, primary cutaneous type
    Peripheral T cell lymphoma, not otherwise characterized
    Angioimmunoblastic T cell lymphoma
    Anaplastic large cell lymphoma, T/null cell, primary systemic type

Hodgkin's lymphoma (Hodgkin's disease)

    Nodular lymphocyte predominance Hodgkin's lymphoma
    Classical Hodgkin's lymphoma
    • Nodular sclerosis Hodgkin's lymphoma
    • Lymphocyte-rich classical Hodgkin's lymphoma
    • Mixed cellularity Hodgkin's lymphoma
    • Lymphocyte depletion Hodgkin's lymphoma

Table 22.2. *Lymph node histology simulating lymphoma*

Follicular histology

Reactive hyperplasia
Rheumatoid arthritis
Toxoplasmosis
Angiofollicular hyperplasia

Diffuse histology

Phenytoin treatment
Dermatopathic lymphadenopathy
Angioimmunoblastic lymphadenopathy with dysproteinaemia
Metastatic carcinoma or melanoma

Others

Sinus histocytosis with massive lymph-node enlargement
Infectious mononucleosis (Epstein–Barr virus infection)
Cat scratch fever
Metastatic carcinoma or melanoma

Hodgkin's disease

Familial clustering and the increased risk that a sibling will develop the disease suggest a possible genetic predisposition. Individuals with the human leucocyte antigen-A1 (HLA-A1) histocompatibility antigen have a marginally increased frequency, and HLA-A12 is more common in young patients with disease of good prognosis. In young patients, Hodgkin's disease appears to be more common in socially disadvantaged groups, whereas in the older population, higher social classes seem to be more at risk.

One possible aetiological factor is infection with the Epstein–Barr virus (EBV). The EBV genome has been detected in up to 40% of cases and Reed–Sternberg cells commonly express the EBV latent membrane protein.

The recent increase in the incidence of human immunodeficiency virus (HIV) and acquired deficiency syndrome (AIDS) has also been associated with an increase in Hodgkin's disease.

Non-Hodgkin's lymphoma

Both congenital and acquired disorders have been identified as predisposing to the development of NHL (*Table 22.3*). The incidence is increased in patients with immune suppression, such as recipients of renal allografts and patients with AIDS (the majority being B-cell in origin).

The majority of cases of Burkitt's lymphoma in equatorial Africa show anti-EBV serology. Other viral agents have been identified as possible causal factors, including human T-cell leukaemia/lymphoma virus 1 and/or 2 (HTLV 1/2) and HIV

Genetic abnormalities are commonly identified, such as the translocation t18:14 in Burkitt's lymphoma and the translocation t14:18 in follicular lymphoma.

Clinical Presentation

Clinical presentation, key points

- Most patients present with painless lymphadenopathy
- Lymph node enlargement may cause obstructive symptoms
- Patients may have 'B' symptoms (fever, sweats, or weight loss)

The most common presentation of both Hodgkin's disease and NHL is painless nodal enlargement. The most common site is the neck, and nodes may fluctuate in size, which delays diagnosis. Nodal compression of anatomical structures may be the presenting feature (more commonly in NHL). Retroperitoneal disease may present as backache, obstructive renal failure, or obstructive jaundice. 'B' symptoms of lymphoma (fever, sweats, and weight loss of more 10% of body weight) are not infrequent. Rarer forms of presentation include pruritus, pyrexia of unknown origin, skin involvement (both by cutaneous lymphoma and by associated rashes such as erythroderma, erythema multiforme, psoriasiform rashes, and bullous eruptions), and bone marrow involvement with associated anaemia, thrombocytopenia, or leucopenia. Wheezing and haemoptysis may be caused by endobronchial involvement, and a pleural effusion may follow direct pleural involvement or obstruction of the lymphatic drainage. Very occasionally, central nervous system (CNS) involvement may be the presenting feature.

Investigations

Investigations, key points

- Baseline blood tests and chest radiography should be performed in general practice
- Biopsy is required for definitive diagnosis
- Staging is important to optimize therapy

Table 22.3. Disorders known to predispose to the development of non-Hodgkin's lymphoma

Congenital
Coeliac disease
Ataxia telangiectasia
Klinefelter's syndrome
Wiskott–Aldrich syndrome
Chédiak–Higashi syndrome
Swiss-type agammaglobulinaemia

Acquired
Chronic immune suppression (e.g. renal transplant recipients)
Acquired immunodeficiency syndrome
Rheumatoid arthritis
Sjögren's syndrome

Investigations of a patient who has suspected lymphoma aim both to establish a precise diagnosis and to stage the patient accurately according to the widely used Ann Arbor staging classification (*Table 22.4*).

Table 22.4. The Ann Arbor staging classification for lymphomas

Stage[a]	Description
I	Involvement of a single lymph node region or a single extralymphatic site or organ (stage IE)
II	Involvement of two or more lymph node regions on the same side of the diaphragm, or of a localized extranodal involvement and one or more lymph node regions on the same side of the diaphragm (stage IIE)
III	Involvement of lymph nodes on both sides of the diaphragm, which may include the spleen (stage IIIS), a localized extranodal site (stage IIIE), or both (stage IIISE)
IV	Diffuse involvement of one or more extralymphatic organ

[a]Suffix A, no constitutional or B symptoms (i.e. fever, night sweats and/or loss of more than 10% of body weight over 6 months).

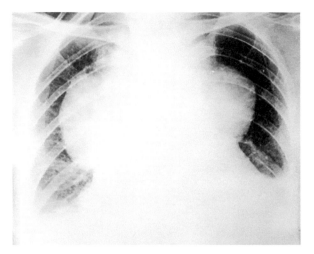

Figure 22.3. *Chest radiograph demonstrating bulky hilar lymphadenopathy in a patient with nn-Hodgkin's lymphoma.*

General practice
Blood tests

The full blood count (FBC) is usually normal in limited stage disease. There may be mild anaemia, a polymorphic leucocytosis, leucopenia, and rarely a haemolytic anaemia. Occasionally, circulating lymphoma cells can be identified. Liver enzymes may be mildly elevated even in the absence of hepatic involvement. Lactate dehydrogenase and β_2-microglobulin are often high in bulky disease. Renal function should also be checked to exclude renal involvement and obstruction.

Radiology

The chest radiograph is an essential investigation. Apart from the detection of mediastinal and bronchopulmonary lymphadenopathy (*Fig. 22.3*), superior vena cava obstruction, pleural effusion, and atelectasis caused by bronchial compression may be identified. Rarely, there may be intrapulmonary involvement or a pericardial effusion.

Hospital
Blood tests

An HIV test with appropriate counselling and consent should be considered if the patient is in a high-risk category.

Biopsy

Cytology alone is insufficient because the diagnosis is based on the morphology of the nodal architecture. Even in relapsed lymphoma it is often important to re-biopsy the lymph node to check for transformation to a higher grade.

Imaging

A computed tomography (CT) scan of the thorax, abdomen, and pelvis is usually sufficient to identify all sites of nodal disease. Occasionally, soft-tissue involvement (such as hepatic or splenic) may be difficult to identify, and additional radiological tests, such as magnetic resonance imaging or fluorodeoxyglucose (FDG)-positron emission tomography may be required. Bone scanning may be useful in demonstrating isolated areas of involvement.

Bone marrow biopsy

A bone marrow trephine and aspirate is required in the staging of all NHL. It should also be carried out on patients with Hodgkin's disease who have advanced disease, B symptoms, or an abnormal FBC.

Lumbar puncture

Clinical suspicion of central nervous system (CNS) involvement requires a lumbar puncture. High-risk groups include patients with lymphoblastic and Burkitt's lymphoma and those with diffuse large B-cell lymphoma who have bone marrow, orbital, base of skull. and testicular involvement.

Investigations prior to starting chemotherapy

A multiple-gated acquisition (MUGA) scan to assess cardiac function and pulmonary function tests may be required if the patient has a history of significant cardiac or respiratory disease, and if the patient is to receive potentially cardiotoxic or pulmonary toxic drugs. If the proposed treatment has the potential to cause sterility (e.g. alkylating agents such as chlorambucil), patients should receive fertility counselling, and males should be offered sperm-banking. The success of egg preservation is not proved, but many centres may offer this service.

Treatment

Treatment, key points

- Hodgkin's disease and 'high-grade' NHL are potentially curable
- Chemotherapy is the mainstay of treatment
- Limited-stage disease may be curable with radiotherapy
- 'Low-grade' NHL is generally incurable, but is indolent in nature
- High-dose therapy and stem cell transplant is generally used in patients who demonstrate a chemo-sensitive relapse

The mainstay of treatment is chemotherapy. Most cases of Hodgkin's disease and high-grade NHL are potentially curable and so an aggressive approach to therapy is usually adopted. Patients with low-grade NHL are rarely curable and palliative treatment is more appropriate, with an aim to control the disease and palliate symptoms without any resultant excess toxicity. Chemotherapy is most often given as an outpatient procedure, by bolus injections, intravenous infusion, or orally. Allopurinol is usually prescribed for the first few courses of treatment to avoid tumour lysis syndrome, and patients are given anti-emetics and prophylactic antibiotics.

Lymphomas are generally radiosensitive, so radiotherapy is often curative in limited disease and also plays a role in the management of bulky and residual disease. Surgery has a limited role in the management of lymphoma. Lymphoma is best treated in specialist centres and patients should be managed by a multidisciplinary team that includes a medical oncologist or haematologist, a radiotherapist, and an expert pathologist.

Hodgkin's disease
Stages Ia- to IIa
A 5-year disease-free survival greater than 80% can be achieved with mantle radiotherapy alone. However, a recent meta-analysis of 23 studies comparing radiotherapy alone with combined radiotherapy and chemotherapy showed that combined modality therapy reduced the 10-year risk of failure by half. There was a small but non-significant increase in overall survival (Specht *et al.*, 1998). Studies that address this issue are ongoing. Poor prognostic factors that appear to predispose to early relapse have been identified (*Table 22.5*).

Stage IIb to IVb
Systemic therapy with combination chemotherapy is the treatment of choice. The most widely used regimens include MOPP (mustine, vincristine, procarbazine, and prednisolone) and ABVD [doxorubicin (adriamycin), bleomycin,

Table 22.5. *Poor prognostic features identified in Hodgkin's disease*

Histology:
lymphocyte depleted
mixed cellularity
Older age
Two sites of disease
Male sex
Bulky disease
High erythrocyte sedimentation rate

vinblastine, and dacarbazine]. The combination VEEP (vincristine, epirubicin, etoposide, and prednisolone) was developed at the Royal Marsden Hospital, London as an effective, relatively non-toxic regimen. Treatment usually lasts for approximately 6 months and CT scans are repeated two or three times during the treatment course to assess response. Radiotherapy is often used in the treatment of initial bulky disease and residual masses following chemotherapy.

Patients with advanced Hodgkin's disease have an overall survival of up to 70%, although this figure is lower in patients with poor prognostic disease. Treatment with newer regimens, such as the Stanford V regimen (Horning *et al.*, 2000) and bleomycin, etoposide, doxorubicin, cyclophosphamide, vincristine, procarbazine, and prednisone (BEACOPP) (Diehl *et al.*, 1998), may improve survival. However, there are concerns over long-term side-effects of these regimens, particularly with regard to second malignancies.

Non-Hodgkin's lymphoma
Low-grade non-Hodgkin's lymphoma
The 10-year overall survival and disease-free survival can exceed 80% following radiotherapy in localized disease. The value of chemotherapy in early-stage disease is less clear.

Advanced-stage low-grade NHL is responsive to both chemotherapy and radiotherapy, but remissions rarely last long. The median survival is approximately 10 years. Treatment in asymptomatic patients can be delayed, since no survival advantage is gained by starting it early. Treatment usually takes the form of chemotherapy and can be a combination regimen such CVP (cyclophosphamide, vincristine, and prednisolone) or single agents such as oral chlorambucil, fludarabine, or prednisolone. In young patients with poor prognostic disease, a more aggressive therapy may be offered, although to date few data suggest a survival advantage. Monoclonal antibody therapy with rituximab (directed against the CD20 antigen on the malignant B cell) is effective even in heavily pretreated patients. Radiotherapy plays an important role in the palliation of symptoms.

High-grade non-Hodgkin's lymphoma
Stage I high-grade NHL is curable with radiotherapy, with a 10-year overall survival of approximately 70%. However, two large randomized studies (from the Eastern Cooperative Oncology Group and the South-Western Oncology Group, *Table 22.6*) showed superior results from combined chemotherapy that involved field radiotherapy in early-stage disease (stages I and II). Patients with stage I or 'non-bulky' stage II disease should receive short-course chemotherapy [e.g. three courses of CHOP (cyclophosphamide, doxorubicin,

Table 22.6. Benefit of combined chemotherapy and radiotherapy in early stage aggressive non-Hodgkin's disease

Study	Regime[a]	5-year progression-free survival	5-year overall survival
[17]SWOG[b]	CHOP × 8	64%	72%
	CHOP × 3 plus radiotherapy	77%	82%
		p = 0.03	p = 0.02

		6-year disease-free survival	**6-year overall survival**
[18]ECOG[c]	CHOP × 8	58%	70%
	CHOP × 8 plus radiotherapy	73%	84%
		p = 0.03	p = 0.06

[a]CHOP, cyclophosphamide, doxorubicin, vincristine, and prednisolone.
[b]Miller et al., 1998.
[c]Glick et al., 1995.

vincristine, and prednisolone)] followed by involved-field radiotherapy. Patients with bulky stage II disease should be treated with a full course of chemotherapy and may benefit from additional radiotherapy. The CHOP regimen is the most widely used, but a number of newer, more intensive, regimens are in clinical use.

Advanced-stage high-grade lymphoma has cure rates of 35–40%. Survival varies depending on the number of poor prognostic features (*Table 22.7*) Again, chemotherapy is the treatment modality of choice. Single-institution studies have reported superior results to CHOP with intensive regimens such as prednisolone, doxorubicin, cyclophosphamide, etoposide, cytarabine, bleomycin, vincristine, and methotrexate (ProMACE–CytaBOM), but to date these results have not been confirmed in prospective randomized studies. The choice of regimen depends on local expertise and the availability of local support services, since many of these newer regimens are associated with significant morbidity. Apart from its use in residual masses, radiotherapy does not play a significant role.

Burkitt's non-Hodgkin's lymphoma

Burkitt's lymphoma is an extremely aggressive form of NHL; rapid diagnosis and treatment is mandatory to offer the patient the best hope of a cure. The risk of tumour lysis syndrome in these patients is high, and good hydration, treatment with allopurinol, and even dialysis may be necessary to avoid renal failure. Chemotherapy regimens are intensive and have a rapid cycle time to avoid regrowth of the lymphoma. Most contain cyclical cyclophosphamide coupled with a number of drugs,

Table 22.7. International prognostic index for large-cell lymphoma

Number of factors[a]	5-year disease-free survival (%)	5-year overall survival (%)
0–1	70	73
2	50	51
3	49	43
4–5	40	26

[a]Poor prognostic factors: older age, Ann Arbor stage, performance status, serum lactate dehydrogenase, number of extranodal sites of disease

including intermediate- to high-dose methotrexate. Intrathecal CNS prophylaxis must also be given.

Patients with limited disease have an excellent prognosis, with at least a 90% cure rate, and may require less intensive therapy. Overall survival in higher stage disease have been reported as between 50 and 70%, but patients with bone marrow and CNS involvement have a poorer prognosis. However, new chemotherapy regimens have been reported to produce superior results.

Mantle-zone non-Hodgkin's lymphoma

Mantle-zone NHL is an unusual form of lymphoma derived from small B-cells that surround the follicle within the lymph node to give a nodular appearance. This disease has

Key points: lymphoma

Non-Hodgkin's lymphoma

67% of cases occur in patients over 60 years of age, but patients of any all age can be affected

Presenting features include:

lymphadenopathy

hepatosplenomegaly

fatigue

weight loss

40% of patients present with tumour outside the lymph glands

Hodgkin's disease

Over 50% of patients are younger than 40 years of age

Clinical features similar to those for non-Hodgkin's lymphomas (but 95% present with lymph gland involvement)

Reproduced from Department of Health Cancer Referral Guidelines, final version March 2000.

Guidelines for urgent referral: haematological malignancies

Blood count and/or film suggestive of leukaemia: anaemia ± abnormal white blood cell counts (high or low) ± low platelet count

Lymphadenopathy (>1cm) persisting for 6 weeks

Hepatosplenomegaly

Bone pain associated with anaemia and raised erythrocyte sedimentation rate (or plasma viscosity)

Bone X-rays reported as being suggestive of myeloma

Constellation of three or more of the following symptoms: fatigue, night sweats, weight loss, itching, breathlessness, bruising, recurrent infections, bone pain

a poor prognosis with a 10-year survival less than 10%. They can be treated with either radical radiotherapy or moderately intensive chemotherapy such as CHOP.

Lymphoblastic non-Hodgkin's lymphoma

Lymphoblastic lymphomas are characterized by the presence of blast cells in the bone marrow and peripheral blood. Most patients present with a mediastinal mass and respiratory symptoms are not uncommon. Despite prolonged treatment with combination chemotherapy, prognosis is poor in this disease, with a long term survival of 40–50%.

Mucosal-associated lymphoid tissue non-Hodgkin's lymphoma

A large proportion of MALT lymphomas are associated with *Helicobacter pylori* infection, and the majority occur in the stomach. Limited stage disease may be cured with *Helicobacter* eradication therapy, although surgery and radiation can also play a role. More disseminated disease should

be treated with systemic therapy such as chlorambucil or CHOP chemotherapy.

T-cell lymphomas

Peripheral T-cell lymphomas comprise approximately 20% of the high-grade lymphomas. The optimal therapy is poly-chemotherapy, but the prognosis is thought to be poorer than for their B-cell equivalents. Cutaneous T-cell NHL can be treated with topical chemotherapy, radiation therapy, photochemotherapy, and systemic chemotherapy. Response rates are very high, but response duration is short. Adult T-cell lymphoma is an aggressive disease for which, despite systemic chemotherapy, the median survival is around 1 year.

High-dose chemotherapy and stem cell transplant

High-dose therapy is usually reserved for poor-risk relapsed Hodgkin's disease and patients with high-grade

Referral proforma: haematological malignancies

Age:

Malignancy suspected

Leukaemia	☐
Lymphoma (Hodgkin's disease or non-Hodgkin's lymphoma)	☐
Myeloma	☐

Symptoms	Yes	No	
Fatigue			
Night sweats			
Weight loss			
Itching			
Pain on drinking alcohol			
Breathlessness			
Bruising			
Recurrent infections			
Bone pain			

Clinical examination	Yes	No	
Pallor			
Lymph nodes:			
neck			
axilla			
groin			
other			
Hepatomegaly			
Splenomegaly			
Bruising and/or petechia			
Stomatitis and/or mouth ulcers			

Investigations

Haemoglobin..

White cell count...

Platelets..

Erythrocyte sedimentation rate..

Chest radiography..

Comments/other reasons for referral:

Reproduced from England Department of Health Cancer Referral Guidelines Consultation Document April 2001.

NHL who have a chemo-sensitive relapse. There is no evidence of benefit in low-grade NHL. The transplant usually involves reinfusion of autologous peripheral stem cells, which obviates the need for a bone marrow harvest. During the procedure the patient is hospitalized for around 3–4 weeks. Treatment-related mortality is up to 5% and the risk of sterilization is significant. Neutropenia places the patient at risk of infection (bacterial, viral, and fungal) and complications of anaemia and thrombocytopenia are not infrequent.

Further Reading

Diehl V, Frankin J, Hasenclever D, *et al*. BEACOPP, a new dose-escalated and accelerated regimen, is at least as effective as COPP/ABVD in patients with advanced-stage Hodgkin's lymphoma: interim report from a trial of the German Hodgkin's Lymphoma Study Group. *J Clin Oncol*. 1998; **16**: 3810–21.

Glick JH, Kim K, Earle J, O'Connell HJ. An ECOG randomized phase III trial of CHOP vs CHOP plus radiotherapy for intermediate grade early stage non-Hodgkin's lymphoma. *Proc Am Soc Clin Oncol*. 1995; **14**: 391.

Horning SJ, Williams J, Bartlett NL, *et al*. Assessment of the Stanford V regimen and consolidative radiotherapy for bulky and advanced Hodgkin's disease: Eastern Cooperative Oncology Group pilot study E1492. *J Clin Oncol*. 2000; **18**: 972–80.

Miller TP, Dahlberg S, Cassady JR, *et al*. Chemotherapy alone compared with chemotherapy plus radiotherapy for localized intermediate- and high-grade non-Hodgkin's lymphoma. *N Engl J Med*. 1999; **339**: 21–6.

Specht L, Gray RG, Clarke MJ, Peto R. Influence of more extensive radiotherapy and adjuvant chemotherapy on long-term of early-stage Hodgkin's disease: a meta-analysis of 23 randomized trials involving 3888 patients. International Hodgkin's Disease Collaborative Group. *J Clin Oncol*. 1998; **16**: 830–43.

23 Skin Cancer and Melanoma

Louise Fearfield, Anna Stevenson, Christopher Bunker, Meirion Thomas and Martin Gore

Malignant Melanoma of the Skin

Incidence and mortality

Malignant melanoma arises from melanocytes and makes up 2% of all cancers. In the UK the incidence of malignant melanoma, particularly thin lesions, is continuing to rise (MacKie, 1995). The highest rates in the world are found in white people living in Queensland in Australia and in New Zealand, with annual incidence figures around 40 new cases per 100,000 population. There are early indications that the rising incidence of melanoma may have slowed. A study from Scotland demonstrated that rates may even be declining for cohorts born after 1950. Furthermore, the rate of increase in mortality due to melanoma appears to have slowed in areas where public education campaigns have been mounted, for example in Scotland and Australia (MacKie *et al.*, 1997).

Epidemiology and aetiology

Melanoma affects white-skinned populations in sunny countries, indoor workers rather than outdoor workers and the higher socioeconomic classes. There is an inverse relationship between the incidence of melanoma and degree of skin pigmentation. Melanoma is 12 times more common in white people and six times more common in those of Hispanic origin than in black-skinned races with the same lifestyle. Males and females are approximately equally affected. Melanoma can present on sun-exposed and non-sun-exposed sites. Females most commonly get melanoma on the lower limbs, whereas males develop melanoma on the trunk. Black-skinned people develop subungual melanoma and acral lentiginous melanoma (on the palms and soles).

Melanoma is rare in childhood and there is a steady increase in incidence from young adulthood up to a peak in the 50s and 60s. Between 8 and 12% of melanoma patients have a proven positive family history of melanoma. Familial traits such as red or blond hair, fair complexion, freckling, sunburn, dysplastic or atypical naevi and abnormally distributed naevi tend to run in these families. Melanoma-susceptibility genes have been looked for in these patients and 30% of familial melanoma patients have germ-line mutations in the CDKN2A gene encoding the tumour suppressor protein p16. The relevance of this mutation in sporadic melanoma remains unclear.

Melanoma may occur in families with predisposition to other cancers and in genetic syndromes such as xeroderma pigmentosa in which there is a predisposition to cutaneous neoplasms. Iatrogenic immunosuppression (e.g. from drugs and phototherapy) and acquired immunosuppression (e.g. from HIV infection) are associated with increased melanoma risk. Congenital melanocytic naevi have a 0–15% risk of becoming melanoma.

Current evidence suggests that intermittent burning sun exposure is an important risk factor for the development of melanoma. The exact role of sunburn is not known, but it may be that sunburn is a marker both of intermittent sun exposure and of genetic susceptibility. The incidence of melanoma among white people is inversely related to latitude of residence with the world's highest incidence in Australia. Migration studies suggest that moving to an area of more intense sun exposure increases melanoma risk. Depletion of the ozone layer and increased recreational sun exposure have also been linked with the increasing incidence. The epidemiological evidence implicating sun exposure in the causation of melanoma is supported by biological evidence that damage caused by ultraviolet radiation, particularly damage to DNA, plays a central part in the pathogenesis of these tumours.

Over the past decade or so, significant controversy has surrounded the use of sunscreen lotions, with several recent studies linking the use of sunscreens to increased melanoma risk. These studies need to be interpreted with care since those people who are most likely to use sunscreens are often those with a phenotype associated with increased melanoma risk and those with sun-seeking behaviour. Also, while it is clear that sunscreens with a high sun protection factor are effective in preventing sunburn, they are often used in a suboptimal manner

Primary prevention and screening

There is enough epidemiological and laboratory evidence to support reducing sunlight exposure as a primary prevention strategy. A reduction in exposure can be achieved with protective clothing, shade and sunscreen lotion with a sun protection factor of at least 15. This is thought to be particularly important in children. Primary prevention programmes have been running for almost 20 years in Australia and have resulted in a large shift in knowledge, attitudes and beliefs about sunlight exposure and tanning, and a major shift in behaviour. In the UK, a study of Sun Awareness Week in 1995 showed significant improvements in attitudes and behaviour.

Detection and treatment of melanoma early in its course is critical for improving outcomes. Screening and education dramatically increase the proportion of melanomas that are diagnosed as 'thin'. In Scotland the percentage of tumours detected less than 1.5 mm thick rose from 38% in 1979–1984 to 54% in 1985–1989. Patients at risk (e.g. those with a previous primary melanoma, a large number of moles some of which are clinically atypical, or a strong family history of melanoma) should be referred to a specialist clinic..

Clinical appearance

A clinical feature that is common to all variants of malignant melanoma is the presence of a changing pigmented lesion. Often the lesion is noted to be different from all the other benign naevi found elsewhere on the patients skin. There are two simple systems that have been devised to aid clinical diagnosis of melanoma by naked-eye inspection. These are the American ABCD categories (*Table 23.1*) and the Glasgow seven point checklist (*Table 23.2*). It is suggested for the Glasgow

Table 23.3. *Types of melanoma and their incidence*

Types	Incidence (%)
Superficial spreading melanoma	80–85
Nodular melanoma	10–15
Lentigo maligna melanoma	5
Acral lentignous and subungual melanoma	2–8

checklist that any lesion in an adult with one major feature should be considered for removal and that the presence of additional minor features should add to the clinical suspicion.

Melanomas can be subdivided into four different types based on histological and clinical appearance (*Table 23.3*). The most common is the superficial spreading melanoma (80–85%), next is the nodular melanoma (10–15%), followed by lentigo maligna melanoma (5%) and acral lentiginous and subungual melanoma (2–8%).

Superficial spreading melanoma

These present more frequently in patients in their fourth or fifth decade. Early presentation is often of an irregularly shaped lesion usually still macular but with variations in brown and black pigmentation (*Fig. 23.1*). The lesions can

Table 23.1. *American ABCD categories*

A	Asymmetry
B	Irregular border
C	Irregular colour
D	Diameter over 1 cm

Table 23.2. *The Glasgow seven-point check list*

Major features
1	Change in size
2	Change in shape
3	Change in colour

Minor features
4	Diameter more than 6 mm
5	Inflammation
6	Oozing or bleeding
7	Mild itch or altered sensation

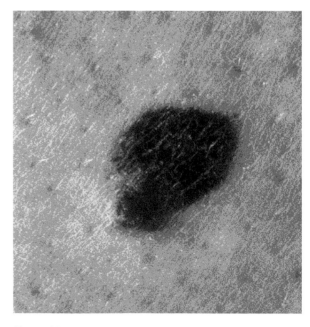

Figure 23.1. *Superficial spreading melanoma.*

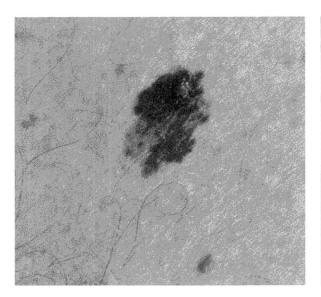

Figure 23.2. *Superficial spreading melanoma with a nodular area within it.*

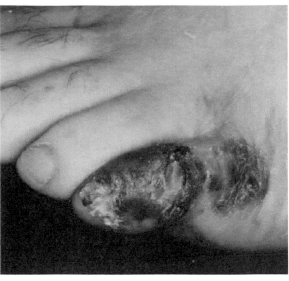

Figure 23.3. *Acral lentiginous melanoma.*

be small (4–5 mm in diameter). Patchy pigmentation loss can occur as a result of partial regression. Elevated palpable areas and a history of bleeding or oozing are seen when the lesion is in its advanced stage.

Nodular melanoma

This variety occurs more frequently in males, in the fifth or sixth decade and on the trunk. These tumours grow rapidly so that often by the time of presentation they are already deep tumours with a correspondingly poor prognosis. Ulceration and bleeding often occur and the tumours themselves can appear quite red, often with a ring of melanin around them (*Fig. 23.2*). This appearance can lead to confusion over the diagnosis. The safest approach is to refer for a biopsy if there is any doubt.

Acral lentiginous melanoma

This type of melanoma, which presents on the palm and soles, is much more common in black and Asian skin than in white skin. They often present on the sole of the foot at a late stage with a correspondingly poor prognosis. Clinically they are usually macular often large pigmented lesions with a raised central area (*Fig. 23.3*).

Subungual malignant melanoma

Any pigmentation of the nail bed must be carefully investigated. Subungual malignant melanomas have a very poor

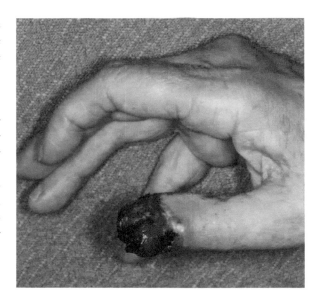

Figure 23.4. *Subungual melanoma.*

prognosis and present late. The melanoma may have been developing for 3 months within the nail matrix before it actually becomes visible to the naked eye. When the nail fold is also pigmented this is known as Hutchinson's sign (*Fig. 23.4*).

219

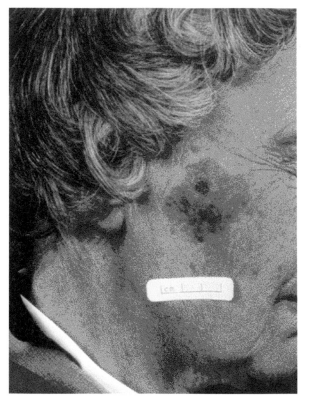

Figure 23.5. *Pigmented macular lesion on the cheek with a darker area within it representing a lentigo maligna melanoma.*

Lentigo maligna melanoma

Most occur on the face and present in the elderly. They are macular, large, pigmented lentiginous lesions, often with variable pigmentation (*Fig. 23.5*). They are rarely invasive but can become so if left.

Dermatoscopy

This technique involves the use of magnification (usually ×10) to examine the surface of pigmented lesions and can help to diagnose early melanomas, but it must not be relied upon. Oil is first put on the lesion to 'clear' the epidermal surface. The instrument is similar to a hand-held ophthalmoscope. This technique in trained hands allows for detailed examination of the distribution of melanin with a sensitivity of 92% and a specificity of 71% in the diagnosis of an early melanoma. It is also helpful in distinguishing lesions such as seborrhoeic keratoses and angiomatous lesions from melanocytic lesions. An early melanoma often has an irregular pigment network, pigmentary pseudopods and blue or milky veins in parts of the lesion, indicating dermal pigment.

Table 23.4. *Histopathological characteristics of each melanoma type*

Type	Histopathological characteristics
Superficial spreading melanoma	Focus of malignant melanoma cells invading the dermis with areas of *in situ* malignant change in the adjacent epidermis
Nodular melanoma	Focus of invasive melanoma cells in the dermis and overlying epidermis with no adjacent epidermal involvement
Acral lentiginous	Extensive area of lentiginous change in the epidermis often surrounding an area of invasive primary melanoma
Lentigo maligna melanoma	Lentiginous replacement of basal epidermal keratinocytes with malignant melanocytes and associated evidence of actinic dermal damage with no dermal invasion

Histology

The unifying feature of all melanomas is the appearance of cytologically malignant melanocytes in the dermis and often the epidermis. Other features that help to confirm that the lesion is a melanoma include the presence of mitoses, ulceration, lymphocytic infiltration and apparent angiogenesis at the base of the lesion. Different histopathological characteristics can be seen in each melanoma type (*Table 23.4*).

Certain pathological features, in particular depth of the melanoma, are used to determine the prognosis of an individual melanoma. Clark's levels (*Table 23.5*) were first developed as a method of predicting prognosis; however, difficulties in interpreting the location of the papillary and reticular levels in the dermis led to differing results. Breslow thickness (*Table 23.6*) has since been established as the most valuable prognostic guide (Breslow, 1970). This is a measurement of thickness from the granular cell layer of the epidermis to the deepest invasive melanocytic cells.

Table 23.5. *Clark's levels*

Clark's level	Histology
I	Intraepidermal or *in situ*
II	Few cells in the papillary dermis
III	Occupation and expansion of the papillary dermis by melanoma cells
IV	Invasion of the reticular dermis
V	Invasion into subcutaneous fat

Table 23.6. *Breslow thickness*

Thickness (mm)	5-year survival (%)
0–0.76	95
0.77–1.69	90
1.7–3.6	80
>3.6	50

The concept of radial and vertical growth phase was introduced to distinguish those melanomas that had no metastatic potential (radial) from those with metastatic potential (vertical). Malignant melanomas in vertical growth phase are those with an obvious dominant clone or aggregate of malignant cells invading the dermis, often with mitoses. Radial growth phase is, however, defined as the presence of only a small number of melanoma cells in the dermis with no obvious dominant clone or aggregate.

Other poor prognostic features include ulceration (even if only microscopic), and the presence of tumour cells in vessels. Other less established prognostic indicators include regression, mitotic rate and lymphocytic infiltrate.

Biopsy

A patient who presents with a suspected melanoma should have an excision biopsy taken. Shave or curette biopsies are absolutely contraindicated. If the diagnosis of melanoma is confirmed, a further excision with wider margins within 6 weeks may be needed depending on the depth of the melanoma and the original excision margin. For lesions less than 0.76 mm, a 1 cm margin (width and depth) is now considered to be adequate. Recent studies have also demonstrated that for melanomas up to 2 mm thick there is no difference in recurrence rates between 1 cm and 3 cm margins. However, for thicker lesions (>2 mm) trials are continuing to try to identify the best width of excision necessary (1 cm versus 3 cm).

Incisional biopsies or punch biopsies are not often used in the diagnosis of melanoma. This is because of speculation as to whether the procedure may aid in the dissemination of the melanoma. However, diagnostic biopsies are still used for large lentigo maligna melanomas or where the surgical field is limited by anatomy.

Lymph node involvement

The presence of metastatic disease in the regional lymph nodes is one of the most important determinants of prognosis. In patients whose nodes are palpable, diagnosis should initially be made by fine needle aspiration cytology rather than excision of a lymph node since excision compromises the efficacy of subsequent lymph node disection. When cytology confirms metastases, a therapeutic lymph node dissection should be performed by a surgeon skilled in the technique to reduce the risk of recurrence. Lymphoedema is the major complication, in particular with inguinal region lymph node dissections, and patients should be well informed before surgery of this risk.

Elective lymph node dissection involves lymphadenectomy in the absence of evidence of regional lymph node involvement. Its use is based on the proposition that micrometastases disseminate sequentially from primary tumours to regional lymph nodes and then distant sites. However, several prospective studies have showed that there is no survival advantage in those patients treated with or without elective lymph node dissection. Despite these results it was still felt that there may be a subgroup of patients with primary stage 1 (no metastases) disease that would benefit from regional node dissection. This theory led to the concept of the sentinel node biopsy.

The aim of sentinel node biopsy is to identify the first lymph node draining the skin in which a melanoma arises. The technique involves intraoperative lymph node mapping with selective lymphadenectomy. It is then possible to determine whether a patient may have regional lymph node disease by examining the excised node. Sentinel node biopsy is an effective method of accurately staging patients; however, the indications for its use are not fully established, since it is not known whether it has any effect on outcome for the patient.

Follow-up

All patients with invasive melanoma should be followed up on a 3-monthly basis for the first 3 years. Thereafter, patients with melanoma less than 1.0 mm thick may be discharged, but the remainder should be reviewed 6 monthly for the next 2 years. Overall, 80% of recurrences occur within the first 3 years, but a few patients (<8%) have recurrence 5–10 years after the initial surgery.

Adjuvant treatment

There is no effective adjuvant therapy for melanoma. Randomized trials of adjuvant chemotherapy, whether delivered locally (isolated limb perfusion) or systemically, have not shown improved survival in patients who are at high risk of relapse. There is, however, great interest in the use of therapies such as interferon alfa and vaccination.

Data from the randomized trials of interferon are conflicting, with some trials suggesting a benefit for high doses of interferon (Kirkwood *et al.*, 1996). In an overview of adjuvant interferon alfa, Wheatley *et al.* (2003) have shown a statistically significant benefit for interferon both in terms of disease-free survival and overall survival. However, these authors emphasize that this analysis is preliminary. The toxicity of interferon is dose-dependent and not insignificant, and therefore most groups in Europe feel that confirmatory data are required before high-dose interferon, or any other schedule, becomes standard adjuvant therapy. Definitive answers will be obtained from trials that are still accruing.

Melanoma is one of the most immunogenic solid tumours and has as a result served as the major model for tumour vaccine development. There are four randomized trials of vaccination in the adjuvant setting using whole cells, ganglioside, shed antigen and a viral lysate of tumour cells. None of these trails has shown a survival benefit for vaccination. However, three of them have demonstrated a significant benefit in those patients who showed an immune response to their vaccinations. It is hoped that continued advances in this area will lead to significant changes in the treatment of melanoma in the next decade.

Patients cleared of lymph node disease or metastatic disease by surgery should be referred to a cancer centre involved in trials of adjuvant therapy. Adjuvant treatment outside such studies is not recommended.

Metastatic disease

Patients with metastatic melanoma have a poor prognosis with a median survival of 6 months, although this does depend on the site involved. Median survival for patients with liver or brain disease is 3–6 months; for those with lung metastases it is 9 months. Some long-term survivors are seen when the disease is confined to skin or lymph nodes. The aim of therapy is palliation rather than cure. All patients should have access to a palliative care team providing expertise in symptom control and psychosocial support.

Surgery can give long-lasting palliation for isolated metastases and is usually most appropriate for skin, soft tissue and solitary brain lesions. Radiotherapy to bone can provide short-term symptomatic control, and radiotherapy to brain metastases has palliative value.

There is no consistent randomized evidence for a significant improvement in overall survival with any systemic therapy but responses to treatment can result in good palliation. Where possible patients should be offered participation in clinical trials. Withholding treatment may be a valid option in the presence of slow-growing asymptomatic metastases

with deferment of treatment allowing quality of life to be maintained. The strongest predictors of outcome are performance status, disease-free interval, number of organs involved and absence of liver involvement.

The single most active drug in metastatic melanoma is Dacarbazine (DTIC), with best responses of 15–20% (Chowdhury *et al.*, 1999). These remissions tend to last only 4–6 months. DTIC is very well tolerated when given with 5-hydroxytryptamine-3 receptor antagonist. Randomized trials have shown no benefit for combination chemotherapy over single-agent treatment in terms of response rate and disease-free or overall survival.

The host immune response is thought to play an important role in the natural history of melanoma. Thus there has been considerable interest in the use of the biological response modifiers such as interferon-alpha (IFN-α), and interleukin-2 (IL-2), biochemotherapy (the combination of immunotherapy with chemotherapy) and vaccines. The response rate to single agent IFN-α or IL-2 is around 15% with some durable responses. IFN-α and IL-2 have been used in combination because of their different mechanisms of action and experimental evidence suggesting synergy. However, no clear advantage for combining the two has been observed.

Chemotherapy and immunotherapy have different mechanisms of action and different toxicity profiles. Recently the term biochemotherapy has come to describe a combination of both IFN-α and IL-2 with chemotherapy. These regimens are toxic with patients suffering myelosuppression, gastrointestinal toxicity, capillary leak syndrome, cardiac toxicity and autoimmune phenomena. Five prospective randomized trials of biochemotherapy have been published but none has demonstrated a convincing survival advantage for biochemotherapy.

Trials of vaccine therapy in metastatic melanoma have also been undertaken. Some studies have shown a significant treatment benefit in those patients showing a host response. Other experimental approaches include gene therapy and some of the newer compounds with novel modes of action such as angiogenesis inhibition and signal transduction blockade.

Single-agent DTIC remains the gold standard treatment for patients with metastatic melanoma and this is therefore the agent against which new treatments should be compared. It is important that patients with metastatic melanoma are managed by a multidisciplinary team with expertise in this disease. While the aim of treatment is palliation, it should be remembered that very occasionally patients live for years following treatment.

Key points

- Tumour stage at presentation is the most significant determinant of prognosis
- For stage I and II, the most important prognostic factor is Breslow thickness
- In metastatic disease, the number of involved lymph nodes correlates with survival
- Median survival for patients with metastatic disease is 6 months
- Patients with metastases to the gastrointestinal tract, liver, brain, pleura or lung have a shorter median survival than those with skin metastases alone
- No adjuvant therapy modality has been shown to increase survival in melanoma
- DTIC is standard therapy for metastatic disease, with a response rate of 15%. In those who respond, quality of life is usually improved; however, no increase in overall survival is seen

Table 23.8. *Aetiological factors for SCC*

Ultraviolet radiation
Ionizing radiation
Genodermatoses
Human papillomavirus
Arsenic
Polycyclic aromatic hydrocarbons
Immunosuppression
Chronic ulcer/sinus tract
Scar
Chronic dermatoses (e.g. lichen planus)

Cutaneous Squamous Cell Carcinoma

Incidence

Cutaneous squamous cell carcinoma (SCC) accounts for about 20% of cutaneous malignancies and the incidence continues to rise (Schiffman, 1975; Ames and Hickey, 1982; Glass and Hoover, 1989). The prevalence of SCC varies greatly between different countries and races. Celtic descendents living in sunny climates such as Queensland are more commonly affected whereas it is an infrequent tumour in dark-skinned people. The most recent population-based incidence figures come from Australia (Marks *et al.*, 1993) and Minnesota, USA (Chuang *et al.*, 1990) (*Table 23.7*). In the UK the incidence for women is 21 per 100,000 person–years at risk, and for men 32 per 100,000.

Epidemiology and aetiology

SCC appears to be more common in males (Marks *et al.*, 1993; Chuang *et al.*, 1990) and its incidence increases

sharply with age (Glass and Hoover, 1989). However, younger persons with predisposing conditions or extensive solar exposure are also at increased risk of developing SCC. SCC occurs most frequently on the skin of the head and neck, followed by the extremities and trunk (Glass and Hoover, 1989). People who burn easily, tan poorly, have light-coloured hair, blue eyes and a fair complexion are at greater risk of developing SCC (and skin cancer in general) (Giles *et al.*, 1988; Aubry and MacGibbon, 1985).

Both environmental and host factors (*Table 23.8*) are important in the development of SCC. However, cumulative ultraviolet radiation is generally the most common cause of SCC of the skin (Vitasa *et al.*, 1990). Cutaneous SCC most often occurs in sun-exposed areas in light-skinned people with a significant history of ultraviolet exposure. Ultraviolet-B light (290–320 nm) is the most carcinogenic wavelength whereas ultraviolet-A light (320–400 nm) augments the effects of ultraviolet-B light and thereby acts as a co-carcinogen. The exact mechanism by which ultraviolet radiation causes SCC is not completely understood and, in some cases, multiple factors contribute to the development of SCC. Ultraviolet radiation is likely to result in mutations within the cellular DNA which do not get repaired, resulting in genetic alterations that ultimately lead to unrestrained growth and tumour formation (Grossman and Leffell, 1997).

Table 23.7. *Annual incidence of SCCs*

	Annual incidence in females	Annual incidence in males	Overall annual incidence
Australia (Marks *et al.*, 1993)	164 cases per 100,000	338 cases per 100,000	—
Minnesota (Chuang *et al.*, 1990)	—	—	39 cases per 100,000

223

The carcinogenic effects of ionizing radiation are well documented (Glucksman, 1958). X-rays are the most common cause; however, grenz rays and gamma-rays can rarely also induce SCC formation.

The genodermatoses are inherited skin syndromes and those directly associated with an increased risk of developing SCC include xeroderma pigmentosum (XP) and oculocutaneous albinism (OCA). Both are inherited as an autosomal-recessive disorder. In XP there is defective DNA repair after ultraviolet exposure and most patients develop their first cutaneous malignancies by the age of 8 years. In OCA , SCC develops in sun-exposed areas owing to a lack of protective melanin being produced.

The human papilloma virus (HPV) has been implicated in the aetiology of SCC of the genital tract and perianal area and of Bowen's disease. HPV types 16 and 18 are the most frequently associated with SCC. Arsenic is also an important aetiological agent in those patients with a history of ingestion or inhalation. Arsenic-induced skin cancer is characterised by the development of basal cell carcinomas, plaques of Bowen's disease and SCCs. Tumours may develop on non-sun-exposed sites and patients often have arsenical keratoses on the palms and soles. Exposure to polycyclic aromatic carbons produced by combustion and distillation of carbonaceous materials also predisposes to the development of SCC, as was first reported in chimney sweeps with the development of scrotal lesions.

Cutaneous SCCs develop in patients on long-term immunosuppressives, such as renal transplant patients (Leigh and Glover, 1995). They appear to behave more aggressively in this group. Cutaneous SCC arises in sun-exposed sites with an average latency period from the time of transplantation to the development of tumours of 1–7 years. These patients require careful and regular skin surveillance, and any suspicious lesions should be biopsied because the SCCs that these patients develop are often fairly banal in appearance.

Precursor lesions

The major precursor lesions to the development of invasive SCC are listed in *Table 23.9*. Actinic keratoses are common

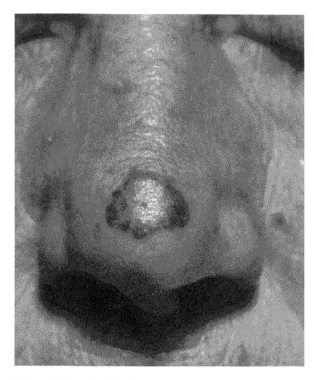

Figure 23.6. *Actinic keratoses on the nose.*

lesions that develop in the chronically sun-exposed patient, most often on the face and hands. They present as erythematous scaly macular lesions (*Fig. 23.6*). They have a very low biologic potential for malignant transformation (Marks *et al.*, 1988). It has also been estimated that 25% of lesions remit spontaneously (Marks *et al.*, 1986). They indicate that the patient has had a significant amount of sun exposure and is at risk of developing non-melanoma skin cancer.

Bowen's disease, erythroplasia of Queyrat and bowenoid papulosis are all forms of SCC *in situ*. National guidelines for the management of Bowen's disease have been published (Cox *et al.*, 1999). They are all usually persistent and progressive, with a small potential for invasive malignancy.

Clinical features

SCC often arises in areas of sun-damaged skin. The lesion may be plaque-like, verrucous, tumid or ulcerated, but there is almost always evidence of induration, i.e. the lesion feels firm between finger and thumb (*Fig. 23.7*). The outline of the tumour is often irregular but it may be rounded, and the surrounding tissue is usually inflamed. The distinction from keratoacanthoma is usually easy, since the rate of growth and domed appearance of keratoacanthomas are characteristic.

Table 23.9. *Precursor lesions for the development of SCC*

Actinic keratoses
Bowen's disease
Erythroplasia of Queyrat
Bowenoid papulosis
Arsenical keratoses
Chronic radiation keratoses

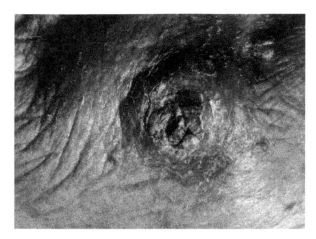

Figure 23.7. *Indurated, keratotic nodule on the cheek, which proved to be an SCC.*

Table 23.11. *Poor prognostic risk factors for SCC*

Recurrence

Depth of invasion (to or below the reticular dermis)

Size (≥2 cm diameter)

Histology (poorly differentiated)

Aetiology (scar, chronic ulcer, sinus tract, radiation dermatitis)

Immunosuppression

Anatomic site (ear)

Perineural invasion (neurotropism)

Rapid growth

On areas such as the lip or genitalia the presenting sign may be of a fissure or small erosion or ulcer that fails to heal and bleeds recurrently. The most common sites for SCC are those exposed to the sun such as the backs of the hands and forearms, the upper part of the face and, especially in males, the lower lip and pinna.

Histology

SCC is a tumour that may arise in any epithelium; in skin it begins when atypical keratinocytes breach the dermal basement membrane and invade the dermis. The cells of SCC vary from large, well-differentiated, polygonal cells with vesicular nuclei and prominent nucleoli through to completely anaplastic cells that provide no cytological evidence of their origin (undifferentiated). SCC has been classified into four main histological patterns (*Table 23.10*). The poorly differentiated pattern is the most aggressive and carries a higher recurrence rate and risk of metastasis.

Prognosis

There are no well-defined prognostic factors identified for SCCs to help to predict which patients are at high risk of relapse. Large studies using multivariate analysis or randomized trials are still needed to address this problem. However Rowe *et al.* (1992) have attempted to address this problem by reviewing all articles written since 1940 on prognostic factors in cutaneous SCC. They have identified nine variables as prognostic risk factors (*Table 23.11*) that are interdependent and thus lesions often have more than one risk factor.

Treatment

Evidence-based guidelines as to the best treatment approach for individual patients are not yet available. However, there are three effective treatments that are currently available for SCC: surgery, local destruction or radiotherapy. Before embarking on the chosen therapeutic option a confirmatory diagnostic biopsy from the centre of the tumour to the margin, including connective tissue, should be taken. As a general rule a very well-differentiated tumour is best treated by surgery or local destruction and a poorly differentiated tumour by surgery or radiotherapy (Mackie, 1998).

It is important to remember that recurrent tumours have a 25–45% metastatic rate, depending on anatomic site, and therefore the best chance to cure SCC is in the primary stage (Rowe *et al.*, 1992). Surgery is the treatment of choice for tumours that can be removed using primary closure, a simple graft or a flap. They should be excised with a 3–5 mm clearance margin. Surgery should also be advised in those patients with metastases, invasion locally into bone or cartilage, or for those lesions that have recurred.

Local destructive therapies including currettage and cryosurgery have been used effectively to treat SCC. However, these methods should be used only for small, low-risk tumours. Successful treatment of tumours with cryosurgery depends on adequate freezing to the correct depth with a margin around it.

Table 23.10. *Histological patterns of SCC*

Conventional (differentiated through to undifferentiated)

Spindle cell

Acantholytic (pseudoglandular, adenoid)

Verrucous

Radiation therapy with fractional dose schedule is also available to treat SCC. With properly selected tumours a cure rate of more than 90% may be obtained with good to excellent cosmetic and functional results (Petrovich *et al.*, 1987). It tends to leave rather fragile scars on the hand and forearm and may be followed by radionecrosis on the trunk. It is therefore best used to treat tumours of the head and neck.

Management and treatment of recurrence

More than 75% of local recurrences occur in the first 2 years after treatment, and therefore patients need frequent follow-up during this period (Dzubow *et al.*, 1982). As most SCCs metastasize to locoregional draining lymph nodes, these nodes should always be palpated when the patient attends for follow up. If palpable nodes are present a fine needle aspirate should be taken to confirm the presence of metastases.

Lymph node metastases can be treated with lymph node dissection, radiotherapy or a combination of the two. Overall the 5-year cure rate for clinical regional disease with all modalities is 34.4% (Rowe *et al.*, 1992). The outlook for patients with distant metastatic disease is poor. Therapeutic options include surgery, radiotherapy, or chemotherapy, either alone or in combination, depending on the site of metastasis and fitness of the patient.

Basal Cell Carcinoma

Incidence

Basal cell carcinoma (BCC) is a slowly growing, locally invasive malignant tumour composed of cells similar to those in the basal area of the epidermis and its appendages. It is the most common cutaneous neoplasm, and the incidence appears to be rising (Gallagher *et al.*, 1995; Gallagher *et al.*, 1990; Miller, 1991). Population-based incidence studies for males and females in Minnesota, Australia and Hawaii are listed in *Table 23.12* (Chuang *et al.*, 1990; Marks *et al.*, 1993; Reizner *et al.*, 1993).

Epidemiology and aetiology

BCC is more common in men than women and it is very rare in blacks (Chuang *et al.*, 1990). The significant aetiological factor is chronic exposure to ultraviolet light, and consequently exposed areas such as the head and neck are the most commonly involved sites (Roenigk *et al.*, 1996). The distribution on the face, including the inner canthus and eyelids, does not, however, correlate well with the area of maximum exposure to light. It is therefore likely that other

Table 23.12. *Incidence figures for BCC*

Country or state	Males (per 100,000)	Females (per 100,000)
Minnesota (USA)	175	124
Hawaii (USA)	576	298
Australia	849	605

Table 23.13. *Risk factors for the development of BCC*

Male sex
Outdoor occupations
Freckling
Scottish or Irish descent
Increasing age
Childhood sunburn
Fair or red hair
Arsenic exposure

regional factors such as the density and type of pilosebaceous follicles are important (Mackie, 1998).

Other hereditary and environmental risk factors are listed in *Table 23.13* (Hogan *et al.*, 1995; Gilbody *et al.*, 1994; Zanetti *et al.*, 1996). BCC can occur in any age group but is rare before the age of 40 years. It can develop at the site of a previous vaccination scar and arise in chronic leg ulcers. Skin areas exposed to ionizing radiation are particularly at risk. BCC can develop in naevus sebaceous and other adnexal hamartomas. BCC also forms part of Gorlin's syndrome or naevoid BCC syndrome, a genetically determined disorder characterized by BCCs, palmoplantar pits and defects in other tissues, such as jaw cysts, abnormalities of the ribs and vertebrae and a variety of less common changes. BCC is also seen in patients with xeroderma pigmentosum.

Clinical features

BCC can be divided into four main clinical subtypes (*Table 23.14*) (MacKie, 1998). The nodular or ulcerative BCC initially presents as a small, translucent or pearly, raised and rounded area covered by a thin epidermis through which a few telangiectatic vessels can be seen (*Fig. 23.8*). As the lesion enlarges, central erosions or ulceration develops. A well-formed rodent ulcer (BCC) often has a sharply demarcated rolled edge (*Fig. 23.9*). Patients often give a history of a 'non-healing' spot that occasionally bleeds and crusts.

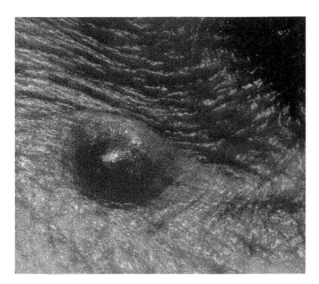

Figure 23.8. *Nodular or cystic BCC.*

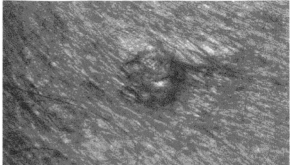

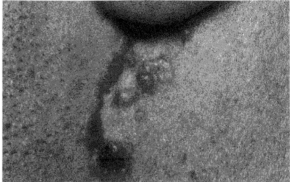

Table 23.14. *Clinical subtypes of BCC*

Nodular or ulcerative (45–60%)
Diffuse (infiltrating and morphoeic) (4–17%)
Superficial (multifocal) (15–35%)
Pigmented variant (1–7%)

Figure 23.9. *Typical BCCs with telangectasia, rolled edges and pearly appearance.*

The diffuse or morphoeic type, as the name suggests, has poorly demarcated clinical margins and is often an indurated slowly growing flat, whitish-pink plaque (*Fig. 23.10*). This type of BCC is typically translucent; a feature best seen after stretching the tumour under a bright light.

Superficial BCCs often present on the trunk as slowly enlarging red patches that have been present for years. They can occasionally become eroded. The clue to the diagnosis is usually made by careful examination of the edge, which is often 'rolled'. This type of BCC is typical of arsenic exposure. The pigmented type of BCC is often similar to the nodular or ulcerated type, with speckled dark brown pigmentation within it (*Fig. 23.11*). Malignant melanoma should also be considered within the differential diagnosis of pigmented BCC.

Histology

BCCs are made up of cells that resemble those of the basal layer of the epidermis and matrix cells of the appendages. The tumour cells have indistinct cytoplasmic borders and

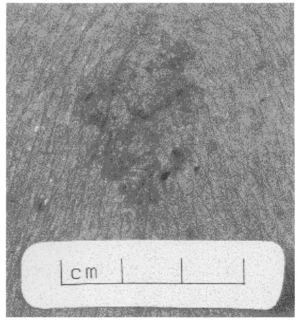

Figure 23.10. *Morphoeic type BCC, a macular lesion with prominent telangectasia.*

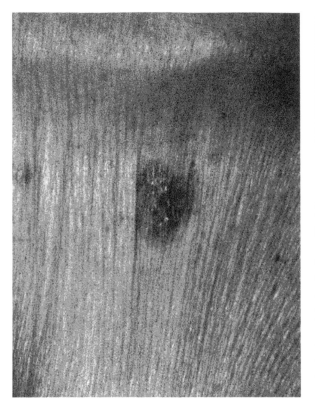

Figure 23.11. Pigmented BCC.

oval, basophilic, darkly staining nuclei. The interaction with the dermis produces the characteristic marginal palisade of tumour cells. In early lesions the tumour buds can be seen arising from the epidermis. In an established tumour the cell masses extend into the dermis and may separate from each other and from their point of origin.

Prognosis

BCCs are generally non-metastisizing but locally destructive tumours. The incidence of metastatic BCC ranges from 0.0028% to 0.1% in large series (Smith and Iron, 1983). There are several prognostic factors used to divide BCCs into 'high-risk' and 'low-risk' tumours (*Table 23.15*) (Telfer *et al.*, 1999).

Treatment

BCC is almost always cured provided treatment is appropriately selected. However, there is a risk of local recurrence and up to 50% of tumours recur after re-treatment of lesions that have been inadequately managed in the first instance

Table 23.15. Poor prognostic factors for BCC

Tumour size (>2 cm)
Tumour site (facial tumours, especially perinasal tumours)
Tumour type and definition of tumour margins (morphoeic BCC)
Recurrent tumours (failure of previous treatment)
Immunocompromised patients

(Menn *et al.*, 1971). Evidence-based guidelines have been published for the management of BCC (Telfer *et al.*, 1999). Management of BCC should therefore be based on these guidelines.

There are three major treatments available for BCC – surgery (excision), local destructive methods and radiotherapy. The primary objective of any excisional procedure is to remove the tumour entirely. The use of currettage before excision of a primary BCC may help to increase the cure rate by more accurately defining the true borders of the BCC. Excision normally extends well into the subcutaneous fat. A 3 mm surgical margin is adequate for well-defined BCC; however, morphoeic and larger BCCs require wider surgical margins. Peripheral excision margins for recurrent BCC of 5–10 mm have been suggested (Burg *et al.*, 1975).

The management of incompletely excised BCC remains controversial since two-thirds that are not re-treated do not recur (Dellon *et al.*, 1985). When deep margins are found to be involved, re-treatment is probably necessary; however, in tumours with lateral margin involvement an expectant policy may be adopted. Re-excision of incompletely excised tumours of an aggressive histological type, previously recurrent tumours and BCC in critical anatomical sites is recommended.

Mohs' micrographic surgery is also recommended for certain BCCs (*Table 23.16*) (Telfer *et al.*, 1999). Mohs' surgery is a method that allows for immediate histological assessment of tumour sections while the patient is undergoing surgery so that no unnecessary tissue is excised. It has also been used in the treatment of SCC.

Table 23.16. Indications for Mohs' surgery for BCC

Site – eyes, ears, lips, nose, nasolabial folds
Histological type – morphoeic, infiltrative, micronodular
Recurrence
Size – >2 cm, especially in high-risk sites
Other situations – perineural spread

Local destructive methods include curettage and cautery or electrodesiccation and cryosurgery. Curettage and cautery is best selected for low-risk, small, well-defined lesions in non-critical sites where good cure rates can be achieved. Tumour size is important because the recurrence rate rises dramatically with increasing tumour size. Cryosurgery is widely used to re-treat solitary and multiple BCCs that are not 'high-risk' tumours.

Radiotherapy is a very useful form of treatment, best performed by clinical oncologists with a special interest in skin cancer. The problem of accurately defining tumour margins, especially in morphoeic BCC, arises. However, careful patient selection can result in very high cure rates of up to 90.3%.

Other less established treatments used in the management of BCC include topical 5–fluorouracil (5FU), intralesional interferon and photodynamic therapy. Topical 5FU is useful to treat patients with multiple superficial BCCs. Intralesional interferon is still an investigative tool that seems to be useful in the treatment of low-risk tumours but not so beneficial for high-risk BCC (Telfer *et al.*, 1999). Photodynamic therapy is currently used only in research, although some success has been reported (Safai and Good, 1977).

Management and treatment of recurrence

Unfortunately there is little effective treatment available when metastasis does occur. Once the tumour has metastasized beyond the regional lymph nodes it is usually fatal, with a reported survival time of 10–14 months (Wieman *et al.*, 1983). Tumour shrinkage can sometimes be obtained with cisplatin-based chemotherapy, but cures are not seen.

References and Further Reading

Ames FC, Hickey RC. Metastasis from squamous cell carcinoma of the extremeties. *South Med J.* 1982; **75**: 920–3.

Aubry F, MacGibbon B. Risk factors of squamous cell carcinoma of the skin. *Cancer.* 1985; **55**: 907–11.

Breslow A. Thickness, cross-sectional areas and depth of invasion in the prognosis of cutaneous melanoma. *Ann Surg.* 1970; **172**: 902–8.

Burg G, Hirsch RD, Konz B, Braun-Falco O. Histographic surgery: accuracy of visual assessment of the margins of basal-cell epithelioma. *J Dermatol Surg Oncol.* 1975; **1**: 21–4.

Chowdhury S, Vaughan MM, Gore ME. New approaches to the systemic treatment of melanoma. *Cancer Treat Rev.* 1999; **25**: 259–70.

Chuang TY, Popescu NA, Su WDP, *et al.* Squamous cell carcinoma. A population based incidence study in Rochester Minnesota. *Arch Dermatol.* 1990; **126**: 185–8.

Chuang TY, Popescu A, Su WPD, *et al.* Basal cell carcinoma. A population based incidence study. *J Am Acad Dermatol.* 1990; **22**: 413–17.

Cox NH, Eedy DJ, Morton CA. Guidelines for management of Bowen's disease. *Br J Dermatol.* 1999; **141**: 633–41.

Dellon AL, DeSilva S, Connolly M, Ross A. Prediction of recurrence in incompletely excised basal cell carcinoma. *Plast Reconstr Surg.* 1985; **75**: 860–71.

Dzubow LM, Rigel DS, Robins P. Risk factors for local recurrence of primary cutaneous squamous cell carcinomas. *Arch Dermatol.* 1982; **118**: 900–2.

Gallagher RP, Hill GB, Bajdik CD, *et al.* Sunlight exposure, pigmentary factors and risk of non-melanocytic skin cancer. I. Basal cell carcinoma. *Arch Dermatol.* 1995; **131**: 157–63.

Gallagher RP, Ma B, McLean DI, *et al.* Trends in basal cell carcinoma, squamous cell carcinoma and melanoma of the skin. *J Am Acad Dermatol.* 1990; **23**: 413–21.

Gilbody JS, Aitken J, Green A. What causes basal cell carcinoma to be the commonest cancer? *Aust J Public Health.* 1994; **18**: 218–21.

Giles GG, Marks R, Foley P. Incidence of non-melanocytic skin cancer treated in Australia. *BMJ.* 1988; **296**: 13–17.

Glass AG, Hoover RN. The emerging epidemic of melanoma and squamous cell skin cancer. *JAMA.* 1989; **262**: 2097–100.

Glucksman A. Carcinogenesis of skin tumor induced by radiation. *Br Med Bull.* 1958; **14**: 178–80.

Grossman D, Leffell DJ. The molecular basis of nonmelanoma skin cancer: new understanding. *Arch Dermatol.* 1997; **133**: 1263–70.

Hogan DJ, To T, Gran L, *et al.* Risk factors for basal cell carcinoma. *Int J Cancer.* 1995; **60**: 482–8.

Kirkwood JM, Strawderman MH, Ernstoff MS, *et al.* Interferon alpha 2b adjuvant therapy of high-risk resected cutaneous melanoma: the Eastern Cooperative Oncology Group Trial EST 1684. *J Clin Oncol.* 1996; **14**: 7–17.

Leigh IM, Glover MT. Cutaneous warts and tumours in immunosuppressed patients. *J R Soc Med.* 1995; **88**: 61–2.

MacKie book Basal cell carcinoma (epithelioma) 15.32–15.37

MacKie RM. Melanoma prevention and early detection. *Br Med Bull.* 1995; **51**: 570–83.

MacKie RM. Epidermal skin tumours: basal cell carcinoma. In: Champion RH, Burton JL, Burns DA, Breathnach SM, eds. *Rook–Wilkinson–Ebling Textbook of Dermatology.* Oxford: Blackwell Science, 1998: 1679–85.

MacKie RM. Epidermal skin tumours: squamous cell carcinoma. In: Champion RH, Burton JL, Burns DA, Breathnach SM, eds. *Rook–Wilkinson–Ebling Textbook of Dermatology.* Oxford: Blackwell Science, 1998: 1687–92.

MacKie RM, Hole DH, Hunter JAA, *et al.* Cutaneous malignant melanoma in Scotland: incidence, survival and mortality,1979–1994. The Scottish Melanoma Group. *BMJ.* 1997; **315**: 1117–21.

Marks R, Foley P, Goodman G, *et al.* Spontaneous remission of solar keratoses: the case for conservative management. *Br J Dermatol.* 1986; **115**: 649–55.

Marks R, Rennie G, Selwood TS. Malignant transformation of solar keratoses to squamous cell carcinoma. *Lancet.* 1988; **i**: 795–7.

Marks R, Staples M, Giles GG. Trends in non-melanocytic skin cancer treated in Australia. The second national survey. *Int J Cancer.* 1993; **53**: 585–90.

Menn H, Robbins P, Kopf A, *et al.* The recurrent basal cell epithelioma. *Arch Dermatol.* 1971; **103**: 628–31.

Miller SJ. Biology of basal cell carcinoma (part 1). *J Am Acad Dermatol.* 1991; **24**: 1–13.

Petrovich Z, Parker RG, Luxton G, *et al.* Carcinoma of the lip and selected sites of the head and neck skin: a clinical study of 896 patients. *Radiother Oncol.* 1987; **8**: 11–17.

Reizner GT, Chuang TY, Elpern DJ, *et al.* Basal cell carcinoma in Kauai, Hawaii: the highest documented incidence in the United States. *J Am Acad Dermatol.* 1993; **29**: 184–9.

Roenigk RK, Ratz JL, Bailin PL, Wheeland RG. Trends in presentation and treatment of basal cell carcinomas. *J Dermatol Surg Oncol.* 1986: 12: 860–5.

Rosso S, Zanetti R, Martinez C, *et al.* The multicentre south European study 'Helios' II. Different sun exposure pattern in the aetiology of basal cell and squamous cell carcinomas of the skin. *Br J Cancer.* 1996; **73**: 1447–54.

Rowe DE, Carroll RJ, Day CL Jr. Prognostic factors for local recurrence, metastasis and survival rates in squamous cell carcinoma of the skin, ear and lip: implications for treatment modality selection. *J Am Acad Dermatol.* 1992; **26**: 976–90.

Safai B, Good RA. Basal cell carcinoma with metastasis. *Arch Pathol Lab Med.* 1977; **101**: 327–31.

Schiffman NJ. Squamous cell carcinomas of the skin of the pinna. *Can J Surg.* 1975; **18**: 279–83.

Smith JM, Iron GB. Metastatic basal cell carcinoma: review of the literature and report of three cases. *Ann Plast Surg.* 1983; **11**: 551–3.

Telfer NR, Colver GB, Bowers PW. Guidelines for the management of basal cell carcinoma. *Br J Dermatol.* 1999; **141**: 415–23.

Vitasa BC, Taylor HR, Strickland PT, *et al.* Association of nonmelanoma skin cancer and actinic keratosis with cumulative solar ultraviolet exposure in Maryland watermen. *Cancer.* 1990; **65**: 2811–17.

Wheatley K, Ives N, Hancock B *et al.* Does adjuvant interferon- for high-risk melanoma provide a worthwhile benefit? A meta-analysis of the randomised trials. *Cancer Treatment Rev* 2003 (in press).

Wieman TJ, Shively EH, Woodcock TM. Responsiveness of metastatic basal cell carcinoma to chemotherapy. A case report. *Cancer.* 1983: 52; **1583–5.**

Wilson BD, Mang TS, Stoll H, *et al.* Photodynamic therapy for the treatment of basal cell carcinoma. *Arch Dermatol.* 1992: **128**; 1597–601.

Zanetti R, Rosso S, Martinez C, *et al.* The multicentre European Helios study 1. Skin characteristics and sunburns in basal and squamous cell carcinomas of the skin. *Br J Cancer.* 1996; **73**: 1440–6.

24 Sarcomas

Ian Judson and Clive Harmer

What are Sarcomas?

Sarcomas are tumours of mesenchymal rather than epithelial tissue. There are many different subtypes, some of which resemble tissues such as fat, muscle, nerve, bone, or fibrous tissue. Unlike the epithelial tissues, which form the common cancers, mesenchymal tissues (at least in the adult) do not constantly divide, as the gut and bronchial mucosa do, or undergo cycles of proliferation, as breast tissue and endometrial tissue do. In addition, mesenchymal tissues are not so exposed to environmental carcinogens. These features may account for the rarity of these tumours. Unfortunately, their very rarity tends to lead to late diagnosis, so many patients present with a long history and a large mass.

Soft-Tissue Sarcomas in Adults

Introduction

Soft-tissue sarcomas (STS) are rare; they account for only 1% of adult malignancies, but for 6% of those in childhood. There are about 1000 new cases in the UK annually.

Presentation

The majority of patients present with a painless swelling that has been increasing in size for several months and that can be surprisingly large, especially if in the thigh, buttock, or abdomen. The quadriceps is the most common site, accounting for 25% of all STS. Any new, enlarging mass deep to the deep fascia should be regarded as a sarcoma until proved otherwise (*Fig. 24.1*). Delays in diagnosis are common and usually involve the failure to investigate enlarging lesions or persistent pain in the absence of trauma. Key features that should be regarded as suspicious for a sarcoma are listed in the box.

Key features suspicious of sarcoma

- Any soft tissue mass deep to the deep fascia is a sarcoma until proved otherwise.

- Any tumour >2.5cm in diameter that is enlarging should be regarded as suspicious.
- A painless soft-tissue mass in the absence of a clear history of trauma requires investigation by computed tomography or magnetic resonance imaging.

Diagnosis

If the diagnosis of a soft-tissue tumour is suspected, appropriate imaging is vital and is the one investigation most commonly delayed. Both computed tomography (CT) and magnetic resonance imaging (MRI) can reveal the problem.

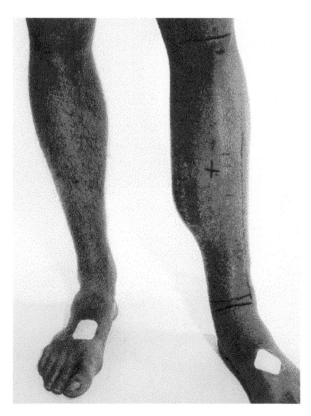

Figure 24.1. *Calf mass caused by a 10cm high-grade liposarcoma in a 23-year-old man. This was treated successfully by pre-operative radiotherapy and compartmental resection.*

Table 24.1. *Simplified classification of characteristic soft-tissue tumours*

Usually aggressive	Usually at least intermediate to high grade	Vary from very low to high grade	Usually slow growing
Synovial sarcoma	Malignant fibrous histiocytoma	Liposarcoma	Alveolar soft-part sarcoma
Epithelioid sarcoma	Fibrosarcoma	Leiomyosarcoma	Myxoid liposarcoma
Angiosarcoma	Malignant peripheral nerve sheath tumour		Epithelioid haemangioendothelioma
Clear-cell sarcoma	Pleomorphic rhabdomyosarcoma		

Their relative merits are unclear, but, although neither can diagnose the problem, they can often differentiate a benign from a malignant lesion.

The next step is a biopsy, preferably made using a cutting needle (e.g. Trucut) to minimize tumour dissemination and difficulties with the subsequent operation. Expert pathology assessment is vital, since errors in diagnosis, including discrimination between benign and malignant disease, are common. These two recommendations underline the fact that, ideally, patients suspected of having a malignant soft-tissue tumour should be referred to a specialist multidisciplinary centre.

Pathology

As a result of their rarity, the pathology of all soft-tissue tumours should be reviewed by a histopathologist with experience and knowledge of this group of diseases. Chemosensitive tumours need to be excluded. The most important and occasionally the most difficult decision is to determine whether the tumour is benign or malignant.

In addition to examining the appearance of the tumour under the microscope, some very sophisticated molecular biology tools are now available that can help to make a precise diagnosis, especially in those tumours associated with children and adolescents.

A very simplified classification of some characteristic soft-tissue tumours is given in *Table 24.1*.

Apart from the variable rates of growth and tendency to metastasize, marked differences occur in patterns of behaviour. For example, epithelioid sarcoma and pleomorphic rhabdomyosarcoma may spread to lymph nodes, but this is otherwise rare. Angiosarcoma commonly involves bones, and myxoid liposarcoma is characterized by the ability to metastasize from a limb to the abdomen. Low-grade liposarcoma and leiomyosarcoma are not infrequently mistaken for benign lesions and may recur or metastasize many years after the original tumour has been removed. Lung metastases from alveolar soft-part sarcoma can reach a certain size and then lay dormant for years. Synovial sarcoma metastasizes fre-

quently, but may be sensitive to chemotherapy. In other words, although these tumours are grouped together for the purposes of initial treatment they behave very differently.

The chemosensitive small round cell tumours [rhabdomyosarcoma, Ewing's sarcoma, and primitive neuroectodermal tumour (PNET)] are dealt with separately, although they do occur in the adult age range.

Management

Summary of primary management

- Diagnosis should preferably be made by a cutting needle (e.g. Trucut) biopsy. An open incision biopsy is rarely necessary.
- The pathology of soft-tissue tumours should be reviewed by an expert. Errors in differentiating benign from malignant disease are common.
- Properly planned, wide excisional surgery, usually with radiotherapy, offers the best chance of local cure. Simply shelling out the tumour increases the likelihood of local recurrence and makes definitive surgery more difficult. Amputation for previously untreated soft-tissue sarcomas is rarely necessary.
- Pre-operative staging should include a computed tomography scan of the thorax, since the lungs are the primary metastatic site for most sarcomas. Large high-grade tumours carry a 50% risk of metastatic disease.
- Good functional results, combined with low rates of local recurrence and amputation, are indicative of good-quality treatment. Patients with soft-tissue sarcoma should be treated in specialist multidisciplinary units.
- Adjuvant chemotherapy has not been shown to give a clear-cut survival benefit, but may prolong the disease-free interval and be beneficial in patients with large high-grade limb primaries.

Operative management

Resection of a sarcoma needs to be planned in the light of detailed anatomical information derived from CT or MRI. Wide excision is vital. This may involve excision of the entire muscular compartment that contains the tumour, although preservation of function must be considered. Sarcomas may spread along fascial planes, a feature that needs to be taken into account in determining the appropriate operation. Excision biopsy is always a mistake and can jeopardize the chance of cure.

Radiotherapy

Patients with high-grade tumours, or a marginal excision, benefit from radical-dose radiotherapy, which reduces the risk of local recurrence. Treatment is given to the original tumour volume and entire compartment. High dose is mandatory (e.g. 50Gy) plus a boost to the tumour bed of 10Gy over 6 weeks. Care needs to be taken to include muscle origins and insertions, given the tendency of sarcomas to spread along fascial planes, and the surgical scar to avoid implantation recurrence. If feasible, a corridor of normal tissue needs to spared when irradiating a limb to reduce the risk of lymphoedema, which can cause significant morbidity. Other late problems are fibrosis and induration, which can be minimized by physiotherapy.

Adjuvant chemotherapy

The role of adjuvant chemotherapy remains unclear, but a recent meta-analysis of primary data from all published randomized trials showed significantly improved progression-free survival and a small improvement in overall survival (amounting to 4% at 10 years), which failed to reach conventional levels of statistical significance. Patients with large, high-grade tumours in the limbs probably do benefit.

Management of metastatic sarcoma

Chemotherapy

The chemotherapy of advanced STS remains unsatisfactory, with response rates of only 25–30%. Doxorubicin and ifosfamide are the most active drugs, but are associated with hair loss and a risk of infection with low white blood cell counts. Good palliation of symptoms can often be achieved, although responses tend to be short-lived.

Pulmonary metastasectomy

Resection of lung metastases is a safe and effective treatment for patients with a limited number of lesions. The best results are obtained in those with a long disease-free interval and fewer than 10 metastases. Operations can be performed via a median sternotomy or lateral thoracotomy depending on the site and number of lesions. Long-term disease control is reported, although the true success of this procedure is difficult to judge, because no controlled trials have been conducted and patient selection occurs before referral.

Follow-up

The main site of metastatic disease is the lungs and relapse most commonly occurs in the first 2 years. Follow-up is advised to identify those patients who can be treated surgically. In the majority of cases lung metastases do not cause symptoms until very late, so radiology is required. Chest radiography together with physical examination of the original tumour site is required every 3 months for the first 2 years, after which the frequency of follow-up can be reduced.

For patients with intrathoracic or retroperitoneal tumours, follow-up is more difficult. Gastrointestinal stromal tumours often spread to the liver and otherwise to peritoneal surfaces. Ultrasound is useful, using CT on suspicion of abdominal masses or persistent symptoms (e.g. colicky pain).

Rhabdomyosarcoma

Rhabdomyosarcoma is the most common soft-tissue tumour in childhood and adolescents. More than half the cases occur in children under 10 years of age and it is rare in adults over 40 years of age. The male to female ratio is 1.3:1. The most common sites of origin are the head and neck, genitourinary tract, and extremities. The disease may spread locally (e.g. to the meninges and central nervous system) and may metastasize to lymph nodes, lungs, bones, bone marrow, and brain. This is an aggressive disease that requires multimodality treatment; the outcome depends on the disease site and the histological subtype.

Table 24.2. Prognostic factors in rhabdomyosarcoma

Good	Poor
Orbit, paratesticular, vagina	Parameningeal, retroperitoneal, extremities
Localized to tissue of origin	Contiguous spread, nodal, or metastatic disease
Complete resection feasible	Unresectable
Embryonal histology	Alveolar histology
Infant or child	Adult
Complete response to chemotherapy	Poor response to chemotherapy

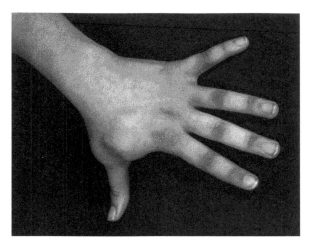

Figure 24.2. *Alveolar rhabdomyosarcoma in a 15-year-old girl with a 6-month history of swelling in the hand.*

Presentation

Like other solid tumours, rhabdomyosarcoma presents with swelling or other local symptoms (*Fig. 24.2*), such as displacement of the eye, vaginal bleeding, or dysuria. In establishing the diagnosis it is advisable to obtain fresh tissue for chromosomal studies.

Embryonal rhabdomyosarcoma

Embryonal rhabdomyosarcoma accounts for about 60% of cases. It occurs mainly in children under 15 years of age, and most commonly affects the head and neck (including the orbit) or the genitourinary tract. 'Embryonal' refers to the spectrum of cell type from primitive round cells to rhabdomyoblasts, which may be thought of as mimicking the stages in muscle embryogenesis. Botryoid rhabdomyosarcoma is characterized by polypoid growth, like a 'bunch of grapes', and is usually found in hollow organs such as the vagina, bladder, or nasopharynx.

Alveolar rhabdomyosarcoma

Alveolar rhabdomyosarcoma is characterized by poorly differentiated, round or oval cells that form irregular spaces and are separated by fibrous septae, to give the appearance of 'alveoli' (*Fig. 24.2*). Sometimes this appearance is absent, but the uniform appearance of the cells is distinct from that of the embryonal variety. Multinucleate giant cells may be observed. Alveolar rhabdomyosarcoma has a significantly worse prognosis than the embryonal type. Molecular biology techniques may aid diagnosis.

Management
Chemotherapy

Patients with embryonal histology may be treated with vincristine plus dactinomycin with the addition of ifosfamide, doxorubicin, and other drugs according to stage and histology. Drugs such as etoposide or carboplatin and high-dose alkylating agent therapy with peripheral blood progenitor-cell rescue may have improved the outlook for some patients with metastatic disease, but the prognosis remains grave for alveolar rhabdomyosarcoma.

Radiotherapy

Rhabdomyosarcomas are highly sensitive to radiotherapy. Chemotherapy plus radiotherapy at a dose of 40–50Gy usually ensures disease control. However, serious long-term problems are associated with the use of radiotherapy in children. These include damage to sensitive organs (such as the bladder, eye, and ear) and endocrine glands (such as the testis, ovary, and thyroid), and the risk of second malignancy and imbalanced bone growth (especially when epiphyses are included in the field). In infants and children with localized tumours and favourable histology, such as embryonal rhabdomyosarcoma of the orbit, chemotherapy alone is likely to be used, although older adolescents and adults can safely be treated with radiotherapy. Conversely, extremity, alveolar histology, and parameningeal tumours require radiotherapy. The outlook for rhabdomyosarcoma in the adolescent or young adult appears to be especially poor, and better treatments are required.

Surgery

Surgery usually follows the initial tumour shrinkage with chemotherapy. Wide excision is recommended for extremity tumours. Surgery is rarely indicated in the case of orbital tumours, and can rarely be radical in other head and neck sites, especially when parameningeal. Paratesticular tumours should be removed using a high inguinal-approach orchidectomy. Careful assessment of regional lymph nodes is required. Bladder-conserving surgery or radiotherapy should be employed for bladder and prostate tumours.

Bone Sarcomas

Osteosarcoma

Osteosarcoma is the most common bone tumour and principally affects long bones, especially epiphyseal sites. The peak incidence coincides with the adolescent growth spurt, although it may occur at any age. Other bone tumours include chondrosarcoma (which is locally aggressive, may

Key points: sarcomas

Sarcomas are rare tumours.

Soft-tissue sarcoma

Can occur at any age – more common over 30 years of age.

Most soft-tissue masses are benign (only 1 in 200 are malignant).

Features of soft-tissue mass suggestive of malignancy include:

  diameter >5 cm

  painful

  increasing in size

  deep to fascia

  recurrence after previous excision

Lumps that are superficial and painless and less than 5cm in diameter and static in size are extremely unlikely to be malignant.

Primary bone tumours

These tumours includes osteosarcoma, Ewing's sarcoma, and chondrosarcoma.

Most common in adolescents.

50% arise around the knee.

Symptoms include pain, which is typically non-mechanical, waking the patient at night.

Bony swelling and limp are usually late features.

Most are diagnosed radiographically.

Reproduced from England Department of Health Cancer Referral Guidelines Consultation Document May 2000.

Guidelines for urgent referral: sarcomas

A soft-tissue mass with one or more of the following characteristics:

  diameter >5cm

  painful

  increasing in size

  deep to fascia

  recurrence after previous excision

Patients with radiological suspicion of a primary bone tumour based on evidence of bone destruction, new bone formation, soft-tissue swelling, periosteal elevation.

metastasize, and is generally resistant to chemotherapy and radiotherapy) and giant cell tumours (which are usually benign but which can be locally destructive and occasionally metastasize).

Presentation

Osteosarcoma presents with bone pain, especially on weight bearing, often associated with soft-tissue swelling. The tumour site is usually warm. Radiographs of the affected bone show a permeative, destructive lesion, often associated with abnormal calcification in the tumour surrounding the damaged bone (hence the term osteogenic sarcoma).

Management

The initial management of osteosarcoma is with chemotherapy. This has been shown to reduce dramatically the incidence of death from metastatic disease and also serves to shrink the tumour pre-operatively, which is of particular benefit in the case of extensive soft-tissue disease. The most active drugs are cisplatin, doxorubicin, and high-dose methotrexate. It is usual to

Referral proforma: sarcomas

Age:

Suspected diagnosis

Soft-tissue sarcoma ☐

Primary bone tumour ☐

History	Yes	No	
Swelling			
Location...			
Pain			
Increase in size			

Clinical examination	Yes	No	
Diameter............cm			
Deep to fascia			

Radiology

Not done ☐

Suspicious of bone tumour ☐

Other ☐

administer three cycles of chemotherapy before and three after an operation. Limb-conserving surgery is generally possible using a specially manufactured endoprosthesis. However, the incidence of prosthetic failure in adolescents is high, owing to the extreme stresses associated with sports. In young children the problem is that of growth, which requires either regular replacement of the prosthesis or insertion of devices that can be lengthened. Remote-control lengthening prostheses have been designed to try and overcome this problem. Radiotherapy is required only if surgical margins are involved or the tumour is inoperable

Metastatic disease

Patients who present with metastatic disease, either in the lungs or in other bones, have a poor prognosis. The late occurrence of isolated lung metastases may be managed by pulmonary metastasectomy, which can be highly successful. Salvage chemotherapy may provide effective palliation, but is rarely curative.

Ewing's sarcoma and related tumours

Ewing's sarcoma is now regarded as one of a family of tumours, all of which share chromosomal translocations that involve the EWS gene on chromosome 22. In the translocations parts of two chromosomes are exchanged, and this causes disease by resulting in certain genes becoming permanently switched on.

The Ewing's family tumours are:

- Ewing's sarcoma of bone;
- soft-tissue Ewing's sarcoma;
- PNET (may arise in bone or soft tissue); and
- Askin's tumour, a PNET of the chest wall.

Presentation

Ewing's sarcoma of bone may present in a similar fashion to osteosarcoma, although the sites of disease are more varied. The tibia is a more likely site than the distal femur, and the pelvic bones are quite commonly affected. Ewing's family tumours are rare, with an incidence in the adolescent group of only 0.6 per million per annum. Soft-tissue tumours may present at a variety of sites, including chest wall and pelvis. Unfortunately, in older patients pelvic tumours tend to be very large before they are diagnosed. Pain is a common feature, and CT or MRI is required, followed by the appropriate biopsy. These tumours tend to metastasize to bone, bone marrow, and lungs, and hence staging investigations include isotope bone scan, bone marrow aspirate plus trephine, and CT scan of the lungs.

Management

The key to treatment is urgent and effective chemotherapy. Aggressive induction combination chemotherapy is used, which comprises doxorubicin, ifosfamide, vincristine, and probably etoposide. Following the initial chemotherapy, which controls symptoms, reduces swelling, and begins to treat occult disease, the tumour is removed if possible. Otherwise radio-therapy is used, which can be administered concurrently with the chemotherapy. If bone resection is involved an endopros-thetic replacement is used, as in the case of osteosarcoma. Chemotherapy may need to be prolonged for up to a year, especially in children. Currently, a trial is under way to address the potential benefit of high-dose chemotherapy for poor prognosis cases, such as those patients who present with lung metastases or those with a poor histological response to drug treatment. The latter is the most important adverse prognos-tic factor, followed by large tumour size and presence of metas-tases. Patients with bone or bone marrow disease do particularly badly.

Conclusions

- Sarcomas are rare tumours that affect children, adolescents, and adults of all ages. They vary dramatically in their manner of presentation and clinical behaviour. The outcome depends on histological subtype, grade, and tumour size. Size is an independent prognostic factor; larger tumours are more likely to metastasize and may be more difficult to remove radically.
- Growing lumps, especially in young people, should never be ignored; unless superficial and mobile they should be assumed malignant. Referral to a specialist centre is encouraged since the wrong operation can jeopardize the chance of cure. Some types of sarcoma require immediate chemotherapy, which further underlines the need to make the right diagnosis as soon as possible.
- Careful follow-up is useful since some patients who have a relapse in the lungs may be treatable surgically. In most cases a chest radiograph and physical examination are all that is required. Follow-up of patients with abdominal sarcomas is more difficult, as is the management of relapse.
- At least half of all patients with adult sarcomas can be cured with local treatment. Chemotherapy is mainly palliative, although adjuvant treatment may be beneficial in some patients.

Further Reading

Details concerning soft tissue and bone sarcomas can be found on the CancerNet website of the National Cancer Institute, USA (see http://cancernet.nci.nih.gov/pdqfull.html and go to Cancer Information Summaries, Sarcomas).

The charity Cancer BACUP has produced booklets on soft tissue and bone sarcomas. They can be contacted at 3 Bath Place, Rivington St, London EC2A 3DR; Tel. 020 7696 9003; Fax: 020 7696 9002; website: www.cancerbacup.org.uk.

25 Head and Neck, and Thyroid Cancer

Peter Rhys Evans and Clive Harmer

Incidence

Head and neck cancer accounts for only 5% of malignant tumours and yet nowhere in the field of human cancer are the effects of progression of the disease more readily apparent, more cosmetically deforming, and more functionally and psychologically disturbing than in this region. It includes a wide range of malignant tumours that arise from multiple diverse structures and tissues.

The most common site is the larynx, but a GP might only expect to see one laryngeal carcinoma every 10 years. Other sites include the lips, the oral cavity and tongue, the pharynx (nasopharynx, oropharynx and hypopharynx), the cervical oesophagus and trachea, and the nasal cavity and sinuses. Tumours of other associated structures, such as the thyroid and salivary glands, the ear, orbit and skull base, and the skin of the head and neck, are also included (*Table 25.1*). Malignant lumps in the neck, whether caused by metastatic disease or lymphomas, are also an essential part of the scope of head and neck cancer. Various statistics relating to head, neck and thyroid tumours are shown in *Fig. 25.1*.

Pathology

Almost 7000 new head and neck cancers are seen annually in the UK, with a male to female ratio of 2:1. It affects patients mainly in the sixth and seventh decades and the regional variation is wide, ranging from about 8 per 100,000 population in the south of England to 13–15 in the north-west, Wales, and Scotland. Although cancers of individual sites within the head and neck are rare, collectively the combined rate for these tumours represents the eighth most common cancer in males (16th in females).

The large majority (80%) of tumours are squamous cell carcinomas, which arise from the surface mucosa of the upper aerodigestive tract as an ulcerative or exophytic mass (*Fig. 25.2*). They grow locally invading adjacent structures and usually spread to the draining lymph nodes in the neck, where they are confined for some period of time. The presence of cervical node metastases is the single most adverse prognostic factor in head and neck cancer, reducing survival by a factor of 50%. Only about 10%, however, eventually metastasize to other organs. Spread to the local nodes depends largely on the effectiveness of lymphatic drainage, with early spread from the nasopharynx, tonsil, and tongue base (where rich lymphatics occur), and rare neck node involvement from the vocal cords (which are virtually free of lymphatics). Metastases from the breast, lungs, and gastrointestinal tract may also appear in the lower neck.

Other tumours include adenocarcinoma, adenoid cystic carcinoma and mucoepidermoid carcinoma, which arise from the major (parotid, submandibular) and minor (oral and nasal cavities, pharynx, and larynx) salivary glands, and

Table 25.1. *Incidence of head and neck cancers in the UK for 1988*

	England	Scotland	Wales	Northern Ireland	UK
Population (millions)	47.4	5.09	2.85	1.57	57.0
Larynx	1926	243	155	52	2376
Oral cavity (total)	1664	294	138	60	2156
lip	243	58	24	17	342
mouth	805	158	63	27	1053
tongue	616	78	51	16	761
Pharynx	1006	122	82	31	1241
Thyroid	792	99	65	23	979

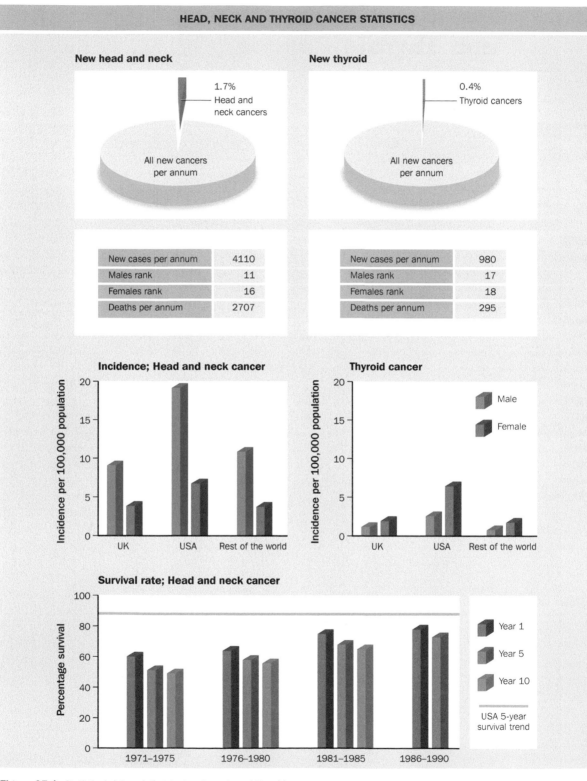

HEAD, NECK AND THYROID CANCER STATISTICS

New head and neck

1.7%
Head and
neck cancers

All new cancers
per annum

New cases per annum	4110
Males rank	11
Females rank	16
Deaths per annum	2707

New thyroid

0.4%
Thyroid cancers

All new cancers
per annum

New cases per annum	980
Males rank	17
Females rank	18
Deaths per annum	295

Incidence; Head and neck cancer

Thyroid cancer

Male
Female

Survival rate; Head and neck cancer

Year 1
Year 5
Year 10

USA 5-year
survival trend

Figure 25.1. Statistical data relating to head, neck and thyroid cancer.

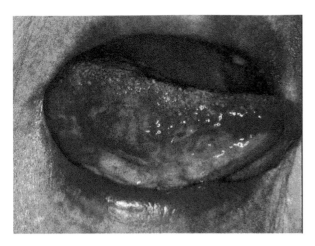

Figure 25.2. *Carcinoma of the lateral border of the tongue (see also Fig. 20.4).*

lymphomas, which usually present as a rubbery neck swelling, and (rarely) sarcomas. Cutaneous tumours include basal and squamous cell carcinomas as well as melanomas, which may also occur rarely as mucosal lesions in the nasal and oral cavities.

Swellings of the thyroid gland are quite common and the great majority are benign. Thyroid cancer is rare and a separate entity that occurs in younger patients and has excellent prognosis for the differentiated papillary and follicular types. Medullary thyroid cancer is less common and may be associated with multiple endocrine neoplasia syndromes. Undifferentiated or anaplastic carcinoma occurs in the elderly and is rapidly progressive. Primary lymphoma also occurs in the thyroid, but is rare.

Aetiology

Tobacco is by far the most important aetiological factor in head and neck cancer; up to 90% of patients with cancers of the oral cavity, oropharynx, hypopharynx, and larynx have used it at some stage in their lives. In patients from the Indian subcontinent the habit of chewing tobacco is an especially important cause of oral cancers. Alcohol has an important synergistic effect when combined with tobacco.

Prevention

Cancer of the head and neck is largely a preventable disease and the benefits of eliminating tobacco and reducing alco-

hol intake are well documented. A well-balanced diet, including fruit and vegetables with supplements of vitamins A, C, and E, probably offer some protective role. The greatest cost benefits are gained by educating children not to take up a tobacco habit and by increasing public awareness of early symptoms. Early detection of small-volume disease, particularly in high-risk groups, significantly improves survival and reduces morbidity associated with extensive surgery.

Clinical Presentation

Inflammatory conditions of the head and neck are very common, but invariably resolve spontaneously or with a course of antibiotics. Any symptoms (such as hoarseness, difficulty with swallowing, a sore throat, a lump in the neck, or ulcer in the mouth) that persists for more than 2–3 weeks should be urgently referred to an ear, nose, and throat (ENT) specialist and cancer considered the cause until proved otherwise. The level of suspicion should be further increased if there is a history of smoking or heavy alcohol intake, particularly if the patient is over 45 years of age, or if there are two or more symptoms. Persistent pain at any site is an indication of advanced disease. A list of the common symptoms are given in *Table 25.2.*

Table 25.2. *Common head and neck cancer symptoms*

Presenting symptom	Suspicious site (%)
Hoarseness	Larynx (80–90)
	Hypopharynx (50)
Neck lump	Oropharynx and nasopharynx (80–90)
	Hypopharynx (50)
	Thyroid (90)
Sore throat/dysphagia	Hypopharynx and oropharynx (80–90)
	Larynx (30–40)
Earache	Oropharynx, tongue (70–80)
Oral pain/ulceration/ visible lesion	Oral cavity, tongue (80–90)
Unilateral deafness	Nasopharynx (50)
Nasal obstruction/bleeding	Nasal cavity/sinuses (80–90)
Lump in parotid/ submandibular gland	Salivary gland (90)

Investigations

General practice

In patients with suspicious ENT symptoms or signs, an initial examination of the appropriate part should be carried out as well as palpation of the neck to detect any obvious lymphadenopathy (*Fig. 25.3*). Examination of the throat may be restricted to the mouth and oropharynx, but a good light source is essential and gentle bimanual palpation can be helpful. Most other tumours are difficult to see (*Fig. 25.4*), and urgent referral for a full ENT examination is essential.

Hospital

Current government legislation (*The New NHS – Modern, Dependable*) guarantees that everyone with suspected cancer will be able to see a specialist within 2 weeks of a GP decision that an urgent referral is necessary and a request for an appointment. These arrangements were guaranteed for breast cancer from April 1999 and for head and neck cancer the implementation date was December 2000, which has been facilitated by Rapid Access ENT Clinics.

Fibreoptic examination carried out in the clinic under local anaesthetic provides a quick and accurate assessment of any lesion in the nasal cavity, pharynx (see *Fig. 25.4*), or larynx, in addition to general ENT examination. Fine-needle aspiration cytology (FNAC) of any swelling in the neck, thyroid, or salivary glands should be carried out at the same clinic visit, if appropriate, to allow rapid confirmation of diagnosis. Routine haematological tests, a chest radiograph, and electrocardiogram are carried out to determine the general physical state of the patient, as well as computed tomography scans of the head, neck, and thorax to assess the extent of the disease and any metastases or second primaries. Additional information may be gained in tumours at some sites with magnetic resonance imaging. A barium swallow and videofluoroscopy may help to assess dysphagia in hypopharyngeal or cervical oesophageal lesions and other swallowing problems.

Pharyngoscopy and microlaryngoscopy under general anaesthetic are then necessary to allow biopsy and assessment of the tumour extent, as well as detection of any second primaries.

Head and Neck Cancer Unit

Head and neck cancer is designated a rare tumour, so a general ENT or oral surgeon sees fewer than 10 new cases each year. In line with government recommendations, all patients should be treated by an appropriate multidisciplinary team of head and neck specialists (ENT and/ or head and neck surgeon, maxillofacial surgeon, plastic surgeon, radiotherapist, and oncologist), which sees at least 80 new patients annually in a cancer unit (and may or may not be part of the local ENT–oral–plastic surgery department). Appropriate referral to a member of the team should be made on suspicion or diagnosis of the cancer. It is preferable that the investigations be carried out by the specialists who will decide and co-ordinate treatment.

Neck lumps

A special word of caution is required for patients who present with a suspicious lump in the neck without any obvious

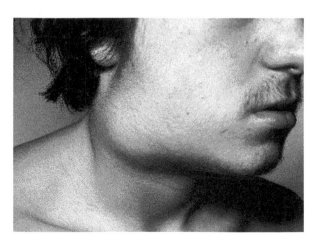

Figure 25.3. *Large node metastasis from an apparently occult primary.*

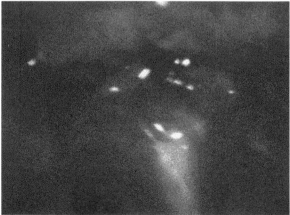

Figure 25.4. *Small asymptomatic carcinoma of the nasopharynx presenting with neck node (Fig. 25.3), but only found on fibreoptic nasendoscopy.*

upper aerodigestive tract symptoms. It is essential that these patients are referred for ENT assessment and FNAC, and not for excision biopsy, because many of them will be found on detailed examination to have small squamous cancers of the pharynx (see *Fig. 25.4*) and unnecessary incisions in the neck may increase the risk of complications.

Thyroid cancer

Thyroid cancer may present as a localized swelling of the gland or a feeling of pressure in the lower anterior neck, or as a solitary and/or cold nodule during investigation for thyroid symptoms. About 50% of papillary cancers have enlarged neck nodes on presentation and the true diagnosis may only be found on FNAC of the node. Ultrasound-guided FNAC is a more accurate diagnostic investigation than radioactive scanning for thyroid swellings. Rapid enlargement of the thyroid in an older patient may suggest anaplastic carcinoma or lymphoma. Thyroglobulin is a helpful serum marker in the follow-up of differentiated thyroid cancer, as is calcitonin in the initial diagnosis of medullary cancer.

Stage and prognosis

The overall 5-year survival for head and neck cancers is good (males 72%, females 54%) when compared with malignant tumours at other sites. Although there have been great advances in treatment over the past 20 years, particularly developments in immediate reconstructive surgery and voice restoration following total laryngectomy, long-term survival has not changed significantly. Restoration of function, quality of life, and 3-year survival figures are very much better, but in the longer term other smoking-related diseases (lung cancer, second primaries, heart disease, and strokes) take their toll.

The tumour, node, and metastasis (TNM) classification is used to designate the stage and extent of the tumour and the presence or absence of nodes and metastases. For squamous carcinoma the treatment, prognosis and 5-year survival depend not only on the stage but also on the site of the tumour, as shown in *Table 25.3*. In the UK the majority (60%) of laryngeal cancers occur on the vocal cords and have an excellent prognosis (90% for stage I and 80% for stage II) because they present early with persistent hoarseness and lymphatic drainage from the cords is poor so that node metastases are uncommon. Cancers of the pharynx, however, have a poor prognosis of 20–40% because of late symptomatic diagnosis and frequent nodal metastases through a rich lymphatic drainage.

The majority of papillary and follicular thyroid carcinomas have an excellent prognosis, particularly in females under

Table 25.3. *Age-adjusted 5-year survival for head and neck cancer (West Midlands Cancer Registry)*

Site	Males (%)	Females (%)
Skin, squamous cell cancer	91	86
Skin, melanoma	43	66
Oral cavity	41	45
Oropharynx	19	37
Nasopharynx	25	20
Hypopharynx	12	11
Nasal cavity/sinuses	32	38
Larynx	56	56
Lymphoma	57	57
Sarcoma	37	52
Head and neck overall	72	54

40 years of age who have small tumours and no metastases (20-year survival, 90–98%). Males and older females fall into the higher risk categories, along with large tumours and metastases (20-year survival, 25–55%). The overall 20-year survival for papillary carcinoma is 90–95% and for follicular carcinoma it is 70–75%. Fortunately, these tumours have a long natural history and are unique in that they can be targeted specifically by radioactive iodine, an important part of the treatment. Medullary carcinoma has a slightly worse prognosis (10- and 20-year survival of 75% and 60%, respectively), but patients with anaplastic carcinoma rarely live longer than 6 months. The similarly presenting lymphomas, however, have a much better prognosis, as with lymphomas at other sites.

The prognosis for malignant salivary gland tumours depends on whether they are high grade (adenoid cystic, squamous cell, and high-grade mucoepidermoid and adenocarcinoma) or low grade (acinic cell, and low-grade mucoepidermoid and adenocarcinoma), and on the stage at diagnosis. Rarer tumours, such as sarcomas, melanomas and neuroectodermal tumours, have an intermediate prognostic outlook, which main depends on the extent at diagnosis.

Treatment

The overall cure rates for cancer treatment in this country are poor compared with specialist centres in most other western countries, where cancer is treated mainly by cancer specialists working in specialist cancer centres rather than by general hospital departments. It is therefore essential that head and neck cancers be treated in a specialist unit; hopefully, results will improve with centralization of cancer care in the UK.

Surgery and radiotherapy, either alone or in combination, are the two main forms of treatment for head and neck cancer. In early disease excellent cure rates are usually achievable with either modality used on its own, but for advanced tumours combined therapy with surgery and post-operative radiotherapy are invariably necessary to obtain optimal results. In many situations, however, organ preservation (tongue, larynx) is an important consideration for quality of life and some compromise may have to be made, with informed consent, between chances of cure and functional preservation.

Treatment of the lymph nodes in the neck (with surgery or radiotherapy, depending on the treatment to the primary) is an integral part of management, even if no nodes are palpable, because of the high risk of occult micrometastases.

Surgery

Surgery offers the most definitive treatment for most cancers of the head and neck, with the purpose of complete excision and immediate reconstruction for larger defects to minimize functional loss. Wide margins of excision are often difficult to achieve because of vital adjacent neurovascular structures, such as the carotid artery and cranial nerves, but post-operative radiotherapy reduces the risk of local recurrence following larger resections.

Advances in reconstructive techniques using pedicled flaps from the chest and free flaps from the forearm, abdomen, shoulder, and small bowel have allowed effective immediate restoration of function and cosmesis using skin, muscle, fascia, mucosa, and bone fashioned appropriately to restore the defect.

Radiotherapy

Radiotherapy is a very effective treatment for smaller volume squamous cancers and for the majority of carcinomas of the tonsil, nasopharynx, and lymphomas, even with large nodal disease. It has the great advantage of preservation of structural function, and is therefore used in most carcinomas of the larynx and tongue base for which the only alternative may be total glossectomy. However, not all carcinomas are responsive to radiotherapy, particularly larger tumours and lymph node metastases, and salvage surgery is often required for recurrent disease. Unfortunately, this is associated with more difficult surgery, a greater risk of complications, and poorer outcome. Primary radiotherapy is not advisable for tumours that involve bone or cartilage because of the risk of radionecrosis.

Chemotherapy

Chemotherapy is not a curative treatment for squamous carcinomas of the head and neck, so its role is mainly palliative for recurrent or advanced disease not appropriate for curative treatment. Some evidence indicates that its use concurrently with radiotherapy may improve survival for certain advanced head and neck tumours, but any use should be in the context of prospective clinical trials.

Specific sites
Thyroid cancer

Surgery is the only definitive treatment for differentiated thyroid cancer and is best undertaken by an experienced head and neck surgeon. Total thyroidectomy with post-operative radioiodine treatment and thyroid-stimulating hormone suppression are mandatory, except for microcarcinomas in young women, for which lobectomy and suppression are effective. Up to 50% of patients may have neck node metastases, which should be treated with selective neck dissection rather than traditional 'berry picking'. External beam radiotherapy is used curatively for thyroid lymphoma, palliatively in anaplastic carcinoma, and post-operatively for unresectable disease.

Oral cavity

Small tumours of the tongue and floor of mouth can be treated either with excision or brachytherapy (radiotherapy implant); larger lesions are best treated with surgery and reconstruction using a free radial forearm flap, with excellent functional results (*Fig. 25.5*). Treatment of the neck is essential except for the small superficial lesions.

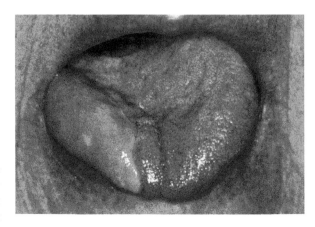

Figure 25.5. *Patient shown in Figure 25.2 3 years after a partial glossectomy and free radial forearm flap for reconstruction, with excellent mobility and contour.*

Key points: head and neck cancer

Risk factors for head and neck cancer (excluding thyroid)

Smoking (>90%)

Alcohol

Poor diet

Socially deprived

Older age

Common symptoms

The common symptoms are given in *Tables 25.2 and 25..4.*

Table 24.4. Common symptoms of head and neck cancer

Cancer	Symptom	Incidence (%)
Larynx	Hoarseness	80–90
	Pain on swallowing	30–40
	Dysphagia	30
Nasopharynx	Lump in the neck	80–90
	Nasal obstruction	60
	Deafness	50
	Post-nasal discharge	40–50
Oral Cavity	Ulceration/visible lesion	80
	Pain	60
	Lump in the neck	20–40
Oropharynx	Persistent sore throat	90
	Lump in the neck	80
	Otalgia	80
Hypopharynx	Dysphagia	80
	Otalgia	60–70
	Hoarseness	50
Nasal cavity	Obstruction/congestion	80–90
	Bleeding	70–80
Thyroid	Thyroid lump	60
	Discomfort in lower neck	80
Salivary	Lump in parotid submandibular gland	90
	Pain	10–20
	Lump in the neck	10–20

Reproduced from England Department of Health Cancer Referral Guidelines Consultation Document May 2000.

Nasopharynx

All tumours, including the neck nodes, are treated with radio-therapy which gives 70–80% locoregional control.

Oropharynx

Functional disturbance of swallowing is a main factor in deciding treatment and many smaller tumours of the tonsil and tongue base respond to radiotherapy; salvage surgery is kept in reserve for any recurrence. For larger tumours combined surgery and reconstruction with post-operative radiotherapy gives a better chance of cure.

Hypopharynx and cervical oesophagus

Low cure rates occur because of late presentation and node metastases. Radiotherapy is only effective for very early tumours and the majority of others (80%) need pharyngolaryngectomy with stomach 'pull-up' or jejunum free-graft reconstruction at some stage. This radical surgery is much more effective if carried out primarily rather than for recurrence, and most patients can subsequently undergo surgical voice restoration (see below).

Larynx

Radiotherapy is effective for most laryngeal cancers, except advanced tumours with airway obstruction or cartilage invasion. Partial laryngectomy with avoidance of permanent tracheostomy is possible for early recurrences, but total laryngectomy may be necessary for advanced disease and most recurrences. The functional disability caused by removal of the voice box should, however, be minimized by restoration of near normal voice with a tracheo-oesophageal speech valve, which is now routinely carried out at the time of total laryngectomy (*Fig. 25.6*). This procedure is unfortunately carried out in only some head and neck units in the UK.

Salivary glands

Experienced surgical excision with facial nerve preservation is the treatment of choice for parotid tumours and also submandibular gland lesions. Post-operative radiotherapy may be advisable for high-grade tumours.

Nasal cavity and sinuses

Small tumours are best excised, but larger lesions may need maxillectomy or craniofacial resection combined with radiotherapy. Palatal prosthesis offers an alternative to surgical reconstruction.

Neck lumps and lymphomas

Malignant tumours of the neck are usually secondary nodal metastases from a squamous carcinoma of the upper aerodigestive tract or primary lymphomas; rarely, they are neuroectodermal tumours. Appropriate investigation usually reveals the site of an apparently occult primary, which is then treated in combination with the neck as detailed above. Incisional biopsies are best avoided and excision of the neck lump is only carried out if the:

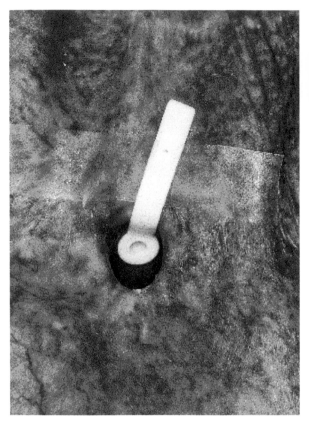

Figure 25.6. *Tracheostomy following a total laryngectomy showing a Blom–Singer tracheo-oesophageal speech valve.*

- preliminary FNAC suggested lymphoma; or
- ENT examination fails to reveal a primary squamous carcinoma site.

If lymphoma is confirmed on histology, further appropriate investigation and treatment are carried out depending on the type determined by immunocytochemistry. For squamous carcinoma nodes with an occult primary a neck dissection is performed with post-operative radiotherapy, if appropriate, and careful follow-up.

Palliative care

Progressive uncontrolled cancer in the head and neck presents some of the most distressing problems for a patient, relatives, and carers. Many do not have metastatic disease elsewhere and the terminal stages may often be accompanied by:

Guidelines for urgent referral: Head and neck cancer

Head and neck cancer: guidelines for urgent referral

Ulceration of oral mucosa persisting for >2–3 weeks

Hoarseness persisting for >2–3 weeks

Dysphagia persisting for >2–3 weeks

Unresolving neck masses for 2–3 weeks

Cranial neuropathies

Orbital masses

The level of suspicion is further increased if the patient is a heavy smoker or heavy alcohol drinker and is over 45 years of age.

Referral proforma: head and neck cancer

Age: Gender   M/F

Cancer area suspected

| Oral cavity | ☐ | Larynx | ☐ |
| Pharynx | ☐ | Thyroid | ☐ |

Other...

Risk factors	Yes	No	
Smoker			
Alcohol			
Poor diet			

Symptoms	Yes	No	
Hoarseness			
Pain on swallowing			
Dysphagia			
Deafness			
Nasal obstruction discharge			
Sore throat			
Otalgia			
Bleeding			

Clinical examination	Yes	No	
Oral ulceration/tumour			
Lump in neck			
Thyroid lump			
Orbital mass			

Other, state...

Comment/other reasons for urgent referral

Reproduced from England Department of Health Cancer Referral Guidelines Consultation Document May 2000.

Referral proforma: head and neck cancer

History		Yes	No	
Rapidly focal progressive deficit	Weakness, heaviness, clumsiness			
	Unsteadiness			
	Numbness, tingling			
	Deafness in one ear			
	Visual disturbance			
Raised intracranial pressure	Headache			
	Nausea, vomiting			
	Double vision			
	Intermittent drowsiness			
Seizures	Focal onset			
	Post-ictal deficit			
	Associated (inter-ictal) focal deficit			
	De novo status epilepticus			
Mental state changes	Short history of cognitive decline (e.g. memory loss)			
	Short history of behaviour and/or personality change			

Examination findings		Yes	No	
Higher mental functions	Alert			
	Orientated			
	Attentive			
	Forgetful			
	Dysphasic			
Cranial nerves	Papilloedema			
	Extraocular muscle palsy			
	Visual field loss			
	Facial weakness			
	Unilateral deafness			
Limbs	Hemiparesis			
	Hemisensory loss			
	Ataxia			

- severe pain that usually requires opiate analgesia;
- airway obstruction, which may need a tracheostomy;
- progressive dysphagia relieved by percutaneous endoscopic gastrostomy or nasogastric tube;
- loss of voice from involvement of the larynx or oral cavity;
- cosmetic deformity from disease and/or treatment;
- infected fungating tumour of the skin or oral cavity;
- leaking fistulae from the mouth or pharynx;
- loss of sight, hearing, taste, and smell;
- gross oedema of the tongue, face, and neck from lymphatic obstruction; and
- potential risk of carotid bleed.

These distressing and disfiguring problems may also inevitably cause intense psychological disturbance from loss of communication, change in body image, loss of self esteem, and loss of attractiveness, particularly to children or grandchildren who do not fully comprehend. Great skill, experience, and empathy are essential to help these unfortunate patients during their last few weeks or months to die with dignity and minimal distress.

References and Further Reading

British Thyroid Association. *Guidelines for the management of thyroid cancer in adults.* London: Royal College of Physicians, 2002.

Vini L, Harmer C. Management of thyroid cancer. *Lancet Oncol* 2002; **3**: 407–414.

Vini L, Harmer C. Thyroid. In: Price P, Silcora K (eds) *Treatment of Cancer.* London: Arnold, 2002, 401–427.

26 Neuro-oncology

Michael Brada

Introduction

Although tumours of the brain and spinal cord are considered relatively rare, brain tumours represent the most common solid tumour in childhood. Intracranial tumours are also the fifth most common tumours in adults of working age, and the brain and spine are frequent sites of metastatic disease. The public, and often medical, perception of brain tumours is that of a devastating incurable malignancy. While malignant gliomas, the most common brain tumours in adults, are incurable, the judicious use of radiotherapy offers effective palliation and generally prolongs good-quality life. Many brain tumours are curable by surgery (meningioma, juvenile pilocytic astrocytoma, and pituitary adenoma) and by combinations of oncological treatments [cranial germ cell tumours, medulloblastoma, primary central nervous system (CNS) lymphoma]. Early diagnosis and appropriate oncological management are therefore important. Various statistics relating to brain and other neurological tumours are shown in *Figure 26.1*.

Clinical Presentation

Patients with cerebral tumours present with features of increased intracranial pressure (headache, vomiting, and papilloedema), local or general brain dysfunction, and epilepsy. Brain dysfunction is expressed as a focal deficit specific to the part of the brain affected. It may range from a focal abnormality and barely perceptible mental deterioration to severe disability and change in consciousness. Epilepsy is a common presenting feature and may be either focal or generalized. Epilepsy of adult onset or presentation with headache and a focal neurological deficit requires immediate further investigations to exclude a tumour.

Gradual personality change and impairment of cognitive function associated with frontal lobe tumours are frequently difficult to detect. Deficits specific to other lobes give more localizing features. Tumours in the pineal region, although rare, are among the most curable of brain tumours and should be diagnosed early. They lie in close proximity to the aqueduct and third ventricle and cause hydrocephalus

through obstruction of cerebrospinal fluid outflow. Compression of the quadrigeminal plate causes paresis of upward gaze with pupils unresponsive to light or accommodation (Parinaud's syndrome), and further tumour extension may affect the mid brain, hypothalamus, and brain stem. Tumours in the brain stem may cause multiple cranial nerve palsies and long tract signs.

Investigations and Referral

Investigations of choice in suspected CNS lesions, including brain tumours, are computed tomography (CT) and/or magnetic resonance imaging (MRI) scans. A CT scan provides an appropriate screening investigation that should be offered to all patients with any symptoms suggestive of brain tumour and to all those who present with epilepsy. An MRI scan should be offered to patients with suspected lesions in the middle cranial fossa and the posterior fossa, as these are poorly visualized on CT because of bony artefact.

Occasionally, imaging is unable to distinguish an acute vascular episode from a space-occupying lesion. Haemorrhage, which may be interpreted as stroke, may also occur in association with a tumour. In such circumstances, an interval scan is advisable.

In the UK there is currently no clear referral path and neurologists, neurosurgeons, general physicians, and oncologists accept patients for further investigations. Neurology and oncology services should be encouraged to organize one-stop brain tumour diagnosis clinics along the lines of breast clinics.

Classification of Brain Tumours

Brain tumours are classified according to the presumed cell of origin into neuro-epithelial tumours, tumours of the meninges, and a mixture of others including lymphomas, germ cell tumours, parasellar region tumours, and metastatic tumours. The current World Health Organization (WHO) classification is given in *Table 26.1*.

The most common primary tumours are of astrocytic origin and meningeal origin. Grade III astrocytomas

NEURO-ONCOLOGY STATISTICS

New neurological cancers

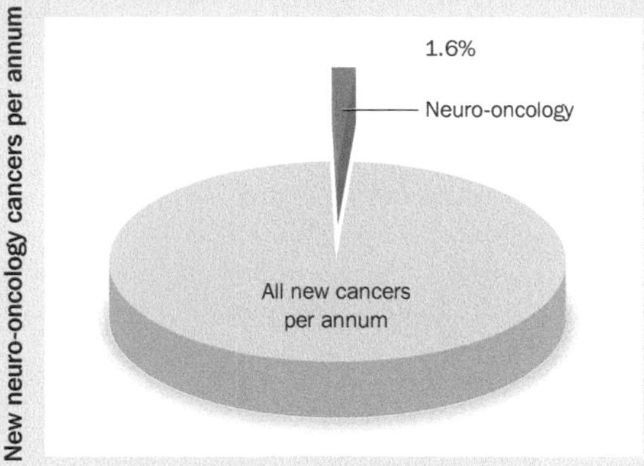

New cases per annum	3910
Males rank	12
Females rank	15
Deaths per annum	3170

Incidence

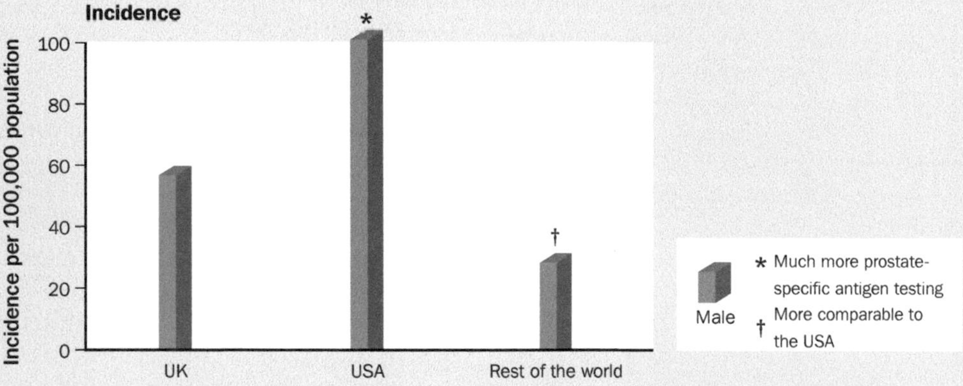

Survival rate

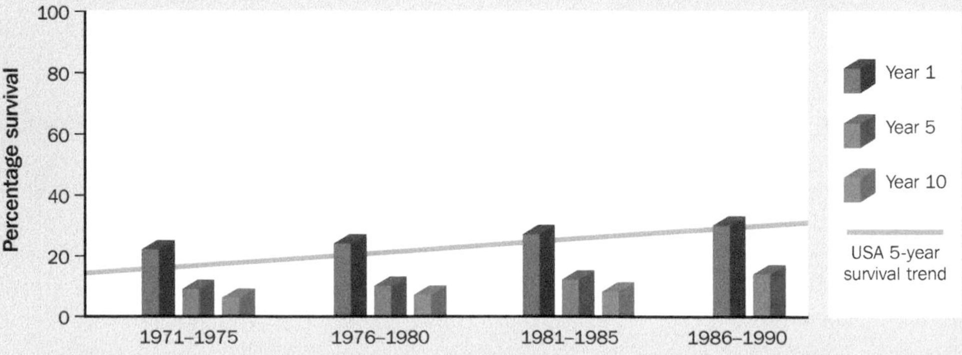

Figure 26.1. *Statistical data relating to brain and other neurological tumours.*

Table 26.1. *WHO classification of brain tumours*

Tumour type	Tumour	WHO malignancy grade
Neuro-epithelial tissue	Astrocytic tumours:	
	diffuse astrocytoma	II
	anaplastic astrocytoma	III
	glioblastoma	IV
	pilocytic astrocytoma	I
	Oligodendroglial tumours:	
	oligodendroglioma	II
	anaplastic oligodendroglioma	III
	Mixed gliomas	
	Ependymal tumours	
	Choroid plexus tumours	
	Neuronal and mixed neuronal–glial tumours:	
	gangliocytoma	I
	dysembryoplastic neuro-epithelial tumour	I
	ganglioglioma	I–II
	central neurocytoma	I–II
	Neuroblastic tumours	
	Pineal parenchymal tumours:	
	pineocytoma	I
	pineoblastoma	IV
	Embryonal tumours:	
	medulloblastoma	IV
	supratentorial primitive neuro-ectodermal tumours	IV
	ependymoblastoma	IV
	ganglioneuroblastoma	IV
Meningeal tumours	Tumours of meningothelial cells:	
	meningioma	I
	atypical meningioma	II
	anaplastic meningioma	III
	Mesenchymal, non-meningothelial tumours: chondrosarcoma and others	
Lymphomas and haemopoietic neoplasms	Primary CNS lymphomas and others	
Germ cell tumours	Germinoma	
	Embryonal carcinoma	
	Yolk sac tumour	
	Choriocarcinoma	
	Teratoma	
	Mixed germ-cell tumours	
Tumours of the sellar region	e.g. craniopharyngioma, pituitary adenoma	
Metastatic tumours		
Unclassified tumours		

(anaplastic astrocytomas) and grade IV astrocytomas (glioblastoma multiforme) are the most common malignant brain tumours.

Management

Initial medical management of brain tumours

Increased intracranial pressure is treated with systemic corticosteroids, and in general it is appropriate to start oral corticosteroids (usually in the form of dexamethasone) prior to a definitive diagnosis. The dose of dexamethasone should be kept to the lowest dose able to improve symptoms and should be under constant review to avoid prolonged and potentially indefinite use, which has attendant side effects. Conventional analgesia and anti-emetics should also be used as necessary. In cases of life-threatening raised intracranial pressure, intravenous mannitol is appropriate and requires hospital admission.

Epilepsy is a relatively common presentation of intracranial tumours. Following the first fit, in the absence of a recognized underlying brain tumour, the current consensus is not to offer any specific treatment. However, because the risk of having further fits is not defined, the family should be instructed in managing a convulsion without the need for emergency medical services. Anticonvulsants are indicated after more than one convulsion and they are appropriate before a definitive diagnosis. The choice is between any of the conventional anticonvulsants (phenytoin, carbamazepine, or sodium valproate).

Tumour-directed therapy and support

Brain tumours are treated with a combination of surgery, radiotherapy, and chemotherapy, although some tumours (such as low-grade gliomas) are appropriately managed by a policy of surveillance with no specific initial treatment. The overall management must pay close attention to symptom control, rehabilitation of disability, and psychological and physical support for both the patient and carers. A summary of treatment approaches and outcome in terms of tumour control (progression-free survival) is given in *Table 26.2.*

Table 26.2. *Prognosis and treatment in a variety of brain tumours*

Tumour type	Primary therapy[a]	Progression-free survival
Pilocytic astrocytoma	S	80–100% at 10 years
Astrocytoma and oligodendroglioma	Observation or other	45–55% at 5 years
Anaplastic astrocytoma and glioblastoma	(S) + RT	40–50% at 1 year
Ependymoma low grade	S (+ RT)	40–60% at 5 years
Ependymoma high grade	S + RT	30–40% at 5 years
Cranial germinoma	RT	80–100% at 10 years
Cranial non-germinomatous germ-cell tumour	C + RT	60–70% at 5 years
Medulloblastoma	S + RT (+ C)	60% at 5 years
Primary central nervous system lymphoma	C + RT	50% at 2–3 years
(radical treatment)		30–40% at 5 years
Pituitary adenoma	S or S+RT	90–95% at 10 years
Craniopharyngioma	S + RT	70–80% at 10 years
Acoustic neuroma	S or SRT	75–85% at 10 years
Chordoma	S + RT	30–60% at 5 years
Chondrosarcoma	S or S + RT	60–80% at 5 years
Benign meningioma	S or S + RT	70–90% at 10 years
Optic nerve and/or chiasmal glioma	RT or C	80–90% at 10 years
Multiple brain metastases	RT	50% at 0.25–0.3 years
Solitary brain metastases	S or SRT	50% at 1 year

[a]S, surgical excision; RT, radiotherapy; C, chemotherapy; SRT, stereotactic radiosurgery or radiotherapy.

Neurosurgery

Surgery is necessary for histological diagnosis and as a palliative or curative procedure to remove the bulk of tumour. In general, it is a curative procedure in accessible benign tumours and a palliative procedure in malignant tumours.

Neurosurgical approaches range from minimally invasive procedures of stereotactic biopsy and endoscopy to a radical surgical excision either through a craniotomy or by complex skull-base approaches. New surgical techniques include high-precision imaging with three-dimensional (3D) image reconstruction, which allow accurate definition of the surgical target and functional imaging, and may reduce surgical morbidity by mapping vulnerable regions. Most surgical procedures are performed under an operating microscope and are aided by computerized 3D image guidance. The choice of approaches to the tumour is not confined to conventional craniotomy and improved access can be achieved through the face, orbit, or oral cavity. Some of the approaches are complex and associated with potentially serious operative morbidity. Clear survival and tumour control benefit has not yet been demonstrated in comparison with more conventional approaches.

Radiotherapy of central nervous system tumours

Radiotherapy is one of the most effective treatment modalities in the management of intracranial tumours. It is curative in cranial germinoma, and is an essential component in the curative treatment of medulloblastoma. It is also an important component for the treatment of benign tumours such as optic chiasma glioma, pituitary adenoma, and craniopharyngioma. Radiotherapy achieves prolongation of disease control and survival in malignant brain tumours. It is also an effective palliative treatment in patients with brain metastases.

The public and medical apprehension of the damaging effects of radiation on the CNS is considerable. While the brain and spinal cord are particularly sensitive to radiation, current treatment is confined to doses that do not exceed the conventional radiation tolerance of the CNS, so the risk of damage is low, probably less than expected from neurosurgical procedures. However, wide-field irradiation in a very young child results in impairment of the development of brain, and radiation should therefore be avoided in this age group. Radiation beyond tolerance doses causes demyelination and necrosis; the risk is related to the overall dose and the dose per fraction. Treatment with radical radiation doses therefore demands the use of small doses per fraction, which means a protracted course of radiotherapy over 5–7 weeks.

Radiotherapy has been at the forefront of the development of radiation technology. High-precision localized irradiation, described as stereotactic radiotherapy or stereotactic conformal radiotherapy, is currently being explored in the treatment of a number of brain tumours. Radiosurgery, which inappropriately suggests a neurosurgical technique, is a variant of stereotactic radiotherapy in which the treatment is given in one dose (single fraction). Stereotactic radiotherapy and radiosurgery can be delivered with an adjusted conventional linear accelerator (sometimes described as the X-knife) or with a multiheaded cobalt unit (described as the gamma knife). There are no clear differences in the radiation delivered and in the clinical results, except that the linear accelerator can give treatment in multiple doses whereas the gamma unit can currently deliver treatment only in single fractions.

Chemotherapy of central nervous system tumours

Chemotherapy has a relatively limited but increasing role in the treatment of CNS tumours. While the concept that the penetration of drugs across the conventional blood–brain barrier is poor has hampered the use of chemotherapy, it is not a bar to the use of effective chemotherapy in chemosensitive tumours.

Chemotherapy is a component of the curative treatment of chemosensitive tumours, such as cranial non-germinomatous germ-cell tumour (teratoma) and primary CNS lymphoma. It is an increasingly important component of adjuvant therapy in childhood primitive neuro-ectodermal tumours, including medulloblastoma. In malignant gliomas, chemotherapy is largely a palliative treatment, with a limited role in the adjuvant setting.

Management of individual central nervous system tumours

Pilocytic astrocytoma

Pilocytic astrocytomas are mostly tumours of childhood and usually occur in the posterior fossa as cystic enhancing masses. They are not infiltrative and are cured by complete surgical excision. Further treatment is generally not necessary unless the tumour is not excisable. Pilocytic astrocytomas affecting the optic chiasm and optic nerves (chiasma gliomas) are not excisable and are treated with local radiotherapy and, in younger children, with primary chemotherapy. The overall cure rate of pilocytic astrocytomas is in the region of 80–100%.

Low-grade gliomas

The term low-grade gliomas is a clinical one and is not an accepted pathological description. The tumours included in this group are astrocytomas (WHO grade II), oligoden-drogliomas, and mixed low-grade oligoastrocytomas. They have in common an indolent presentation, usually with epilepsy alone, and a CT or MRI appearance of non-enhancing masses that frequently show diffuse infiltration.

The natural history of low-grade gliomas is that of a slow and sometimes imperceptible progression over a number of years, which culminates with transformation into a more aggressive tumour. This can frequently be confirmed histologically as a transformation to a malignant glioma.

In general, the recommendation is that the diagnosis should be histologically confirmed, although in some situations this is not necessary. The options for subsequent management lie between observation alone with medical treatment of epilepsy, surgical excision (which can range from debulking surgery to radical tumour excision), radiotherapy, and primary chemotherapy. Evidence-based data are insufficient to favour any specific treatment approach and no particular therapy has shown survival benefit.

The overall principles of management can be summarized as follows. Patients without neurological deficit and with adequately controlled epilepsy do not require further treatment other than surveillance with regular imaging. In the presence of a mass effect or neurological deficit because of a compressing mass, surgical decompression is appropriate. Radiotherapy is generally reserved for progressive unresectable disease, and for malignant transformation.

Some low-grade gliomas respond to chemotherapy. The anaplastic variant of oligodendroglioma is particularly chemoresponsive (response rate in the region of 70–80%) and nitrosourea-containing chemotherapy is effective at the time of recurrence. Chemotherapy as adjuvant treatment is being tested in randomized trials. In other low-grade gliomas, particularly oligodendroglial, chemotherapy is an experimental treatment option.

Although the overall prognosis of patients with low-grade glioma is good, with a median survival in the range of 5–10 years, this tumour is not curable by any of the currently available treatments and progression to a more malignant form and ultimate resistance to therapy are invariable. Age and performance status are the major determinants of survival, with young and fit patients having the best prognosis.

Ependymomas

Ependymomas are neuro-epithelial tumours (gliomas) that arise from ependymal surfaces. They are the most common gliomas of the spinal cord. In the brain they occur more frequently in the posterior fossa (floor of the fourth ventricle), especially in children and young adults. The primary treatment of ependy-moma is by complete surgical excision, followed by local radiotherapy to reduce the relatively high risk of local recurrence. Ependymomas are generally not chemosensitive.

Malignant gliomas

The principal malignant astrocytic tumours are anaplastic astrocytoma (WHO astrocytic grade III) and glioblastoma multiforme (WHO astrocytic grade IV). They frequently present with a rapid onset of neurological deficit and may be clinically mistaken for a cerebrovascular accident, particularly because they increase in incidence with age.

The overall management depends on the degree of neurological disability, the overall performance status, and age. Older patients (≥65 years) with unequivocal diagnosis on imaging and severe deficit do not necessarily require a biopsy because management is palliative and detailed histology is unlikely to alter the treatment plan. Although there is a small rate of mistaken diagnosis (e.g. primary CNS lymphoma), in practice this is of limited consequence. Most patients require histological diagnosis, which is obtained by either a stereotactic biopsy or through debulking surgery. Most gliomas are infiltrating malignant tumours that are not curable surgically and generally not excisable without risk of neurological damage.

Following a surgical procedure, radiotherapy is the mainstay of treatment. Radical radiotherapy over a period of 6 weeks prolongs survival and improves quality of life in a proportion of patients. However, it is not a curative treatment and is associated with side effects, of which tiredness is the most debilitating. A short course of palliative radiotherapy may be of value in older patients with particularly marked disability and adverse prognosis.

Chemotherapy, particularly using nitrosoureas (alkylating agents), is known to produce clinical and radiological responses, but the survival benefit in an adjuvant setting remains minimal. Chemotherapy is generally used at the time of recurrence as palliative treatment. The response rate of anaplastic astrocytomas is in the region of 20–35%; that of glioblastoma is 5–15%. Responses are of limited duration.

The median survival of patients with malignant gliomas is 9–12 months with rare long-term survivors. The main determinants of prognosis are age, performance status, and tumour histology. Young, fit patients with anaplastic astrocytoma (grade III) have a median survival in the region of 3–5 years, while older disabled patients have a median survival of less than 6 months. The treatment should therefore be tailored to prognosis. Patients in the poor prognostic group should be offered limited or no surgery and supportive care with or without short palliative radiotherapy. Patients with a favourable prognosis should be treated with surgery followed by conventional radiotherapy. Adjuvant chemotherapy is generally not recommended. All patients and families with malignant glioma require intensive community support.

Embryonal tumours

Embryonal tumours comprise supratentorial peripheral neuro-ectodermal tumours, medulloblastomas, and ependymoblastomas. Medulloblastoma is the most common brain tumour in childhood and presents with cerebellar deficit with or without hydrocephalus. Treatment is by radical surgery (as complete a resection as possible) followed by radiotherapy to the whole craniospinal axis and boost to the site of original disease in the posterior fossa. Adjuvant chemotherapy is recommended in patients with adverse prognostic features. It is not routinely given to patients with good prognosis (complete excision and no evidence of spread); its role is being tested in randomized studies.

Patients with medulloblastoma have an overall 5-year survival in the region of 60%, with the majority of 5-year survivors being cured. The main determinants of outcome are the extent of disease (presence or absence of residual and metastatic disease in the CNS).

Cranial germ-cell tumours

Cranial germ-cell tumours, which are histologically identical to testicular and ovarian germ-cell tumours, comprise germinomas (equivalent to seminoma) and non-germinomatous germ-cell tumours (equivalent to testicular teratoma). Although rare they are curable and it is therefore important to recognize them. They usually occur in the pineal or suprasellar regions and are more common in boys in their late teens. The diagnosis is by serum tumour markers (α-fetoprotein and human chorionic gonadotrophin) and by histological confirmation if markers are negative. Cranial germinomas are cured by low-dose irradiation, while non-germinomatous tumours are treated with chemotherapy followed by irradiation. With this policy, the cure rate of patients with germinomas is in the region of 80–100%, and long-term survival of patients with non-germinomatous tumours is in the region of 60–70%.

Primary central nervous system lymphoma

Non-Hodgkin's lymphoma localized to the CNS occurs in association with immune deficiency (acquired immmunodeficiency syndrome and following organ transplantation) and as sporadic primary CNS lymphoma (PCL), which is more common in the elderly. The treatment of sporadic PCL is primary chemotherapy followed by cranial irradiation, which usually results in complete clinical and radiological remission. Such intensive treatment should be reserved for patients who are fit with good performance status and reasonable life expectancy. The prognosis following radical treatment is equivalent to that for stage IV systemic non-Hodgkin's lymphoma, with a 30–40% 5-year survival. Patients with poor performance status have an adverse prognosis regardless of the treatment. They tolerate intensive therapy poorly and have high treatment-induced morbidity and mortality. The usual treatment is palliative radiotherapy or simple palliative chemotherapy, and the median survival is less than 1 year.

Benign cranial tumours

The primary treatment for benign pituitary adenoma is surgery. Residual or recurrent (progressive) non-functioning tumours and secreting tumours not cured by surgery and medical therapy are treated effectively with localized low-dose radiotherapy. The long-term control rate following partial excision and radiotherapy and after radical surgery is 90–95% at 10 years.

Craniopharyngiomas are suprasellar tumours of childhood, although they can occur at any age. Radical resection is associated with serious morbidity, and the usual recommended treatment policy is conservative surgery to relieve pressure on the optic apparatus (and hydrocephalus) followed by localized radiotherapy. With this policy, the tumour control rate is in the region of 80% at 10 years.

Meningiomas are treated primarily by surgical resection. Convexity tumours are usually excisable with no need for further therapy. Meningiomas in the region of the skull base are less accessible, although through-skull-base surgical approaches they are more readily excisable. Residual or recurrent skull base meningiomas are treated with localized irradiation usually in the form of a fractionated stereotactic radiotherapy. The control rate of skull base meningiomas following surgery and radiotherapy is in the region of 80–90% at 10 years. Localized treatment in the form of radiosurgery is offered in some centres, but the long-term results are not yet known.

Acoustic neuromas have traditionally been treated by surgical excision. Radiation techniques with fractionated stereotactic radiotherapy or radiosurgery appear equally effective with regard to long-term tumour control (90% at 10 years) with low toxicity.

Skull base tumours

Skull base tumours include chordomas and chondrosarcomas. They are appropriately treated with surgery, although

Key points: brain tumours

Age: rare below 30 years of age, but the most common solid tumour of childhood. Relatively evenly distributed thereafter (with peak at 60–69 years of age)

Patients with brain tumours typically present with one or more of the following clinical features:

progressive neurological deficit (e.g., progressive weakness, sensory loss, dysphasia, ataxia) developing over days to weeks

seizure disorder

raised intracranial pressure (headache, vomiting, papilloedema)

cognitive and/or personality (mental state) changes

Prevalence among patients presenting with brain tumours:

focal neurological deficit	50%
seizures	25–30%
headaches	25–35%
papilloedema	23–50%
mental changes	16–20%

The probability of having a brain tumour in the following situations is as follows:

new-onset seizure (any type) in adults	2–6%
new-onset status epilepticus	10%
headache of non-migrainous type	2%

Reproduced from England Department of Health Cancer Referral Guidelines Consultation Document May 2000.

Guidelines for urgent referral: brain tumours

Any patient with progressive neurological deficit developing over days to weeks (e.g., weakness, sensory loss, dysphasia, ataxia, visual disturbance)

Adult patients with new onset seizures characterized by one or more of the following:

focus seizures

prolonged post-ictal focal deficit

status epilepticus

headache

Patients with headache, vomiting, and papilloedema

Patients with headache and either seizures or focal neurological symptoms and/or signs

Patients with non-migrainous headaches of recent onset (or with a change in pattern), if accompanied by features suggestive of raised intracranial pressure (e.g., morning headache, vomiting)

complete excision may not be achievable because of difficult access and the involvement of critical structures. The prognosis for chordoma is relatively poor regardless of surgery and subsequent adjuvant treatment with radiotherapy. Chrondrosarcomas are generally indolent tumours with a 10-year control rate in the region of 80–90%, regardless of the primary treatment modality.

Brain metastases

The aim of treatment for patients with brain metastases is palliative. Patients with multiple brain metastases receive effective palliation with a short course of whole-brain radiotherapy. Brain metastases in patients with chemosensitive tumours (e.g. lymphoma or testicular tumours) can be treated with primary chemotherapy. The median survival of patients with multiple brain metastases is 3–4 months.

Patients with solitary lesions confirmed on MRI, no other metastatic disease, and a controlled primary tumour can achieve prolonged disease control and survival with more aggressive local treatment approaches. These include surgical resection or single-fraction radiosurgery, which can be considered a non-invasive alternative to surgery. Radiosurgery has no proven role in patients with multiple brain metastases and is not associated with survival benefit.

Spinal Tumours

The tumours that most frequently affect the spinal cord are secondary deposits; they are usually extradural. Primary intradural tumours are relatively uncommon. Of these, the most common intradural extramedullary tumours are meningiomas and nerve sheath tumours, while spinal ependymomas and astrocytomas represent the majority of intramedullary tumours.

Clinical presentation

The main symptoms of spinal tumours are local pain at the site of the lesion and impairment of neurological function at or below the affected spinal level. Pain caused by bone or spinal root involvement is localized to the level of the lesion and may predate other symptoms by months or years. The pain may be worse on coughing or straining and can intensify at night. Spinal cord compression by the tumour causes segmental loss of power and tendon reflexes.

The importance of early detection of spinal cord compression by metastatic tumour is to preserve neurological function, as the likelihood of retaining mobility is related to the degree of dysfunction at the time of therapeutic intervention.

Treatment

Spinal meningiomas are treated by primary surgery. Intraspinal ependymomas limited to a few segments can also be excised. More extensive ependymomas are treated by a combination of surgical decompression and radiotherapy. Spinal astrocytomas are generally not excisable and are temporarily controlled with adjuvant radiation.

Spinal cord compression from metastatic disease should be recognized early, and treatment should be considered in the context of the extent and activity of the malignant disease. In general, chemosensitive tumours (lymphomas and germ cell tumours) are treated with primary chemotherapy. Cord compression from metastatic breast, lung, or prostate cancer is treated with primary radiotherapy and adjuvant systemic treatment, with surgery reserved for progressive dysfunction not controlled with radiation. Surgical decompression may be the appropriate first treatment for posterior tumours.

Conclusion

Although the diagnosis of brain tumours fills patients and clinicians with foreboding, there are many curable tumours, particularly if recognized early, and there is effective treatment, whether palliative or curative, available for malignant tumours. The diagnosis of brain and spinal tumours requires a high index of suspicion and easy access to CT and/or MRI imaging with rapid referral to neuro-oncology services.

Further Reading

Copy to come

27 Children's Cancer

Aurelia Norton, Kathy Pritchard-Jones and Nina Patel

The clinical behaviour of the majority of children's cancers is different from that of typical adult epithelial cancers. Their histological appearance suggests an origin in embryonic tissues (*Fig. 27.1*). They are generally much more sensitive to chemotherapy, and overall cure rates are now approximately 70%. The role of the general practitioner (GP) within the management of childhood cancer can often be difficult, since the majority of children and adolescents with cancer are treated in regional cancer centres.

Incidence and Prevalence

Malignancy is rare in childhood, with an annual incidence of approximately 1 in 10,000 children under 15 years of age, so the average GP probably sees only one or two cases in his or her career. However, it is the most common cause of childhood death after accidents and congenital abnormalities. Furthermore, with the increasingly intensive treatment of relapse, cancer in childhood is becoming a 'chronic disease' that a child may live with for many years. The most common group of diagnoses are the leukaemias, the majority of which are acute lymphoblastic leukaemia. The second largest group is the brain tumours, followed by soft-tissue

sarcomas and the lymphomas (*Table 27.1*). Improved treatment since the 1980s, with the use of multiagent chemotherapy combined with other modalities of treatment, such as radiotherapy and surgery, means that 70% of children diagnosed with cancer will be long-term survivors (*Fig. 27.2*). Hence, in the year 2000 as many as one in 1000 young adults were survivors of childhood cancer.

Aetiology

Genetic predisposition is an important factor in the aetiology of some childhood cancers, either as a germ line mutation in a phenotypically normal child or as part of a congenital malformation syndrome. A wide range of constitutional chromosomal abnormalities predispose to childhood malignancy, of which Down's syndrome is the most well recognized (*Table 27.2*).

The aetiology of leukaemia in childhood is becoming clearer, and it is thought that genetic and environmental factors play an important role. Leukaemia develops in stem cells, which proliferate in a microenvironment that supports clonal expansion and is devoid of stringent architectural barriers. As a result, it is believed that fewer genetic events are required to

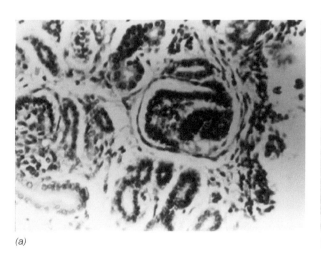

(a)

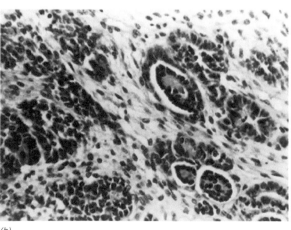

(b)

Figure 27.1. (a) Human foetal kidney. (b) Triphasic Wilms' tumour.

Table 27.1. *Annual incidence of childhood cancers in UK (National Registry Data)*

Diagnostic group	Disease	Annual rates per million	Approximate number of cases in the UK per year
Leukaemia		43.4	452
	Acute lymphoblastic leukaemia	35.3	366
	Acute non-lymphoblastic Leukaemia	6.5	69
	Chronic myeloid leukaemia	0.9	9
	Other and unspecified	0.7	7
Lymphomas		11.8	141
	Hodgkin's Lymphoma	4.5	56
	Non-hodgkin's lymphoma	7.0	81
	Other and unspecified	0.3	3
Brain and spinal cord		30.7	336
	Ependymoma and choroid plexus	3.1	32
	Astrocytoma	12.8	141
	PNET	6.2	67
	Other glioma	3.9	43
	Other specified	2.9	34
	Unspecified	1.8	20
Sympathetic nervous system		9.4	87
	Neuroblastoma	9.3	86
	Other	0.1	1
Retinoblastoma		4.6	41
Renal tumours		7.9	75
	Wilm's tumour	7.7	73
	Renal cell carcinoma	0.1	2
Hepatic tumours		1.2	12
	Hepatoblastoma	1.0	9
	Hepatic carcinoma	0.3	3
Bone tumours		5.0	63
	Osteosarcoma	2.6	33
	Ewing's sarcoma	2.0	25
	Other and unspecified	0.4	4
Soft tissue sarcomas		9.5	101
	Rhabdomyosarcoma	5.5	57
	Fibrosarcoma	1.0	12
	Other specified	2.3	26
	Unspecified	0.6	7
Gonadal and germ cell		4.3	46
	Intracranial/intra-spinal germ cell	1.2	14
	Other extragonadal germ cell	1.1	10
	Gonadal germ cell	1.8	20
	Other and unspecified	0.2	2
Carcinoma and melanoma		4.0	50
	Adrenocortical carcinoma	0.1	1
	Thyroid carcinoma	0.5	6
	Nasopharangeal carcinoma	0.2	6
	Malignant melanoma	1.4	18
	Skin carcinoma	0.7	9
	Other carcinoma	1.0	13
Other and unspecified		0.9	1
Total		132.6	1414

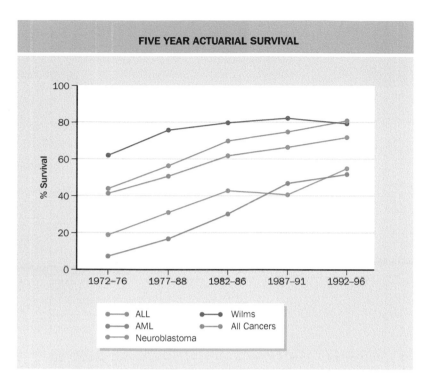

FIVE YEAR ACTUARIAL SURVIVAL

% Survival (y-axis: 0, 20, 40, 60, 80, 100)

x-axis: 1972–76, 1977–88, 1982–86, 1987–91, 1992–96

Legend: ALL, AML, Neuroblastoma, Wilms, All Cancers

Figure 27.2. *5-year actuarial survival in four childhood cancers. (National Registry Data.)*

produce malignancy. In childhood leukaemia, twin concordance rates are about 5%, while in infant leukaemia they are as high as 50–75%. It is postulated that a single cell undergoes a genetic mutation prenatally and as this abnormal clone expands it 'metastasizes' to the second twin via the common placental circulation. This preleukaemic clone requires a second event, possibly infection, to produce overt leukaemia. Several recent, large epidemiological studies suggest that infection may play a role in the aetiology of childhood leukaemia because of the phenomenon of population mixing, as evidenced by clustering, seasonality, and population density. The theory postulates that certain communities are immunologically isolated and as new families move into the area exposure to novel infections occurs.

The association of Epstein–Barr virus (EBV) with the development of Burkitt's lymphoma best demonstrates the role of viral infection in cancer aetiology. Infection early in life with EBV may maintain certain pre-B- and B-cell populations in a proliferative state, making them more susceptible to genetic change and tumour formation.

Very few childhood cancers to date have a definite link to environmental causes, but there is evidence that exposure to ionizing radiation either pre- or post-natally increases the risk of some malignancies. Radioiodine released into the atmosphere following the Chernobyl nuclear disaster led to a marked increase in thyroid cancer in children in the Ukraine, with a relatively short lag time of only 5 years. Some drugs are linked to an increased incidence of childhood malignancy. Diethylstilbestrol, which was used in the 1960s to prevent spontaneous abortion, is associated with clear cell carcinoma of the vagina in female offspring. Ironically, some of the cytotoxic drugs used to treat cancer actually increase the risk of a primary second cancer. The worst culprits are the alkylating agents, such as cyclophosphamide and drugs that inhibit DNA topoisomerases, such as etoposide. These two agents predispose particularly to secondary acute myeloid leukaemias, which have a different lag period and cytogenetic abnormality, according to the preceding drug. Other agents have been implicated, but these implications have not been substantiated.

Clinical Assessment and Differential Diagnosis of the Child with Suspected Cancer

It is often difficult to diagnose childhood cancer in its early stages because the symptoms and signs are usually non-specific, mimicking more common childhood disorders (*Table 27.3*). Confusion may arise as some malignancies can mimic non-accidental injury, especially neuroblastoma, which can present with

Table 27.2. *Examples of recognized gene disorders and syndromes predisposing to childhood cancer*

Recognized gene disorder or syndrome	Gene/chromosome if known	Tumour predisposition	Prevalence in childhood cancer population
Down's syndrome	Trisomy 21	Leukaemias	0.8% (2% acute lymphoblastic leukaemia)
Neurofibromatosis type 1	NF1 gene 17q	Brain tumours, soft-tissue sarcomas, leukaemias	0.5% (30–50% optic nerve gliomas)
Immune deficiency syndromes (ataxia telangiectasia, Fanconi's syndrome, X-linked xeroderma pigmentosa, Bloom's syndrome)	Multiple	Lymphomas	0.1% (<1% of childhood lymphoma)
13q deletion syndrome/ retinoblastoma	RB1 13q14	Retinoblastoma Sarcomas Pinealoblastomas	1% (40% of retinoblastomas have a germ line mutation)
Wilms' tumour, aniridia syndrome, genitourinary abnormalities and mental retardation (WAGR)	WT1gene 11p13	Wilms' tumour Nephroblastoma	1–2% of all Wilms' tumours
Beckwith–Weidemann syndrome and hemihypertrophy	11p15.5	Wilms' tumour Hepatoblastoma Adrenocortical carcinoma Rhabdomyosarcoma	3% of Wilms' tumours
Li–Fraumeni syndrome	p53 gene, 17p	Breast cancer Sarcomas Brain tumours Leukaemias	0.7%
Gorlin's syndrome Naevoid basal cell carcinoma	PTCH gene	Medulloblastoma Skin cancers	<1%

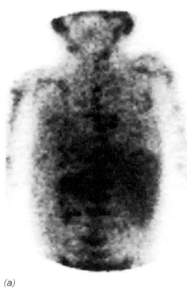

(a)

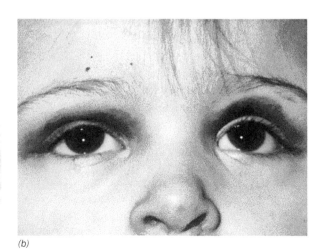

(b)

Figure 27.3. *(a) 131-meta-iodobenzylguanidine scan in a child with stage IV neuroblastoma. (b) Periorbital ecchymoses in a child with neuroblastoma.*

Table 27.3. Common presenting signs and symptoms of childhood malignancy, with possible differential diagnoses

Signs and symptoms	Differential diagnosis	Possible malignancy	Investigations
Paleness and fatigue, frequent, or prolonged infections	Anaemia Immune deficiency	Leukaemia Lymphoma	Full blood count and film
Recurrent fever with bone pain	Infection Trauma	Leukaemia Bone tumours Neuroblastoma	Full blood count and film Radiography Referral
Lymphadenopathy not responding to antibiotics or asymmetrical	Infection	Lymphoma Leukaemia	Full blood count and film Chest radiography
Bleeding and easy bruising	Coagulation disorder Platelet disorder Non-accidental injury	Leukaemia Bone marrow infiltration	Referral
Abdominal mass	Constipation Renal cyst Full bladder	Wilms' tumour Neuroblastoma Hepatoblastoma Lymphoma	Blood pressure Referral
Morning headache, squint, convulsions, behaviour or personality changes, and visual disturbance	Migraine Sinusitis	Brain tumour	Fundoscopy Referral
Weight loss, failure to thrive, diarrhoea or constipation	Infection Cystic fibrosis Hirchsprung's disease	Lymphomas Neuroblastoma Abdominal tumour (e.g. sacrococcygeal tumour) Rhabdomyosarcoma Ewing's sarcoma	Blood pressure Examination of the abdomen Full blood count Chest radiography
Limping or chronic pain	Juvenile arthritis Infection Trauma/NAI	Bone tumours Leukaemias Neuroblastoma	Full blood count Radiography Referral
Recurrent cough, wheeze, shortness of breath, superior vena cava (SVC) syndrome [obstruction of venous drainage via the SVC]	Infection Asthma	Lymphoma Leukaemia Other mediastinal tumours	Chest radiography Full blood count and film Referral
Proptosis	Infection	Leukaemia Neuroblastoma Rhabdomyosarcoma Histiocytosis	Referral
White 'red reflex'		Retinoblastoma	Referral
Horner's syndrome		Neuroblastoma	Referral
Precocious puberty		Adrenocortical carcinoma	Referral
Chronic drainage from ear or nose	Infection	Rhabdomyosarcoma Histiocytosis	Referral
Vaginal discharge or bleeding	Infection NAI	Yolk sac tumour Rhabdomyosarcoma	Referral

Table 27.4. Vaccination programme following standard dose chemotherapy

Time from end of treatment	Previously completed vaccination programme up to age 18 months	Not completed primary vaccination programme
During and until six months off treatment	None	Continue with primary vaccination schedule as close to on time as possible, using non-live vaccines e.g. *inactivated* polio vaccine
From six months after completion of treatment (single vaccination of each)	Diphtheria, tetanus and accellular pertussis (DTP) Inactivated polio (IPV) Measles, mumps, and rubella (MMR) Meningococcal C HIB	Diphtheria, tetanus and accelular pertussis Inactivated polio (IPV) Measles, mumps and rubella (MMR) Meningococcal C HIB
At 13 years of age	BCG if not previously immunized Rubella if not had MMR	BCG if not previously immunized Rubella if not had MMR

If previous BCG vaccination, tuberculin test and consider revaccination

Vaccination programme following high dose chemotherapy/bone marow transplant		
Time since transplant	Autograft or allograft	Unrelated donor
12 months	DT × 3 at monthly intervals Inactivated polio × 3 at monthly intervals Meningococcal C × 3 at monthly intervals HIB × 3 at monthly intervals	
15 months	Conjugate pneumococcal vaccine	
18 months	MMR	DT × 3 at monthly intervals Inactivated polio × 3 at monthly intervals Meningococcal C × 3 at monthly intervals HIB × 3 at monthly intervals
21 months		Conjugate pneumococcal vaccine
24 months	Polysaccharide pneumococcal vaccine	MMR
30 months		Polysaccharide pneumococcal vaccine

BCG is not recommended after bone marrow transplant

Notes
1. Following an unrelated bone marrow transplant, no immunizations should be given until the individual has been off cyclosporin A for atleast six months or is 18 months from transplant, which ever is longer.
2. Siblings of children undergoing treatment for cancer should receive inactivated polio vaccine.
3. Influenza vaccine is recommended annually in autumn for all patients receiving chemotherapy, and for those still within six months of completion of chemotherapy. In children who have had high dose chemotherapy, influenza vaccine should be administered every autumn for as long as the patient remains clinically immunocompromized or is considered to be at risk from influenza virus infection..

bilateral periorbital bruising (*Fig. 27.3*), or leukaemia that presents with widespread frequent bruising and a limp. This can be an extremely difficult situation for both the GP and the parents. However, if non-specific signs and symptoms persist, parents and/or patients often worry about the possibility of a serious illness, such as malignancy, and they may express their worries directly to the GP. At this stage a relatively high index of suspicion is important to prevent any delay in the diagnosis (many parents have concerns in this area, having seen their GP several times in the weeks before the final diagnosis).

The first steps in the diagnostic pathway are to obtain the history and perform a detailed physical examination. It is very important to take a detailed family history, including parents, siblings, and first cousins, with particular attention

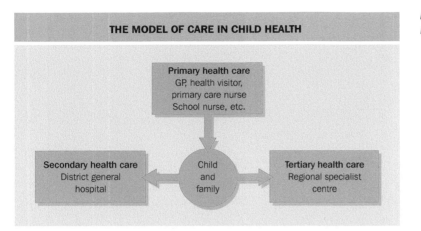

Figure 27.4. *The model of care in child health.*

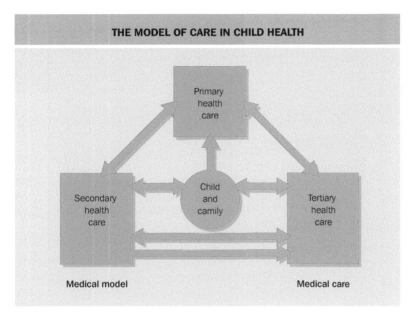

Figure 27.5. *Ideal UK management model of care in paediatric oncology.*

to any occurrence of malignancy in a family member under the age of 40–50 years and to certain familial and genetic diseases, such as autoimmune diseases, neurofibromatosis, and Down's syndrome. Certain presenting complaints raise the index of suspicion of malignancy in a child. Many paediatric malignancies are associated with the presenting signs and symptoms shown in *Table 27.3*, but some presentations with more unusual signs and symptoms make early diagnosis even more difficult. The paediatric malignancy most commonly associated with unusual signs and symptoms is neuroblastoma, which may present with Horner's syndrome, spontaneously resolving skin nodules, or periorbital ecchymoses (*Fig. 27.3*).

Investigations

Although many investigations are now available to evaluate a child with suspected malignancy, it is important that as few investigations as possible are used to confirm it. With this in mind, if a diagnosis of malignancy is suspected, a child should be referred initially to a general paediatrician at the earliest possible stage. This is to carry out preliminary investigations in an appropriate setting, such as a full blood count, erythrocyte sedimentation rate, lactate dehydrogenase, plain radiography, ultrasound scans, computed tomography scans, and magnetic resonance imaging. If these initial investigations confirm the suspicion, then a paediatric oncology unit

INDIVIDUALIZED SYMPTOM GUIDELINES IN ADVANCED ACUTE LYMPHOBLASTIC LEUKAEMIA		

Name: John Smith **Hospital No:** 2222

Last weight: 50kg

Central venous access: Portacath

For all symptoms assess causative factors and influences – physical, psychological, social, and spiritual

SYMPTOM		ACTION
Pain	Disease-related:	Assess and establish cause
	marrow infiltration	Analgesia:
	orbital recurrence	opioids
	bone/pain	Co-analgesia:
	soft tissue/organ infiltration	oral antibiotics
	infection	corticosteroids
		?radiotherapy
Constipation	Drug-induced	Assess bowel action
	Poor appetite and fluid intake	Regular aperients
		Diet and fluids as appropriate
Nausea and vomiting	Central nervous system disease-related	Assess oral intake and causative factors
	Drug-induced	Anti-emetics

Figure 27.6. *Guidelines for a child with acute lymphoblastic leukaemia.*

should be involved to make a tissue diagnosis and evaluate the stage of the disease. Invasive investigations to make a tissue diagnosis (e.g. biopsies and bone marrow aspirates) should be carried out only in centres that perform these procedures regularly and are familiar with how to handle the specimen for full histopathology and molecular studies.

Treatment

All paediatric malignancies, including the most common, should be managed by paediatric oncology centres. Evidence supports the centralization of services. Survival is improved in acute myeloid leukaemia, and children with Wilms' tumour are less likely to be overtreated if managed by a tertiary centre rather than a district general hospital. In many cases treatment involves different modalities, such as chemotherapy, radiotherapy, and surgery, and this needs to be co-ordinated with the appropriate health care professionals. All the major paediatric oncology centres in the UK are members of the United Kingdom Children's Cancer Study Group (UKCCSG). This organization is responsible for co-ordinating national and international trials in an effort to improve the treatment of childhood cancers. Clinical trials continuously evaluate new strategies compared with standard current treatments. Such trials aim at reducing long-term side effects and improving cure rates. The approach is to stratify patients into risk groups using their age, stage, histology, and molecular genetics to tailor chemotherapy to the patients' needs. Reducing the use of external beam radiotherapy in the paediatric group is important because of its significant long-term sequelae. Alternative approaches include systemic delivery of radioactive molecules targeted to the tumour cells [e.g. 131-meta-iodobenzylguanidine (MIBG) is taken up specifically by neuroblastoma] or the use of stereotactic methods to deliver radiotherapy more precisely and so spare surrounding normal tissues.

Although a child at times undergoes very intensive treatment, it is important not to forget his or her educational and psychosocial development, as well as the impact of the diagnosis and treatment on the entire family. It is not uncommon for siblings to feel neglected and for parents to suffer from stress-related symptoms. The diagnosis of cancer in a child usually results in added financial stress because of loss of income and added travelling and childcare costs. At such stressful times, families benefit from the expertise of the tertiary centre's multidisciplinary team, which includes social workers and psychological support, along with an appropriate liaison with local services, including the child's GP.

Key points: children's cancers

1 in 550–600 children is affected by the age of 15 years – which is similar to the rate for Down's syndrome, diabetes, or meningitis in childhood.

The estimated number of new cases diagnosed each year by individual tumour type is shown in *Table 27.1*. Acute leukaemia accounts for about one-third or all childhood cancers, and brain and central nervous system tumours account for about 20–25%.

Since the creation of the UKCCSG in the 1970s the majority of childhood cancer sufferers have been treated in regional cancer centres. This, combined with the rarity of the disease in this patient group and the increasing complexity and intensity of treatment, means that the average GP has very little contact with the child and the family during the active treatment phase. Yet, the GP is often called upon by the paediatric community nurses or the district nurses to prescribe fluids to flush intravenous devices while the child is receiving treatment. If the child's sibling or a school friend has a suspected chickenpox or measles rash, it is often the GP who is called upon for confirmation so that adequate steps can be taken to protect the child with cancer. About 6–12 months after the completion of cancer therapy, with the guidance of the regional centre, the parents are asked to return to the GP to recommence the child's immunization programme (*Table 27.4*).

Over the past 15 years significant inadequacies in the service provision for the management of childhood cancer survivors have become apparent. It is important that the role of the GP in the management of this group of patients is clearly defined, and a care package delivered within the primary health care setting. The holistic model of care is the ideal (*Figs 27.4* and *27.5*).

In the initial stages following the diagnosis the family may lose confidence in the GP. It is important at this stage to rebuild the bridge with the family by being attentive and an effective communicator to gain or regain professional confidence. Although the GP's role is minimized during the child's active treatment, his or her role in providing support, empathic listening, and general understanding towards the family group helps to rebuild family confidence.

Care of the Dying Child

Sadly, despite the improvements in cancer care over the past decade, approximately 30% of children with cancer still die from their disease. As a result of the improved treatment of relapse, cancer is now considered a chronic illness since children often live with their cancer for many years before succumbing. The palliative treatment phase, during which cure is no longer thought possible, may last for many months and sometimes years. For much of this time, the child may live a relatively normal life, but eventually treatment is required for an increasing number of symptoms. Hence management of death and dying falls firmly within the remit of cancer care. The rarity of childhood cancer itself makes it uncommon for a GP to face the situation of a dying child. The GP must cope with the challenge of working in true partnership with the parents and the child. This difficult time is made easier if the GP has maintained contact during all phases of the child's treatment.

Effective symptom management in palliative care is placed high on the agenda. It is the role of the professionals to make sure that a co-ordinated package of appropriate palliative care is delivered in the home environment to enable a child to die peacefully and comfortably at home. It is at this time that the GP becomes an important link between the family and the cancer centre, and eases both the practical and emotional burden of the family. Despite the difficulties that may be encountered by professionals during this period, it is essential that a good and caring relationship be established and maintained with the dying child and his or her family. This is important, because the family will require support from their GP for many years to come.

For good symptom control in the palliative phase of the child's illness, an innovative practice of individualized patient symptom and medication guidelines has been developed by the clinical nurse specialists at the Children's Unit of the Royal Marsden NHS Trust. Interdisciplinary professionals, who include the clinical nurse specialist, a specialist registrar with an interest in palliative care, and a pharmacist, compile these guidelines. All the known and predicted symptoms of the disease are simulated for the individual child. The drug dosages, including safe dose escalations, are calculated for the weight of the child. Such guidelines provide a comprehensive pathway of care that can be delivered at home, which gives confidence to the child, parents, and professionals (*Figs 27.6* and *27.7*).

Importantly, the tolerance of children to suggested prescribed dosages and dosage escalations may be very different

Table 27.5. Associations with childhood tumours

Childhood tumour	Association
Leukaemia	Down's syndrome
Central nervous system tumours	Neurofibromatosis type 1
Wilms tumour	Aniridia, hemihypertrophy, Beckwith–Wiedemann syndrome
Soft-tissue sarcoma	Li–Fraumeni syndrome (e.g. relatives with pre-menopausal breast cancer)
Hepatoblastoma	Familial adenomatous polyposis coli
Retinoblastoma	May be familial or heritable (mainly bilateral tumours)

Notes on individual childhood cancers

Leukaemia
Children usually present with a relatively short history (weeks rather than months) with pallor, fatigue, irritability, fever, bone pain ± bruising. 70% have hepatosplenomegaly. 50% have lymphadenopathy. Differential diagnosis includes infectious mononucleosis and other rare conditions (e.g. idiopathic thrombocytopenia, aplastic anaemia, metastatic neuroblastoma, juvenile rheumatoid arthritis).
Brain tumours
Common presenting features are given in *Table 27.6*.

Table 27.7. Common presenting features of various childhood cancers – Brain tumours

Brain tumours
Headache
Vomiting
Changes in personality and/or mood
Squint
Behaviour out of character
Deterioration in school performance
Growth failure
(Rapidly increasing head circumference
in infants)
Lymphomas
Hodgkin's disease – usually presents with non-tender cervical
    lymphadenopathy; natural history is long (months); only a
    minority have systemic symptoms.
Non-Hodgkin's lymphoma – lymphadenopathy and/or disease in
    mediastrinum or abdomen; rapid progression of symptoms.
Neuroblastoma
Majority have symptoms of metastatic disease, which may be indis-
    tinguishable clinically from acute leukaemia.
Infants under 1 year of age may have localized abdominal or
    thoracic masses; very young infants (age <6 months) may have
    rapidly progressive intra-abdominal disease.

Wilms tumour (nephroblastoma)
Unilateral abdominal mass ± pain
Haematuria
Soft-tissue sarcoma
Mass at almost any site, for example:
    head and neck (proptosis, nasal obstruction)
    genitourinary tract (urinary obstruction, bloodstained vaginal
    discharge); limbs, trunk (most often asymptomatic mass)
Bone tumours
Limbs are the most common sites
Persistent localized bone pain
Plain radiography usually helps
Retinoblastoma
White pupillary reflex
Squint
General tumours
Testicular/paratesticular masses can be difficult to differentiate –
    any non-transilluminable mass associated with the testis is
    significant
Ovarian tumours can be associated with precocious puberty

Reproduced from England Department of Health Cancer Referral Guidelines for Suspected Cancer Consultation Document April 2000.

Guidelines for urgent referral: children's tumours

Fatigue

In a previously healthy child combined with one or more of the following:

    lymphadenopathy

    hepatosplenomegaly

    clinical evidence of anaemia

Bone pain

Especially if it is diffuse or persistently localized, limits activity, or requires analgesia.

Lymphadenopathy

Lymphadenopathy with one or more of the following characteristics:

    painless

    firm and/or hard and >3cm in diameter

    unresolved after a course of antibiotics or progressively enlarging

    associated with signs of generalized ill health, fever, and/or weight loss

    involves axillary or supraclavicular nodes

    seen as mediastinal mass or hilar mass on chest X-ray

Headache

Headache of recent origin with one or more of the following features:

    increasing frequency or severity (e.g. causing nocturnal awakening)

    associated with behavioural change or deterioration in school performance

    associated with neurological signs (e.g. squint, ataxia)

    associated with vomiting

Soft-tissue mass

Soft-tissue mass that has one or more of the following characteristics:

    diameter >3cm

    shows rapid or progressive growth

    fixed or deep to fascia

    associated with regional lymph node enlargement

Reproduced from the Department of Health Referral Guidelines for Suspected Cancer Document 2000.
http://www.doh.gov.uk/pub/dosc/doh/guidelines.pdf

in the palliative setting. The result of good practice is reflected in the improvement of the child's daily living activity and quality of life within the confines of the palliative phase of the disease.

The GP's role should not be viewed as ending on the death of the child, which should, rather, be seen as the beginning of another facet of care for the family. Bereavement support should be regarded as an integral part of comprehensive care within the primary health care setting.

Future Trends

The future holds an exciting prospect in the management of childhood and adolescent cancer care. It is becoming evident that, with the advent of good supportive measures, much more drug therapy will be given on an outpatient basis, which has major implications for care in the community. The formation of primary care groups (PCGs) in the late 1990s and their continuing development into the

Referral proforma: children's tumours

Age:

Diagnosis suspected

Leukaemia	☐	Soft tissue sarcoma	☐
Brain tumour	☐	Bone tumour	☐
Lymphoma	☐	Retinoblastoma	☐
Neuroblastoma	☐	Hepatoblastoma	☐
Wilms' tumour	☐	Uncertain/other	☐

Symptoms	Yes	No	
Fatigue/malaise/lethargy			
Bone pain			
Headache			
Behavioural change			
Deterioration in school performance			
Haematuria			

Examination	Yes	No	
Lymphadenopathy			
Soft-tissue mass			
Fever			
Abdominal mass			
Hepatomegaly			
Splenomegaly			
Neurological signs specify..			
Pallor/signs of anaemia			
Other			

Specify...

Comments/other reasons for requesting urgent referral

Reproduced from England Department of Health Cancer Referral Guidelines Consultation Document May 2000.
http://www.doh.gov.uk/pub/docs/doh/refpaed.pdf

INDIVIDUALISED MEDICATION SYMPTOM CARE GUIDELINES

Last weight: 50kg

Child preference to suspensions or tablets of oral drugs: Tablets

For all symptoms assess causative factors and influences – physical, psychological, social and spiritual

Symptoms	Drugs	Dose	Route
Pain	Codeine phosphate	Currently on 25mg every 4 hours	Oral
	Oral morphine	5mg every 4 hours, to start if pain not controlled on codeine phosphate (max. 10mg every 4 hours)	Oral
	Prednisolone	10mg daily Increase to 20mg twice daily for 3 days as directed	Oral
	Diamorphine (divide the total dose of oral morphine by 3 to obtain equivalent analgesic dose of parenteral diamorphine; no upper limit to diamorphine dose)	10–20mg over 24 hours Dose increment as necessary	Intravenous
		1.5–3.0mg start bolus dose	Intravenous
Nausea and vomiting	Cyclizine	12.5mg three times a day	Oral
		50mg over 24 hours	Intravenous
	Haloperidol	0.25mg twice daily to start (maximum 0.5mg twice daily)	Oral
	Methotrimeprazine	5mg over 24 hours (maximum 10mg over 24 hours)	Intravenous
Constipation	Lactulose	Currently on 10ml twice daily	Oral
	Co-danthramer	Currently 2.5ml daily To increase twice daily if necessary	Oral

Caution:

No more than three drugs in a syringe driver at any one time because of increased risk of drug precipitation.

Caution:

Hyoscine hydrobromide can exacerbate restlessness.

Caution:

When increasing doses of cyclizine and diamorphine in the syringe driver, amount of dilutant may need to be increased.

Figure 27.7. Example of the drugs used in the symptom care guidelines for acute lymphoblastic leukaemia.

21st century will influence and change the global delivery of health care for all diseases, including cancer care. It may be that, with the formation of PCGs, supportive care for long-term survivors of childhood cancer can be a collaborative venture between the regional centre and the local hospital. This pathway could enable delivery of a true holistic care package in the community setting for these young adults.

Further reading

Gibson F, Evans M. *Paediatric Oncology: Acute nursing care*. London: Whurr Publishers; 1999.

Goldman A. *Care of the Dying Child*. Oxford University Press; 1998.

Mycroft J, Crabtree S, Patel N, Williams J. *Pharmaceutical Guidelines for Symptom Control for Children with Advanced Cancer*. The Royal Marsden NHS Trust, Wolfson Children's Cancer Unit. [Available from the Unit]

Pinkerton CR, Plowman PN. *Paediatric Oncology. Clinical practice and controversies*. London: Chapman and Hall; 1992.

Pinkerton CR, Michalski AJ, Veys PA. Clinical Challenges in Paediatric Oncology. London: ISIS Medical Media; 1999.

Pinkerton CR, Cushing P, Sepion B. *Childhood Cancer Management: A practical handbook*. London: Chapman and Hall; 1994.

Stiller C *et al*. United Kingdom National Registry of Childhood Tumours, England and Wales 1981–1990. In: DM Parkin *et al*. (eds). *International Incidence of Childhood Cancer*, Vol II. Lyon: IARC Scientific Publication No. 144 IARC, 1998: 365–7.

28 HIV-Associated Cancer

Chris Boshoff

Incidence

A substantial burden of human cancer worldwide is attributable to infection. Viral infections account for approximately 15% of all human cancers. Cervical cancer, hepatocellular carcinoma, and Kaposi's sarcoma (KS), all caused by viruses, are some of the most important tumours in sub-Saharan Africa and therefore also in immigrants to the UK from these countries.

The interface between infection and malignancy is highlighted by the cancers prevalent in acquired immunodeficiency syndrome (AIDS; *Table 28.1*). Individuals infected with the human immunodeficiency virus (HIV) are specifically prone to cancer caused by viruses, such as the Epstein–Barr virus (EBV; lymphomas), papillomaviruses (squamous carcinomas of skin and anogenital carcinoma), and Kaposi's sarcoma-associated herpesvirus (KSHV; lymphomas, multicentric Castleman's disease, and KS). The tumours that have an increased incidence in HIV-infected individuals for which a virus is not yet described (see *Table 28.1*) could still have a viral aetiology (unknown or known virus infection). Carcinogenesis is a multifactorial process and not all persons infected with oncogenic viruses develop a cancer; in fact, only a fraction of infected individuals develop a tumour, particularly in the absence of immunosuppression. The incidences of certain tumours with a known viral aetiology (e.g. nasopharyngeal and hepatocellular carcinoma) do not increase with AIDS, which indicates that viral infection and immunosuppression, without co-factors, are not enough to precipitate the specific cancer. However, efficacious immunization against the primary infection would virtually eliminate the occurrence of the tumour with which the virus is associated. A successful vaccine against hepatitis B virus is available, whereas vaccines against EBV and human papillomaviruses are currently in clinical studies.

Incidence, key points

Cancer is a major complication of HIV infection.

Kaposi's sarcoma (KS) and non-Hodgkin's lymphoma are the two most common neoplasms in HIV-infected patients.

Both KS and the majority of lymphomas associated with AIDS are caused by herpesviruses.

Anti-retroviral treatment often leads to the resolution of KS lesions.

Table 28.1. Tumours increased in patients with acquired immunodeficiency syndrome

Cancer type	Relative risk	Viral link
Kaposi's sarcoma	310	Kaposi's sarcoma-associated herpesvirus
Non-Hodgkin's lymphoma	113	Epstein–Barr virus (EBV)
Angiosarcoma	36.7	?
Anal cancer[a]	31.7	Human papillomavirus
Leukaemias other than lymphoid and myeloid	11.0	?
Hodgkin's disease	7.6	?EBV
Leiomyosarcoma and other soft tissue sarcomas[b]	7.2	?EBV
Multiple myeloma	4.5	?
Primary brain cancer[c]	3.5	Papovaviruses
Testicular seminoma or malignant germinoma	2.9	?

[a]Anal carcinoma is increased in homosexual men, even prior to HIV infection.
[b]EBV sequences described in smooth-muscle tumours from children with AIDS, including monoclonal EBV episomes in some cases.
[c]Predominantly malignant glioma or astrocytoma. The detection of papovavirus sequences in brain tumours remains unconfirmed.

Aetiology and Pathology

Kaposi's sarcoma

For over 100 years, KS remained a rare curiosity to clinicians and cancer researchers, until it shot to prominence as the sentinel of what we now call AIDS. In 1872, the Hungarian dermatologist Moriz Kaposi published the case histories of five middle-aged and elderly male patients in Vienna with idiopathic multiple pigmented sarcomas of the skin.

Classic KS occurs predominantly in elderly male patients of southern European ancestry. A high frequency is also seen in Israel and other Middle Eastern countries. This form of the disease is generally not as aggressive as the form originally described by Kaposi, for unknown, possibly immunological, reasons. Patients usually present with purplish lesions on the skin of the lower legs, and these lesions can ulcerate. Almost all patients with classic KS in the UK are of Middle Eastern, Mediterranean, or Jewish origin.

In some equatorial countries of Africa, KS has existed for many decades, long preceding HIV (known as endemic KS). This form is found in younger patients as well as the elderly; the male:female ratio is >3:1. It is generally a more aggressive disease than classic KS, although less so than African AIDS-associated KS. In particular, endemic KS in African children is often associated with lymph node involvement only and no skin lesions. Children from Africa occasionally present with this form of KS in the UK.

KS is also known to develop after an organ transplant (post-transplant or iatrogenic KS). Patients of Mediterranean, Jewish, or Arabian ancestry are also clearly over-represented among immunosuppressed patients who develop KS after a transplant in the UK.

In 1981, the US Centers for Disease Control and Prevention became aware of an increased occurrence of two rare diseases in young homosexual men from New York City and California: KS and *Pneumocystis carinii* pneumonia. This was the beginning of the AIDS epidemic, and AIDS KS is today the most common form of KS. Most patients with KS in the UK are HIV-positive homosexual men.

Studies of AIDS case surveillance support the pre-AIDS data on the existence of a sexually transmissible KS co-factor: KS occurs predominantly in homosexual and bisexual men with AIDS, less commonly in those who acquire HIV through heterosexual contact, and rarely in AIDS patients with haemophilia or in intravenous drug users.

Histopathologically, KS consists of sheets of spindle-shaped tumour cells (called KS spindle cells) with prominent angiogenesis and an inflammatory infiltrate. The spindle cells express markers of endothelial cells and the tumour is therefore believed to be of endothelial origin.

Kaposi's sarcoma-associated herpesvirus (KSHV, also called human herpesvirus-8) is thought to be the cause of KS. This is a gammaherpesvirus distantly related to the EBV. KSHV is found in all the different epidemiological forms of KS. The prevalence of this virus in healthy individuals in the UK is <5%, but it is found in up to 50% of HIV-infected individuals, in whom it is thought to be predominantly sexually transmitted. The seroprevalence of KSHV in the different HIV risk groups correlates with the incidence of KS: in the developed world, KSHV is found predominantly in HIV-positive homosexual men and not in HIV-positive patients with haemophilia or HIV-positive intravenous drug users or heterosexuals. In Mediterranean countries the prevalence of KSHV in the general population is around 10–20% and in sub-Saharan African countries the prevalence is up to 60%. The prevalence of KSHV correlates with the incidence of KS among different ethnic groups in the UK. KSHV is transmitted from mothers to their children in Africa and, as in Mediterranean Europe, the prevalence of antibodies to KSHV increases steadily with age.

Herpesviruses are usually controlled by the immune system, so that only a fraction of blood cells remain latently infected throughout life. KSHV infects circulating B-lymphocytes and it is thought that the immunosuppression induced by HIV or immunosuppressive drugs after an organ transplant leads to an increased KSHV viral load with subsequent infection of endothelial cells and KS formation.

Non-Hodgkin's lymphoma

In the developed world, people diagnosed with AIDS are about 60 times more likely than the general population to have some type of non-Hodgkin's lymphoma (NHL) and a thousand times more likely to have Burkitt's lymphoma or central nervous system (CNS) lymphoma. Up to 10% of HIV-infected individuals develop NHL. The risk increases with increased levels of immunosuppression. HIV-associated lymphomas are atypical and patients often present with extranodal disease such as involvement of the digestive tract, bone marrow, or skin. The most common type is B-cell immunoblastic lymphoma, followed by primary CNS lymphoma and a Burkitt's-type small cell lymphoma.

EBV is found in nearly 50% of large cell lymphomas in HIV-infected patients and in 100% of primary CNS lymphomas. Since EBV is clonal in these lymphoma cells, it is thought to be the aetiological agent that drives the proliferation of lymphoma cells. EBV, the prototype of gamma-herpesviruses, is a highly transforming virus and EBV-infected B-lymphocytes are highly immunogenic and elicit powerful cytotoxic T-cell responses. However, despite these two important characteristics, only a fraction of EBV-infected individuals actually develop EBV-associated tumours and, despite the interactions between autologous EBV-infected B-cells and CD8+ T-cells, EBV persists in B-cells. These two apparent paradoxes are solved by the down-regulation of all viral proteins associated with growth transformation, which include those known to elicit cytotoxic T-cell responses, in persistently infected B-lymphocytes. During this latent state, only EBV nuclear antigen 1 (EBNA-1) is expressed in these cells. EBNA-1 is essential to maintain the stability and proliferation of the viral episome (unintegrated viral DNA) and does not evoke an immune response.

Hodgkin's disease

In HIV-positive patients, Hodgkin's disease usually presents atypically at a late stage with extranodal dissemination. The predominant forms are of mixed cellularity and lymphocyte-depleted, which are relatively rare in the HIV-uninfected population.

EBV is present in nearly 50% of Hodgkin's disease biopsies. However, the exact role, if any, of EBV in Hodgkin's disease pathogenesis remains unclear.

Multicentric Castleman's disease

Castleman's disease is a rare and usually polyclonal lymphoproliferative disorder found in both HIV-negative and, more frequently, HIV-infected individuals. The systemic variety is designated multicentric Castleman's disease (MCD) and is usually of the plasma-cell type. Interestingly, patients with MCD are at an increased risk of developing KS and certain B-cell lymphomas. Systemic MCD is associated with fever, night sweats, spleen and liver involvement, and often a poor prognosis.

KSHV is nearly universally present in HIV-positive individuals with MCD. Among MCD cases in immunocompetent hosts the presence of KSHV is restricted to about 40% of cases. In MCD, KSHV is present in large immunoblastic-like cells in the mantle zone. These cells are monoclonal and are not present in KSHV-negative cases. KSHV-positive MCD appears to have a particularly poor prognosis, especially in HIV-infected patients.

Aetiology and pathology, key points

KS-associated herpesvirus (KSHV) is the cause of Kaposi's sarcoma and certain lymphoproliferations.
KSHV is a rare infection in the general population of the UK.
EBV is present in nearly 50% of systemic and 100% of CNS lymphomas associated with HIV.

Clinical Presentation

AIDS-associated KS usually starts with purplish skin or mucosal lesions. These can progress rapidly to multiple skin lesions, followed by systemic involvement, including lung, liver, and spleen. This can result in breathlessness or jaundice.

Lymphomas present with systemic B-cell symptoms, including weight loss and night sweats, although these symptoms are also caused by HIV infection. Otherwise patients present with local symptoms (e.g. related to bowel or cardiopulmonary involvement). Primary CNS lymphomas present with either focal CNS symptoms or signs of increased cranial pressure. Patients who present with AIDS-related lymphoma usually have other signs of immunodeficiency, such as mucosal or skin candidiasis.

Diagnosis and Investigations

Kaposi's sarcoma
General practice

KS is usually a clinical diagnosis, confirmed by a biopsy for histopathology. Patients who present with KS and who are not of Mediterranean, Middle Eastern, or Jewish descent should have an HIV test. Various clinical staging systems are used, but the most important prognostic indicator in HIV-infected patients is CD4+ cell count and HIV viral load. Any case of suspected KS should be referred to a specialist centre as soon as possible.

Hospital

Routine clinical staging includes a chest radiograph, ultrasound, or computed tomography (CT) scan of the abdomen and pelvis. In HIV-infected patients, suspicious lesions in the liver, lung, or spleen need to be confirmed by needle biopsy to distinguish them from other malignant or infective causes.

Non-Hodgkin's lymphoma
General practice
HIV-infected patients are usually severely immunosuppressed by the time they develop NHL, and therefore NHL is very rarely the presenting feature of HIV infection. In suspected cases of lymphoma, a lymph node biopsy is usually the first investigation. However, in HIV-infected patients, NHL often presents without lymph node involvement and systemic investigations are therefore warranted. In the UK, HIV testing is usually recommended in suspected cases of NHL or Hodgkin's disease in 'high-risk groups' including young men (especially if it is known that they are homosexual), intravenous drug users, and African–Caribbean patients. Any case of suspected lymphoma (HIV-related or not) should be referred to a specialist centre as soon as possible.

Hospital
Routine investigations for systemic NHL include CT scans, bone marrow aspirate, and trephine biopsy. In cases of suspected CNS lymphoma a CT scan or magnetic resonance imaging scan is performed. Up to 50% of patients have multiple brain lesions. These investigations do not always differentiate between NHL and other AIDS-related CNS diseases, such as toxoplasmosis or progressive multifocal leukoencephalopathy. If the diagnosis is uncertain, patients are treated for 14 days with antitoxoplasmosis chemotherapy as a therapeutic trial. A stereotactic brain biopsy is performed if the therapeutic trial fails. Although biopsies have a high diagnostic yield for HIV-associated intracranial lesions, the complication rate is also relatively high. The diagnosis of CNS lymphoma can also be confirmed by cerebrospinal fluid examination for EBV by the polymerase chain reaction. Recently, other imaging techniques, such as positron emission tomography and single-photon emission CT scan with thallium-201 have been used to distinguish CNS NHL from toxoplasmosis.

Diagnosis and investigations, key points

Suspected cases of AIDS-associated Kaposi's sarcoma and NHL should be referred to a specialist centre as soon as possible.

AIDS-associated NHL often presents atypically with systemic symptoms, rather than with lymph node enlargement.

Routine imaging techniques often do not distinguish primary CNS lymphoma from other CNS diseases related to the HIV infection, such as toxoplasmosis.

Management

AIDS-related cancer presents specific therapeutic problems because the underlying immunosuppression compromises optimal therapies. The risk of overwhelming infection and sepsis is therefore a real problem with most treatment modalities.

Kaposi's sarcoma
The introduction of highly active anti-retroviral therapy (HAART) to treat HIV infection has resulted in responses from AIDS-associated KS lesions. It is thought that immune reconstitution achieved with this therapy leads to the recovery of cytotoxic T-cell responses against KSHV, with the subsequent resolution of KS lesions. Anti-HIV treatment is therefore currently the first-line therapy to manage AIDS-associated KS.

In AIDS-associated KS patients who are already on HAART, isolated skin lesions are treated with radiotherapy. For more extensive disease or systemic involvement, cytotoxic therapy is used. Liposomal daunorubicin is one of the most active agents, and patients usually do not suffer hair loss with this treatment. Long-term control is seldom achieved without managing the underlying immunosuppression. Similarly, post-transplant KS is managed by reducing immunosuppressive therapies; in cases of aggressive KS, this does occasionally mean sacrificing the donated organ.

Novel anti-angiogenic therapy is currently also used as experimental treatment for KS. Other experimental approaches include retinoic acid derivatives and immune modulators, such as interleukin-12.

Non-Hodgkin's lymphoma
Cytotoxic therapy is used to treat systemic NHL. However, because of the additional risk of infection with a compromised bone marrow and immune reserve, chemotherapy regimens are usually tailored to individual cases according to performance and immune status. A few HIV-infected patients with NHL have undergone successful syngeneic or allogeneic bone marrow transplantation.

AIDS-associated primary CNS lymphoma is usually treated with cranial radiotherapy with or without systemic chemotherapy. At some centres, intraventricular reservoirs are placed for intraventricular cytotoxic therapy such as methotrexate. However, the prognosis is extremely poor and few patients survive for longer than 6 months. It appears that combined radio- and chemotherapy is appropriate for a small subset of patients, which translates into meaningful palliation not strikingly dissimilar from that seen in non-

AIDS patients. Novel therapies to manage these patients are needed. One such approach is to use the anti-HIV agent zidovudine in combination with ganciclovir (as an anti-EBV treatment) and interleukin-2.

Conclusions

Cancer is a major cause of morbidity and mortality in HIV-infected individuals. In many African countries, KS is now the most common cancer overall because of the AIDS epidemic. The two most common malignancies in HIV-positive patients, that is KS and NHL, are caused by herpesviruses. Effective HIV-1 therapies may have a direct or indirect impact on the development of AIDS-associated malignancies. Indirect protection against the occurrence of these tumours may result from a boost of the immune system by antiretroviral therapies. The treatment of HIV-associated NHL, and in particular primary CNS lymphoma, remains unsatisfactory and novel therapies are warranted.

Management, key points

KS can respond to highly active antiretroviral therapy.

Localized KS is treated with radiotherapy.

Advanced KS is treated with chemotherapy (e.g. liposomal daunorubicin).

Systemic NHL is treated with combination chemotherapy, but poor bone marrow reserve and immune function compromise optimal therapy.

Primary CNS lymphoma has a very poor prognosis, and active treatment is not always indicated.

Further Reading

Boshoff C, Weiss R. AIDS-related malignancies. *Nat Rev Cancer* 2000; **2**: 373–82.

Boshoff C. Kaposi's sarcoma-associated herpesvirus. In: *Cancer Surveys: Infections and Human Cancer*, Vol. 33. Newton R, Beral V, Weiss RA (eds). New York: Cold Spring Harbor Press, 1999; 157–90.

Chamberlain MC, Kormanik PA. AIDS-related central nervous system lymphomas. *J Neurooncol*. 1999; **43**: 269–76.

Newton R, Beral V, Weiss RA. Human immunodeficiency virus infection and cancer. In: *Cancer Surveys: Infections and Human Cancer*, Vol. 33. Newton R, Beral V, Weiss RA (eds). New York: Cold Spring Harbor Press, 1999, 237–62.

Sitas F, Carrara H, Beral V, *et al*. Antibodies against human herpesvirus-8 in black South African patients with cancer. *N Engl J Med*. 1999; **340**: 1863–71.

Tulpule A, Levine A. AIDS-related lymphoma. *Blood Rev*. 1999; **13**: 147–50.

SECTION 5

Information

29 Interpreting Data and Evidence

Douglas Russell

When looking at figures about cancer there are some caveats for those not used to interpreting such data. Figures can be actual and accurate or provisional or estimates. Even figures that are confirmed by cancer registries can be inaccurate since they are often several years out of date or confounded by other factors.

Standardization: Comparing Apples with Pears?

Figures may be raw data or adjusted to 'standard populations'. This is particularly important when comparing rates of incidence or mortality. In general, three types of standardization are in common use: the European standard population, the world standard population and US figures, which up to 1998 were adjusted to the 1970 US standard population and from 1999 are adjusted to the 2000 US standard population. There are significant differences between these standards. For example, the world standard population has a much higher percentage of younger people than the other two.

Ethnicity and Other Factors

In a population, genetic, environmental and socioeconomic factors are all-important influences of the incidence and mortality of cancer. Access to health care systems is also a potential confounding factor that affects comparisons between countries and between regions within a country. The degree of difference in access of coverage by health care insurance, and indeed type of health care insurance, can all have varying impact on figures.

Cancer Registry Data

The UK has a good record on the completeness and quality of cancer registration data. Scotland appears particularly well served, because of the use of a generic primary care clinical information system that can allow episode–record linkage

across primary and secondary care, meaning that very few patients are lost to follow up.

The USA does not have a nation-wide cancer registry, and the quality of case reporting varies among state cancer registries. Thus, in compiling US cancer estimates researchers use population data collected by the US Bureau of the Census and cancer incidence rates collected by the National Cancer Institute's Surveillance, Epidemiology, and End Results (SEER) program (Landis *et al*, 1998). The Healthy People 2010 website has a map showing the progress that individual states have made to meet the required cancer registry standards.

In Europe the depth and detail of cancer registries varies and it is not unusual for a country to be represented by the figures from a cancer registry or registries covering one or more regions.

The UK is divided into several Cancer Registry regions. They are:

- East Anglia;
- Merseyside and Cheshire;
- Northern Ireland;
- North Western Cancer Registry and Centre for Cancer Epidemiology;
- Scottish Cancer Intelligence Unit;
- South and West;
- Thames;
- Trent;
- Wales; and
- West Midlands.

Coding Systems

Cancer figures tend to use either the International Classification of Diseases Codes (ICD), revision 9 or 10. In comparing year-on-year figures, beware of pitfalls consequent on a change of coding system. For example, the England and Wales ONS (Office for National Statistics) firm data for most cancer sites in their Health Statistics Quarterly 04 Winter 1999 do not identify non-Hodgkin's lymphoma (ICD-9 200 and 202), which are all given in ICD-10. The estimated figures for 1995 based on previous ICD-9 data predicted that non-Hodgkin's lymphoma represented 4% of all new male cancers and 3% of all new female cancers – 8240 patients in total.

GP systems tend to use the Read code system, which was developed by a GP, Sir James Read, and is now licensed for use in the NHS. There are different versions of this system. The latest version, with a greatly expanded range of clinical terms, is designed to be relational, as opposed to previous versions, which were hierarchical. It is hoped that the newer version will be more acceptable to hospital clinicians and to professions other than medicine.

Mapping between coding systems can be problematic. The Read system can be mapped to ICD-9 or ICD-10, but reverse mapping is not practical. For primary care the main issue is for all clinicians in teams to agree and standardize on the clinical terms they use for key epidemiological data, otherwise aggregation of data is virtually impossible.

Survival Data

Survival figures can be crude or relative. Crude figures are the actual number of people still alive from a given cohort after a particular period time. However, patients who have cancer die of other diseases and this can be adjusted for by taking into account deaths from other causes by age group; this results in relative survival data.

A further complication is that survival varies with socioeconomic status and, thus, aggregate figures may disguise considerable variation within populations.

Detailed information for England and Wales 1971–1995 by deprivation and NHS region is available (Coleman M *et al.*), and a website has similar detail for Scotland.

Evidence

New disciplines of critical appraisal have become part of the general medical education curriculum. In 1990 the British Royal College of General Practitioners introduced a paper on critical appraisal as part of the membership examination.

The emergence of clinical effectiveness, evidence-based medicine and a proliferation of guidelines for treatment and referral have been seen by some as a reductionist approach ('cook-book medicine'). Where very strong evidence exists, it might indeed be possible to delegate certain health care elements to technicians rather than professionals.

The Cochrane database has a library of appraised literature and evidence, and publications such as *Clinical Evidence* contain detailed analyses of current evidence.

In appraising evidence and in implementing guidelines reference is made to grades of evidence. Slight variations exist in the systems used. One definition is quoted here.

Level of evidence

- Level Ia – evidence obtained from meta-analysis of randomized controlled trials
- Level Ib – evidence obtained from at least one randomized controlled trial
- Level IIa – evidence obtained from at least one well-designed controlled study without randomization
- Level IIb – evidence obtained from at least one other type of well-designed quasi-experimental study
- Level III – evidence obtained from well-designed, non-experimental, descriptive studies, such as comparative studies, correlation studies and case studies
- Level IV – evidence obtained from expert committee reports or clinical experiences of respected authorities

Grades of recommendations

- Grade A – at least one randomized controlled trial as a part of the body of literature of overall good quality and consistency addressing specific recommendation (evidence levels Ia and Ib)
- Grade B – the availability of well-conducted clinical studies but no randomized clinical trials on the topic of recommendation (evidence levels IIa, IIb and III)
- Grade C – evidence obtained from expert committee reports or opinions or clinical experiences of respected authorities; indicates absence of directly applicable clinical studies of good quality (evidence level IV)

The Clinical Outcomes Group papers on improving outcomes in specific cancers use a slightly different scale (though with the same effect).

1. Grade 1 (strong evidence) – randomized controlled trial or systematic review of randomized controlled trials
   - Grade IA – calculation of sample size, and accurate and standard definition of outcome variables

- Grade IB – accurate and standard definition of outcome variables
- Grade IC – none of the above
2. Grade II (fairly strong evidence) – prospective study with a comparison group (non-randomiszed controlled trial or good observational study)
   - Grade IIA – calculation of sample size, and accurate, standard definition of outcome variables and adjustment for the effects of important confounding variables
   - Grade IIB – one of the criteria for grade IIa is met
3. Grade III (weak evidence) – retrospective study
   - Grade IIIA – comparison group, calculation of sample size, and accurate, standard definition of outcome variables
   - Grade IIIB – two of the criteria for grade IIIa are met
   - Grade IIIC – none of the criteria for grade IIIa is met
4. Grade IV (weak evidence) – cross-sectional study

Making Recommendations

Recommendations after appraisal are now usually allocated to one of the following categories:

- beneficial – interventions for which effectiveness has been demonstrated by clear evidence from controlled trials;
- likely to be beneficial – interventions for which effectiveness is less well established than for those listed as 'beneficial';
- trade off between benefits and harms – interventions for which clinicians and patients should weigh up the beneficial and harmful effects according to individual circumstances and priorities;
- unknown effectiveness – interventions for which there are currently insufficient data or data of inadequate quality;
- unlikely to be beneficial – interventions for which lack of effectiveness is less well established than for those listed under 'likely to be ineffective or harmful'; and
- likely to be ineffective or harmful – interventions whose ineffectiveness or harmfulness has been demonstrated by clear evidence.

In challenging professions and professionals, society asks what does the professional bring that the technician does not? Professions are, by definition, closed shops that are self-selecting and self-regulating (for now at least) and that set their own standards.

What do we do when there is no adequate evidence? Society needs professionals where there is no overwhelming evidence, and there is a requirement for the exercise of judgement. Clinical trials are the bedrock of cancer research and if evidence from trials does not exist then we must rely on the considered opinion of respected experts. A part of cancer care falls into this category, even though the discipline probably has the strongest tradition of randomized controlled clinical trials of any medical speciality.

In spite of this, it is interesting to note that some GPs remain cautious about referring patients to centres conducting clinical trials (weak evidence), fearing their patients will be allocated to 'the wrong arm of the study' (Ellis *et al.*, 1999).

The UK Cancer Research Campaign (now Cancer Research UK) has highlighted the need for more randomized controlled trials for new treatments in children (Lashford, 1998–1999). The same volume contains a useful article on emerging ethical issues in clinical trials (Secher, 1998–1999).

Further Reading

Clinical Evidence. London: BMJ Publishing Group, 2000.

Ellis PM, Hobbs MK, Rikard-Bell GC, Ward JE. General practitioners' attitudes to randomised controlled trials for women with breast cancer. *Med J Aust*. 1999; **171**: 303–5.

Landis SH, Murray T, Bolden S, Wingo PA. Cancer statistics 1998 in CA. *Cancer J Clin*. 1998; **48**: 6–29.

Lashford L. *CRC Scientific Yearbook 1998–1999*. 39-40.

Secher D. *CRC Scientific Yearbook 1998–1999*. 35-6.

30 Sources of Information and Support for Cancer Patients

Val Speechley

Since 1990, and particularly since 1995, the need to provide good-quality, accurate, accessible, and timely patient information has been recognized and endorsed by government, organizations that represent patients, and those formed of partnerships between patients and professionals.

The Calman–Hine report (1995) was the first document from the Department of Health to state clearly the responsibility of health care professionals with regard to information giving:

> Patients, families and carers should be given clear information and assistance in a form they can understand about treatment options and outcomes available to them at all stages of treatment from diagnosis onwards.

This same report acknowledged 'the central and continuing element' that is the primary care team.

The focus on patient information has continued (NHSE, 1996, 1998) and the document from the NHS Information Authority, *Towards Cancer Information Strategy*, looks to set standards for information services in both primary and secondary care, and proposes to link recommendations to specific timescales.

In addition to government initiatives, reports from patient partnership organizations (National Cancer Alliance, 1996; BACUP, 1996) provide a different perspective, but a similar message, while recognizing that provision of information is only one aspect of the support needed by patients and their carers.

There is now a large body of research to inform health care professionals of the potential benefits of information provision (Van Der Molen, 1999). This considers the role of information as a coping strategy, to enable understanding of cancer and its treatment, to facilitate shared decision-making, and to increase compliance. The majority of studies reviewed here indicate that information giving has a positive outcome.

Access to information has become easier for many with the boom in information technology and the internet. However, for a large proportion of patients and carers the main source of information is their doctor, nurse, radiographer, or other health care professional; also, second to face-to-face communication, written materials are the next most universally popular medium for information (BRMB International, 1999).

Much work has been undertaken on the need for patients and carers to be supported throughout the experience of cancer (National Cancer Alliance, 1996; Van Der Molen, 1999, 2000a, 2000b). Support is an all-embracing term that has informational, emotional, psychological, practical, and social aspects. Some fall naturally within the family or professional spheres, while others may be gifted by fellow patients. Wherever the support originates from it has been identified as essential.

Providing the information and support needed by people affected by cancer in a busy practice with finite resources is not an easy task. It can best be achieved by tapping into the services of existing organizations, mainly in the voluntary sector. Many of these produce information that is of a high standard and free to cancer patients. Increasingly, this information can also be accessed on the Internet.

Support can often be provided by referral to a local self-help group. In addition to sharing common experiences, many well-established groups offer counselling and complementary therapies using suitably qualified practitioners.

National and local organizations can supply posters or other publicity materials to display in waiting areas, alerting both patients and professionals to what is available.

Using this Chapter

The list of organizations in this chapter does not include all the sources of information and support that exist in the cancer field. However, the main charities and some other useful contacts are listed under the headings of general information and support, complementary therapy, and disease- or topic-specific organizations (in the order of the chapters in this book) and the range of services offered by each is covered briefly. Some have national (England, Wales, Scotland, Northern Ireland) or regional offices, the details of which can be obtained from the main contact number.

General National Information and Support Organizations

CancerBACUP

Helps patients, their families, and friends cope with cancer. Trained cancer nurses provide information, emotional support and practical advice by telephone, e-mail or letter. Over 50 publications on cancer, its treatment, and practical issues of coping. A one-to-one counselling service is available in Scotland. Translation services.

3 Bath Place

Rivington Street

London EC2A 3JR

Tel: 020 7613 2121

Freephone: 0808 800 1234

Website: www.cancerbacup.org.uk

Cancer Black Care

For people with all types of cancer and their families, relatives and friends. Drop-in centre and telephone support available. Centres in London, Birmingham and Manchester. Counselling is offered. Twi, Yoruba, Hindi, Turkish and other ethnic groups' languages spoken.

16 Dalston Lane

London E8 3DL

Tel: 020 7249 1-97

Website: www.cancerblackcare.org

Cancer Care Society

Offers free, confidential counselling, emotional support, and practical help to anyone whose life has been touched by cancer. Series of self-help groups that allow people in similar circumstances to meet each other, as well as walk-in centres, which provide, free, one-to-one counselling, complementary therapies, befriending, and an information library. Centres in Romsey, Hampshire, and in Merthyr Tydfil, Wales. New centres due to open in Dereham, Norfolk, and Mountain Ash, Wales. Runs a group counselling session in Romsey.

11 The Cornmarket

Romsey

Hampshire SO51 8GB

Tel: 01794 830300

Fax: 01794 518133

e-mail: info@cancercaresoc.org

Website: www.cancercaresoc.org

Chai-Cancer Care (Jewish support and health centre)

Provides reassurance, support, and friendship to Jewish cancer patients and their families, telephone helpline, weekly support meetings, general information service, hospital and hospice visiting, spiritual guidance, and public lectures. A wide range of complementary therapies is available for patients and well people, as well as wellbeing screening clinics for men and women.

Shield House

Harmony Way

off Victoria Road

London NW4 2BZ

Helpline: 0808 808 4567

Tel/Fax: 020 8202 2211

e-mail: info@chai-lifeline.org.uk

website: www.chaicancercare.org

GaysCan

National helpline offering confidential help and support to homosexual men living with cancer and to their partners and carers.

7 Baron Close

Friern Barnet

London N11 3PS

Tel: 020 8368 9027 (10.00AM to 8.00PM)

e-mail: gayscan@blotholm.dircon.co.uk

GEMMA

A national friendship network of disabled and non-disabled lesbians and bisexual women, all ages. Quarterly newsletter, available in large print, tape, and Braille.

BM Box 5700

London WC1N 3XX

Irish Cancer Society

Lectures and talks are provided to the workplace, schools, public, and professional organizations. Range of literature. Cancer Helpline to discuss personal enquiries on the free telephone.

5 Northumberland Road

Dublin 4

Republic of Ireland

Cancer helpline 00353 (1) 800 200 700

Fax: 00353 (1) 668 7599

(Freephone in Republic of Ireland)

Lymphoedema Support Network

Offers quarterly newsletters, information, fact sheets, practical advice and support to patients with primary and secondary lymphoedema.

St Luke's Crypt

Sydney Street

London SW3 6NH

Tel: 020 7351 4480

Helpline: 0707 122 4760

e-mail: adminlsn@lymphoedema.freeserve.co.uk

Website: www.lymphoedema.org/lsn

Macmillan Cancer Relief

Macmillan Cancer Relief (incorporating Cancerlink) [provides information and support for people living with cancer, including access to a UK network of cancer self-help and support groups. Tanslation service and telephone for those who are hard of hearing.

Funds the Macmillan Nursing Services, including Macmillan Paediatric Nurses, for home care and hospital support. The patient grants department provides financial help towards the cost of a wide range of things for people with cancer. Applications are made by a social worker, health visitor, or home care nurse.

89 Albert Embankment

London SE1 7UG

Cancer line: 0808 808 2020

e-mail: cancerline@macmillan.org.uk

Website: www.macmillan.org.uk

Marie Curie Cancer Care

Provides nursing care for people with cancer, through 10 in-patient Marie Curie Centres. A nationwide network of Marie Curie nurses is available to nurse patients in their own homes. (All services to patients are free.) Also runs its own Research Institute and the Education Department provides training courses and conferences for health professionals on cancer and related topics.

89 Albert Embankment

London SE1 7TP

Tel: 020 7599 7777

Fax: 020 7599 7788

e-mail: info@mariecurie.org.uk

Website: www.mariecurie.org.uk

National Cancer Alliance

An independent national membership organization of cancer patients, their families, friends, leading cancer experts, and other health professionals. Campaigns for better cancer services in the UK.

PO Box 579

Oxford OX4 1LB

Tel: 0870 770 2648

Fax: 0870 770 2649

e-mail: nationalcanceralliance@btinternet.com

Website: www.nationalcanceralliance.co.uk

Tak Tent Cancer Support Scotland

Offers information and support for cancer patients, families, friends, and associated professionals. Specific help is available for those between 16 and 25 years of age. Network of support groups in West and Central Scotland, counselling service, and telephone helpline.

Flat 5, 30 Shelley Court

Gartnavel Complex

Glasgow G12 0YN

Tel: 0141 211 0122

e-mail: tak.tent@care4free.net

Website: www.taktent.org.uk

Tenovus Cancer Information Centre

Provides information and advice on all cancer related concerns. Contact by Freephone Cancer Helpline, letter, or personal visit.

Velindre NHS Trust

Velindre Hospital

Velindre Road

Whitchurch

Cardiff CF14 2TL

Freephone Cancer Helpline: 0808 808 1010

Tel: 029 2019 6100

Fax: 029 2048 9919

e-mail: tcic@tenovus.com

Website: www.tenovus.com

Ulster Cancer Foundation

Provides a cancer information and counselling service, support groups throughout the province, volunteer befriender visits, breast cancer fitting service, and hospital-based nurse counsellors.

40–42 Eglantine Avenue

Belfast BT9 6DX

Freephone Cancer Helpline: 0800 783 3339

Tel: 028 9066 3281

Fax: 028 9066 0081

e-mail: info@ulstercancer.org

Website: www.ulstercancer.org

Complementary Care Organizations

Bristol Cancer Help Centre

Aims to meet the needs of cancer patients and their families by offering a holistic approach to help with the physical, emotional, psychological, and spiritual problems experienced by people diagnosed as having cancer.

Grove House

Cornwallis Grove

Clifton

Bristol BS8 4PG

Helpline Tel: 0117 980 9505

Tel: 0117 980 9500

Fax: 0117 923 9184

e-mail: info@bristolcancerhelp.org

Website: www.bristolcancerhelp.org

British Holistic Medical Association

Aims to educate doctors and other health care professionals so that patients are treated as individuals. Publishes a quarterly magazine, *Holistic Health*, for members, also self-help cassettes, and books. Holds annual conferences. Send self-addressed envelope for information.

59 Lansdowne Place

Hove

East Sussex BN3 1FL

Tel: 01273 725951

e-mail: admin@bhma.org

Website: www.bhma.org

Institute for Complementary Medicine

Runs the British Register of Complementary Practitioners and can supply names of reliable practitioners of various kinds of complementary medicine, such as homeopathy, relaxation techniques, and osteopathy. Also has contact with other support groups. Please send self-addressed envelope and two first-class stamps for information, stating area of interest.

PO Box 194

London SE16 7QZ

Tel: 020 7237 5165

Fax: 020 7237 5175

e-mail: info@icmedicine.co.uk

Website: www.icmedicine.co.uk

New Approaches to Cancer

Promotes the holistic attitude to cancer, through a positive attitude to self-help. Local groups throughout the UK.

St Peters Hospital

Guildford Road

Chertsey

Surrey KT16 0PZ

Tel: 01932 879882

e-mail: help@anac.org.uk

Website: www.anac.org.uk

Disease-Specific Support Organizations

Gastrointestinal cancer

British Colostomy Association

An information and advisory service, giving comfort, reassurance, and encouragement to patients. Emotional support on a personal and confidential basis by helpers who have long experience of living with a colostomy. Free leaflets and list of local contacts available. Can arrange visits in hospital or at home on request.

15 Station Road

Reading

Berkshire RG1 1LG

Freephone: 0800 328 4257 or 0118 939 1537

e-mail: sue@bcass.org.uk

Website: www.bcass.org.uk

British Liver Trust

Aims to promote and fund research into liver disease. Supports, informs, and helps people affected by liver disease. Provides information for patients and health professionals in all aspects of liver disease, including primary liver cancer.

Central House

Central Avenue

Ransomes Europark

Ipswich IP3 9QG

Tel: 01473 276327

E-mail: info@britishlivertrust.org.uk

Website: www.britishlivertrust.org.uk

Colon Cancer Concern

Provides an information service with access to specialist nurses, funds research into new treatments for bowel cancer, and also provides education for the public and health professionals. Campaigns for better treatments and screening programmes.

4 Rickett Street

London SW6 1RU

Infoline: 08708 506050

e-mail: queries@coloncancer.org.uk

Website: www.coloncancer.org.uk

Ileostomy and Internal Pouch Support Group

Offers a wide range of advisory services through local groups and national advisers. If you write to the association, please include a large, stamped, self-addressed envelope.

PO Box 132

Scunthorpe

Lincolnshire DN15 9YW

Freephone: 0800 018 4724

e-mail: ia@ileostomypouch.demon.co.uk

Website: www.ileostomypouch.demon.co.uk

Oesophageal Patients Association

Leaflets, telephone advice, and support, before and during treatment. Visits, where possible by former patients, to people with oesophageal cancer.

16 Whitefields Crescent

Solihull

West Midlands B91 3NU

Tel: 0121 704 9860

e-mail: opa@ukgateway.net

Website: www.opa.org.uk

Lung cancer

Roy Castle Lung Cancer Foundation

Provides a free telephone helpline that gives information and details of local support. Hospital-based Lung Cancer Support Nurses in Glasgow, Edinburgh, Newcastle, Liverpool, and Birmingham. Lung cancer information and support groups currently in: Glasgow, Edinburgh, Newcastle, Liverpool, Coventry, Leeds, Birmingham and London. New groups planned. Information booklets available free to lung cancer patients, website providing comprehensive information regarding lung cancer.

200 London Road

Liverpool L3 9TA

Freephone: 0800 358 7200 (office hours)

Website: www.roycastle.org

The Mesothelioma Information Service

An information line for health professionals, patients, carers and others involved in supporting people with mesothelioma. An information booklet is available on receipt of an A5 SAE.

The Mesothelioma Information Service

Yorkshire Centre for Clinical Oncology

Cookridge Hospital

Cookridge

Leeds LS16 6QB

Tel: 0113 206 6466

Breast cancer

Breast Cancer Care

Offers information and support to those affected by breast cancer. A national helpline is run by specialist breast care nurses and trained volunteers. Provides information booklets, factsheets, and a website. Volunteer services provide one-to-one emotional support for women and men with breast cancer and their partners. Volunteer support and outreach networks for women from minority ethnic communities, lesbian and bisexual women, women from socially deprived communities, and younger women. Aftercare service includes prosthesis fitting, telephone support groups for younger women and women with secondary breast cancer, and support services for those living with breast cancer. Regional services provide local information, aftercare services, and local volunteers in Scotland and the North of England.

Kiln House

210 New Kings Road

London SW6 4NZ

Freephone: 0808 800 6000

Tel: 020 7384 2984

Website: www.breastcancercare.org.uk

Urology (bladder, prostate, testicular, renal cancer)

Kidney Cancer UK

Aims to raise public awareness of kidney cancer and the needs of patients and carers. Seeks to empower patients and carers by providing reliable, up-to-date information. Offers support through regular meetings, a regular newsletter, and telephone and internet communication.

11 Hathaway Road

Tile Hill Village

Coventry

West Midlands CV4 9HW

Tel: 024 7647 4993

e-mail: kidneycanceruk@hotmail.com

Website: www.kcuk.org

Prostate Cancer Support Association

A national information and support service for men with prostate cancer.

'Stonycroft'

Beechcroft

Chislehurst

Kent BR7 5DB

Helpline: 0845 601 0766

Website: www.prostatecancersupport.co.uk

Urostomy Association (Central Office)

Assists patients both before and after surgery for the removal of the bladder. Advises on appliances, housing, work situation, or marital problems. 27 regional branches hold meetings on a regular basis. Arranges hospital and home visits on request.

'Buckland'

Beaumont Park

Danbury

Essex CM3 4DE

Tel: 01245 224294

Fax: 01245 227569

e-mail: ua@centraloffice.fsnet.co.uk

Website: www.vagbi.org

WCT Phoneline for Men with Cancer

Provides support and information for men with cancer. Trained ex-patients, and/or their partners, offer an opportunity to talk to someone who has been through a similar experience.

Bellis House

11 Westwood Road

Southampton

Hampshire SO17 1DL

Tel: 023 8077 5611

Fax: 023 8067 2266

e-mail: wct@wessexcancer.org

Website: www.wessexcancer.org

Gynaecology (cervical, uterine, ovarian cancer)

Gynae C

Supports women with gynaecological cancer. Provides a confidential national helpline, information, and advice. A newsletter is available on request. Run by women who have had a gynaecological cancer themselves. A free service – but a self-addressed envelope is welcome for the newsletter.

1 Bollingbroke Road

Swindon

Wiltshire SN2 2LB

Tel: 01793 322005

e-mail: gynae_c@yahoo.com

Website: www.communigate.co.uk/wilts/gynaec

Hysterectomy Support Network

Telephone network of individuals. Sells a range of publications, including a leaflet on hysterectomy. For further information, please send a stamped addressed envelope.

c/o Women's Health

52 Featherstone St

London EC1Y 8RT

Helpline: 0845 125 5254

e-mail: health@womenshealthlondon.org.uk

Website: womenshealthlondon.org.uk

Ovacome

Nationwide support group for all those concerned with ovarian cancer, involving sufferers, families, carers, and health professionals. Aims to share personal experiences, link sufferers, provide information on treatments, screening and research, and raise awareness of the condition.

St Bartholomew's Hospital

West Smithfield

London EC1A 7BE

Tel: 07071 781861

e-mail: ovacome@ovacome.org.uk

Website: www.ovacome.org.uk

RV Club

Telephone contact for help and support (non-medical) for those with vulvectomy operations (operations of the vulva) from one who's been there.

10 Cross Street

Upton

Pontefract

West Yorkshire WF9 1EJ

Tel: 01977 640243

Leukaemia and myeloma

IMF-UK

Provides a range of information booklets on multiple myeloma and AL amyloidosis. Patient and family seminars throughout the UK and Ireland. Quarterly journal style publication *Myeloma Today*.

9 Gayfield Square

Edinburgh EH1 3NT

Freephone: 0800 980 3332

e-mail: theimf@myeloma.org.uk

Website: www.myeloma.org.uk

Leukaemia Care Society

Promotes the welfare of those persons (and their families) who suffer from leukaemia and allied blood disorders. Offers support, friendship, information, leaflets, financial assistance, and caravan holidays.

2 Shrubbery Avenue

Barbourne

Worcester WR1 1QH

Tel: 0800 169 6680

e-mail: enquiries@leukaemiacare.org.uk

Website: www.leukaemiacare.org.uk

Leukaemia Research Fund

Produces a series of free information booklets and leaflets for patients and their families (Hodgkin's disease and other lymphomas, myeloma, myelodysplasia, the myeloproliferative disorders, aplastic anaemia, and the leukaemias). All the information is also available on the website. Accepts general enquiries in writing, by telephone or e-mail.

43 Great Ormond Street

London WC1N 3JJ

Tel: 020 7405 0101

e-mail: info@lrf.org.uk

website: www.lrf.org.uk

Lymphomas

Lymphoma Association

Provides emotional support and information for lymphoma patients and their families (Hodgkin's disease and non-Hodgkin's lymphoma). Literature and videos available, and quarterly newsletters. National network of helpers with experience of the disease, with whom enquirers may be linked usually by telephone. Local groups in many areas.

PO Box 386

Aylesbury

Buckinghamshire HP20 2GA

Helpline: 0808 808 5555

Tel (administration): 01296 619400

e-mail: support@lymphoma.org.uk

Website: www.lymphoma.org.uk

Children's cancer

ACT

Aims to make information available to all parents and professionals about services for families throughout the country, including statutory, voluntary, and self-help groups. Responds to telephone and written enquiries. Also campaigns on behalf of families who care for children with life-threatening or terminal conditions to encourage the development of children's palliative care services, and promotes models of good care.

Orchard House

Orchard Lane

Bristol BS1 5DT

Tel: 0117 922 1556

e-mail: info@act.org.uk

Website: www.act.org.uk

CLIC

Offers help to children with cancer or leukaemia and their families through a well-established 'model of care', including home-care nursing, individual financial assistance, special holidays, and 'home-from-home' family accommodation. Also contributes to paediatric oncology research to improve diagnostic techniques and treatments for childhood cancer. TOPS supports teenages with cancer.

6 Emma-Chris Way

Abbey Wood

Bristol BS34 7JU

Tel: 0117 311 2600

e-mail: clicr@clic-charity.demon.co.uk

Website: www.clic.uk.com

Neuroblastoma Society

Publishes a booklet, which is given to all parents, and newsletters. Provides a befriending service and raises funds to sponsor British research.

18 Harlesden Road

St Albans

Hertfordshire AL1 4LF

Tel: 07727 851818

e-mail: nsoc@ukonline.co.uk

Website: web.ukonline.co.uk/nsoc

The Rainbow Centre for Children

Offers free and professional support and help to children with a life-threatening illness and their families, as well as bereavement support for children and their families when a sibling or parent dies. Provides art and play therapy for children, also counselling, homoeopathy, and some massage for children and their families. Provides home or hospital visits within a 60 mile radius of the Centre, and offers telephone advice and counselling.

27 Lilymead Avenue

Bristol BS4 2BY

Tel: 0117 985 3343

Fax: 0117 985 3353

e-mail: contact@rainbow.fsnet.co.uk

Retinoblastoma Society

Provides written and Braille information for patients and professionals. Links families in the same situation and area, to give moral support and practical help. Creates an opportunity for parents to exchange information and share experiences. Distributes a newsletter 2–3 times per year with contributions from parents and professionals.

St Bartholomew's Hospital

West Smithfield

London EC1A 7BE

Tel: 020 7600 3309 (ansaphone)

Fax: 020 7600 8579

e-mail: rbinfo@rbsociety.org.uk

Website: www.rbsociety.org.uk

Sargent Cancer Care for Children

Supports those under 21 years of age who have cancer, and their families, at home and in hospital from the day of diagnosis. Also provides grants for travelling, extra clothing, heating, and other hardship grants. Provides counselling and advice through a UK-wide network of Sargent social workers, attached to all major cancer treatment centres. Two holiday homes for family respite breaks.

Griffin House

161 Hammersmith Road

London W6 8SG

Tel: 020 8752 2800

Fax: 020 8752 2806

e-mail: care@sargent.org

Website: www.sargent.org

United Kingdom Children's Cancer Study Group

Co-ordinates the management, in all its aspects, of the majority of children with cancer in the UK (excluding leukaemia). Provides an information booklet for parents of children with cancer. Also produces *Contact*, a national magazine for childhood cancer families.

Dept of Epidemiology and Public Health

University of Leicester

22–28 Princess Road West

Leicester LE1 6TP

Tel: 0116 252 3280

Fax: 0116 252 3281

e-mail: ukccsg@le.ac.uk

Website: www.ukccsg.org

Head, neck, and thyroid cancer

Let's Face It

An international mutual-help organization that deals with facial disfigurement. Helping those who are facially disfigured, their loved ones, the professionals who care for them, and the communities in which they live, to understand and solve the problems of living with this disability (from cancer, burns, trauma, and congenital).

72 Victoria Avenue

Westgate-on-Sea

Kent CT8 8BH

Tel: 01843 833724

e-mail: chrisletsfaceit@aol.com

Website: www.letsfaceit.force9.co.uk

National Association of Laryngectomee Clubs (NALC)

Promotes the welfare of laryngectomees within the British Isles. Encourages the formation of clubs to assist rehabilitation through speech therapy, social support, and monthly meetings. Advises on speech aids and medical supplies. Provides a range of literature, audio tapes, and videos.

Ground Floor

6 Rickett Street

Fulham

London SW6 1RU

Tel: 020 7381 9993

Fax: 020 7381 0025

The British Thyroid Foundation

Provides support and clear information. Promotes a greater awareness of thyroid disorders among the general public and the medical
profession. Helps to set up regional support groups. Raises funds for
research.

PO Box 97

Clifford

Wetherby

West Yorkshire LS23 6XD

Tel: 07702 588889

Sarcoma

ROHBTS

Offers a combination of emotional and practical help to families
going through the trauma of having a child or adult suffering from
bone cancer, wherever they are treated. Operates a telephone tree
and runs a holiday home for patients and their families.

The Brick House

Lower Wood Road

Ludlow

Shropshire SY8 2JQ

Tel: 01584 856209

Skin cancer and melanoma

Wessex Cancer Trust MARC's Line

Provides information and support for people with melanoma and
related cancers of the skin, their families, members of the public,
and professionals. Also provides information leaflets on skin cancers
and information on sun protection.

Resource Centre

Dermatology Treatment Centre

Level 3, Salisbury District Hospital

Salisbury

Wiltshire SP2 8BJ

Tel: 01722 415071 (9.00AM to 4PM, Monday to Friday
or ansaphone)

Website: www.wessexcancer.org

Neuro-oncology

United Kingdom Brain Tumour Society

Provides support and information for people affected in any way by
brain tumours and other tumours of the central nervous system.
Raises awareness and encourages research.

BAC House

Bonehurst Road

Horley

Surrey RH6 8QG

Tel: 01293 781479

e-mail: info@ukbts.org

Website: www.ukbts.org

Malignancy associated with human immunodeficiency virus

The Terrance Higgins Trust

Provides information, advice, and help to all those concerned about
AIDS and HIV infection. Practical help includes 'buddies' for people
with AIDS, welfare, housing and legal advice, counselling, and
support groups. Has four regional centres.

52–54 Grays Inn Road

London WC1X 8JU

Tel: 020 7831 0330

Helpline: 020 7242 1010 (Midday to 10PM)

e-mail: info@tht.org.uk

Website: www.tht.org.uk

Palliative Care Services

Hospice Information Service

Publishes a directory of hospice services that gives details of
hospices, home care teams, and hospital support teams in the UK
and the Republic of Ireland. For details of local services, including
hospice services for children, write or telephone. The directory is
available on receipt of a large self-addressed envelope and three
first-class stamps. Information is also available on overseas hospices.

St Christopher's Hospice

51–59 Lawrie Park Road

Sydenham

London SE26 6DZ

Tel: 0870 903 3903

Fax: 020 8776 9345

e-mail: info@hospiceinformation.info

Website: www.hospiceinformation.info

Psychological Support and Bereavement

British Association for Counselling and Psychotherapy

Provides a list of counsellors divided into counties, giving counsellor's qualifications, type of problems counselled, and probable cost;
also provides an information sheet with counselling guidelines.

BACP House

35–37 Albert Street

Rugby CV21 2SG

Tel: 0870 443 5252

e-mail: bacp@bacp.co.uk

Website: www.bacp.co.uk

Compassionate Friends

A nationwide self-help organization of parents whose child of any age, including adult, has died from any cause. Provides personal and group support. Publishes a quarterly newsletter, a postal library, and range of leaflets. This is a befriending, not counselling, system, which works through a system of county contacts and group leaders, located throughout the country.

53 North Street

Bristol BS3 1EN

Tel: 0117 953 9639 (Helpline 9.30AM to 10.30PM every day of the year)

Tel (fax and administration): 0117 966 5202

e-mail: info@tcf.org.uk

Website: www.tcf.org.uk

CRUSE – Bereavement Care

Offers a comprehensive service of counselling by trained and selected people, advice on practical matters, and opportunities for social support, available to all people bereaved by death through one of its 180 branches. Publishes a wide range of supportive information and advisory literature, and a monthly magazine. Arranges training courses for those who work either in a professional or lay capacity with the bereaved. Please send self-addressed envelope for further information.

Cruse House

126 Sheen Road

Richmond

Surrey TW9 1UR

Tel: 020 8939 9530

CRUSE Bereavement Line: 0870 167 1677

CRUSE Youth Line: 020 8940 3131

e-mail: info@crusebereavementcare.org.uk

Website: www.crusebereavementcare.org.uk

Institute of Family Therapy

Offers counselling for families, including those in which a family member has serious illness or disability, or in which there has been bereavement. Fees are on a sliding scale and the client decides what he or she can pay. This can be a minimal donation.

24–32 Stephenson Way

London NW1 2HX

Tel: 020 7391 9150

Fax: 020 7391 9169

e-mail: ift@psyc.bbk.ac.uk

Lesbian and Gay Bereavement Project

Telephone helpline for people bereaved by the death of a same-sex partner. A recording gives the number for a member on duty that evening. Also offers a free will form and notes in return for a self-addressed envelope. As well as giving telephone advice and support, project members can speak on same-sex loss to nurses, social workers, and others concerned with death and dying.

Healthy Gay Living Centre

40 Borough High Street

London SE1 1XW

Helpline: 020 7403 5969

Social Support

British Red Cross Society

Helps vulnerable people through services in local communities, in particular medical loan (e.g., wheelchairs), transport and escort (help home from hospital), and health and social care (provision of short-term carers, befrienders). Please contact your local branch for details.

9 Grosvenor Crescent

London SW1 7EJ

Tel: 020 7235 5454

e-mail: information@redcross.org.uk

Website: www.redcross.org.uk

Carers UK

Provides information and support to people who are caring at home. Publishes a range of free leaflets. Branches and local offices throughout the country – for details of a local contacts, contact the National office.

Ruth Pitter House

20–25 Glasshouse Yard

London EC1A 4JT

CarersLine: 0808 808 7777 (freephone)

Other enquiries: 020 7490 8818

e-mail: info@ukcarers.org

Website: www.carersonline.org.uk

Counsel and Care

Offers an advice service for older people, their relatives, and professionals; information leaflets, grants to help people remain in or return to their homes.

Twyman House

16 Bonny Street

London NW1 9PG

Tel: 0845 300 7585 (calls at local rate) (Monday to Friday 10.30AM to 4.00PM)

e-mail: advice@counselandcare.org

Website: www.counselandcare.org

Crossroads Caring for Carers

Provides care workers who come into the home to give the carer a break. There are over 200 autonomous schemes throughout England and Wales with eight divisional offices.

10 Regent Place
Rugby
Warwickshire CV21 2PN
Tel: 01788 573653
Helpline: 0500 179546
Website: www.crossroads.org.uk

DIAL UK (Disablement Information and Advice Lines)

The national association for the DIAL network of over 100 disability information and advice services which are run and staffed by people with direct experience of disability.

Park Lodge
St Catherine's Hospital
Tickhill Road
Balby
Doncaster DN4 8QN
Tel: 01302 310123
e-mail: dialuk@aol.com
Website: www.dialuk.org.uk

SPOD

Provides information and advice on problems in sex and personal relationships that disability can cause. General leaflets and reading lists are available, and individual advice given on request. A publications list is available.

286 Camden Road
London N7 0BJ
Tel: 020 7607 8851

Further information

The most comprehensive source of information and support organizations throughout the UK is The Cancer BACUP Directory of Cancer services 2003. Published by Class Health, price £21.99.
Class Health

Barb House
Barb Mews
London W6 7PA
Te;: 020 7371 2119
Fax: 020 7371 2878
e-mail: post@class.co.uk
Website: www.class.co.uk

This list is not exhaustive, but is a useful starting point for anyone interested in more information.

Journals

Health Statistics Quarterly. Office of National Statistics UK.

Clinical Evidence. A six monthly journal by the BMJ publishing group together with the American College of Physicians and American Society of Internal Medicine

Websites

CancerBACUP: http://www.cancerbacup.org.uk/.

Cancer Research UK: http://www.cancerresearchuk.org

National Cancer Institute of the United States of America: http://www.nci.nih.gov/.

START Europe against cancer: http://www.cancereurope.org/.

The European Code Against Cancer: http://www.telescan.nki.nl/code/

Books and Reports

Mihill C. *Shaping Tomorrow: Issues Facing General Practice in the New Mill*ennium. London: BMA Publications.

NHS Centre for Reviews and Dissemination. *Effective Health Care Bulletins*. York: NHS Centre for Reviews and Dissemination University of York Effective Health Care. http://www.york.ac.uk/inst/crd/ehc.

Further reading

BACUP. *The Right to Know*. 1996.

BRMB International Ltd. *Developing Information for Cancer Patients*. A report prepared for Macmillan Cancer Relief, 1999.

Calman, Hine. *A Policy Framework For Commissioning Cancer Services – report by the expert advisory group on cancer to the chief medical officers of England and Wales*. 1995. London: Department of Health, November 1996.

National Cancer Alliance. *Patient Centred Cancer Services? What Patients Say?* 1996.

NHSE. *Patient Partnership: Building a Collaborative Strategy*. 1996.

NHSE. *Information for Health: An Information Strategy for the Modern NHS 1998–2005*. 1998.

Van Der Molen B. Relating information needs to the cancer experience. 1. Information as a key coping strategy. *Eur J Cancer Care*. 1999; **8**: 238–44.

Van Der Molen B. Relating information needs to the cancer experience. 2. Jenny's story: a cancer narrative. *Eur J Cancer Care*. 2000a; **9**: 41–7.

Van Der Molen B. Relating information needs to the cancer experience. 3. Themes from six narratives. *Eur J Cancer Care*. 2000b; **9**: 48–54.

31 Glossary

Andy Webb

Clinical

Adjuvant

Adjuvant therapy (mainly hormonal or chemotherapy) is given after a complete surgical resection to improve long-term survival. For example, the use of tamoxifen in women who have had their breast cancer removed.

Brachyradiotherapy

Delivery of radiotherapy using a localizing technique, such as bronchial brachyradiotherapy delivered using a bronchoscope.

CHART (continuous hyperfractionated accelerated radiotherapy)

Radiotherapy delivered several times daily without break.

High-dose chemotherapy

Chemotherapy used at five or more times the conventional dose to overcome potential chemoresistance in residual disease. It is sometimes combined with total body irradiation. This therapy is myleoablative and requires support with peripheral stem cells or bone marrow cells from the patient (autograft) or from a matched relative (allograft).

Neoadjuvant

Therapy (mainly hormonal or chemotherapy) given before removal of operable cancer. For example, chemotherapy given before removal of an operable breast lump to reduce the need for mastectomy.

Paraneoplastic syndrome

Signs or symptoms that may occur in a patient with cancer that are not directly caused by the local effects of the tumour cells. For example, the syndrome of inappropriate anti-diuretic hormone (SIADH), which is commonly seen in patients with small cell lung cancer.

Performance status

A quick and easy-to-use assessment of the patient's functional ability. Two scales are regularly used; the Karnovsky scale, which ranges from 0 to 100%, and the Eastern Cooperative Oncology Group (ECOG) scale, which ranges from 0 to 4.

Positron emission tomography (PET)

An imaging technique that picks up a metabolic image and may be more sensitive than conventional anatomical imaging. The most commonly used isotope is fluoro-2-doxyglucose (FDG) and the PET scan shows areas of high glucose uptake, such as in neoplastic tissue.

Response criteria

Complete response (CR): the disappearance of all known disease determined by two evaluations not less than 4 weeks apart.
Partial response (PR): 50% or more decrease in the sum of the products of the largest and perpendicular diameters of lesions, measured to determine the effect of therapy by two evaluations not less than 4 weeks apart.
Progressive disease (PD): 25% or more increase in the size of one or more measurable lesions or the appearance of new lesions.
Stable disease (SD): no change in lesion size that fulfils criteria for partial response or progressive disease.

Stereotactic radiotherapy

Precise delivery of high-dose radiotherapy to a localized lesion using stereotactic equipment. For example, radiotherapy to solitary brain metastasis.

Tumour marker

A protein that can be measured in serum or urine and that tends to increase and decrease with tumour activity. For example, CA125 in ovarian cancer.

Toxicity grading

Therapy induced toxicities are graded 1–4 according to specific criteria. Grades 3 and 4 toxicities are severe and potentially life threatening, and normally require modification of future therapy (e.g., dose reduction).

Drug Mechanisms

Alkylating agents

This class of chemotherapeutic agents has a mechanism of action that results in a covalent bond between the two strands of the DNA (called cross-linking). More common agents in this class include cyclophosphamide, ifosfamide, chlorambucil, melphalan, lomustine, and carmustine.

Antimetabolites

Several vital biochemical pathways involved in the formation of nucleic acids are used in the formation of both DNA and RNA; the antimetabolites interfere with these pathways, often by acting as an inhibitor of a rate-limiting enzyme. Common examples include methotrexate and raltitrexed (folic acid analogues), 5-fluorouracil, cytarabine and gemcitabine (pyrimidine analogues), and mercaptopurine (purine analogue).

DNA topoisomerase inhibitors

Topoisomerases are a group of enzymes involved in the coiling and uncoiling of the large DNA molecules; this coiling allows the DNA molecules to both fit in the nucleus and yet be efficiently accessed when a region is required.

Topoisomerase I inhibitors include irinotecan and topotecan (camptothecan analogues).

Topoisomerase II inhibitors include anthracyclines such as doxorubicin and epirubicin, and epipodophyllotoxins such as etoposide.

Antimicrotubules

These act by binding to tubulin, an essential protein in the formation of microtubules, which in turn form the mitotic spindle that is essential to the division of a cell. Agents include the vinca alkaloids such as vincristine and vinblastine, and the taxanes such as paclitaxel and docetaxel.

Biological response modifiers

A diverse group of agents, often naturally occurring in humans, that utilize a variety of mechanisms of action to upregulate immunological pathways rather than the traditional methods of cytotoxic agents that cause tumour cell death. Agents in this group include interferons, interleukins, and cis-retinoic acid.

Novel agents

Included in this group are the anti-angiogenesis agents, the mode of action of which is to inhibit the neovascularization that a tumour requires to grow, and the 'small molecules' involved in disrupting intracellular messenger pathways.

Platinum agents

Platinum-containing complexes have a mechanism of action similar to that of the alkylating agents that react with DNA to form intrastrand and interstrand crosslinks, thereby interfering with repair and DNA replication. The most common agents in this class are cisplatin, carboplatin, and oxaliplatin.

Genetics

Allele
Alternative forms (sequences) of a gene.

Gene
The basic unit of heredity. It is the DNA sequence, which contains the information to make a specific protein.

Genotype
The allelic constitution of an individual.

Germline
The genetic information in every cell (including the gametes), which is inherited from the parents.

Mutation
An alteration in the DNA sequence of a gene.

Penetrance
The chance that a disease will occur as a result of the presence of a predisposing mutation.

Phenocopy
An individual who has the disease, but does not have the disease-predisposing mutation.

Phenotype
The physical or biochemical effect of the genotype.

Sporadic
A cancer case occurring in a person who is not a mutation carrier.

Histology

Borderline malignancy
A tumour in which there are some but not all the characteristics of malignancy, and there is no stromal invasion.

Carcinoma in situ
Also known as intraepithelial neoplasia, precancerous condition, or dysplasia. It is best defined as the state in which one or several cells and their progeny have acquired the potential to invade and metastasize, but have not yet exercised the option.

Grade
The histolopathological appearance of tumour in terms of its degree of differentiation; low-grade tumours are well differentiated, high-grade tumours tend to be anaplastic.

TNM

Pathological staging of tumours using tumour, node, and metastasis status.

Molecular Biology

Angiogenesis

The development of new blood vessels within tumours that supply their accelerated growth. Therapies that target new vessel formation are under development.

Antibody therapy

Antibodies that bind to specific tumour epitopes and lead to immunological cell killing. The antibodies can also be linked to various toxins.

Antisense therapy

The use of single chains of DNA with a sequence complementary to a target region of messenger RNA (sense strand), thus blocking protein production.

Apoptosis

A particular mode of cell death in which the cell shrinks and breaks up into small particles that can be detected by light microscopy. These particles are called apoptotic bodies. This form of cell death is triggered by a number of stimuli, including chemotherapy and radiotherapy.

Gene therapy

The deletion or insertion of DNA as an anti-cancer therapy. A vector is required for effective delivery.

Microarray analysis

This technique enables simultaneous screening of tumour tissue to express thousands of genes in a semi-quantitative fashion.

Northern blot analysis

A technique to determine the presence of specific mRNA sequences in cells.

Polymerase chain reaction (PCR)

Method by which a given segment of DNA is amplified many times by the continuos synthesis of complementary strands.

Southern blot analysis

A technique to detect specific DNA sequences in cells.

Western blot analysis

A procedure analogous to southern and northern blot analyses that allows the detection of specific proteins.

Pharmacology

Dose-limiting toxicity (DLT)

The toxicity seen at a particular dose level that precludes further dose escalation. Most commonly the parameters used are grade 4 (i.e. severe or life threatening) haematological toxicity and grade 3 or 4 non-haematological toxicities.

Maximum tolerated dose (MTD)

The dose at which a fixed proportion of patients (e.g., one-third) are expected to experience dose-limiting toxicity (DLT). A common trial design used to estimate the MTD is to treat three to six patients at a given dose level, with recruitment of new patients for increasing levels. The MTD is the highest dose at which one or none of the six patients experiences a DLT, but is immediately below the level at which usually two or (sometimes three) patients experience a DLT.

Pharmacokinetics

The study of the mechanisms involved in the absorption, distribution, biotransformation, and elimination of a pharmaceutical agent. This includes the kinetics (i.e., the rates at which a drug is absorbed and eliminated and the concentrations achieved at the sites of distribution) and the physiological and biochemical pathways by which these processes occur.

Pharmacodynamics

The study of the biochemical and physiological effects of a drug and its mechanisms of action to show the relationship between the concentration of the drug at its site(s) of action and the magnitude and type of effects (therapeutic and toxic) produced.

Phase I trials

Phase I trials are performed to determine the maximum tolerated dose (MTD), and in some cases the schedule of a pharmaceutical agent or drug combination. This type of study uses both pharmacokinetic and pharmacodynamic parameters to escalate the dose. In the assessment of agents under trial for potential future use in cancer, patients with advanced malignancies of various types that are resistant to standard treatment are included. Assessment of the efficacy of the study drug is therefore a secondary aim in this type of trial design.

Phase II trials

The role of a phase II trial is to assess response of an agent in individual tumour types. The dosage and schedule of the drug being investigated are derived from the results of phase I trials. In this study design the patient group is that with a tumour that is most likely to respond and who have progressed on standard treatment. There is no internal control group in this trial type and so the response rate is the primary endpoint. Comparative survival and symptomatic benefit cannot be determined.

Phase III trials

Phase III trials are clinical trials using relatively large populations to assess the relative efficacy of a treatment in a given condition. The treatment being assessed may be a single agent, a combination of drugs, or a particular regimen. The agent in question is compared with another standard treatment by assigning (optimally randomizing) the patients to either of the treatments. The endpoints measured may include survival time, time to progression, response rate, and symptomatic response. It may also assess the role of interpatient variables (e.g. age, sex, etc.) on these endpoints and on drug concentrations and toxicities by performing pharmacokinetics on a limited number of patients (called population pharmacokinetics).

Phase IV studies

Essentially this is post-market surveillance, with ongoing assessment of the drug, in particular with respect to toxicity and previously unknown drug interactions. The pharmaceutical company that retails the particular agent most often performs this research.

Toxicology

Toxicology is the study of the adverse effects of chemicals on living organisms. This can involve the biochemical and physiological pathways that are affected and the clinical implications to the patient.

Statistics

Accuracy

The accuracy of a test is the proportion of individuals whose status is correctly identified by the test. (This terms relates to the study of a test's performance in individuals of known status for the disease or condition under examination.)

Hazard ratio

The hazard ratio is the relative event rate. Thus, if one group has a death rate of 2% per month and another has a death rate of

1% per month, then the hazard ratio of the first to the second would be 2.

Hypothesis testing

Clinical trials are designed to differentiate between different possible hypothetical situations. Two such situations might be that there is no difference between two treatments or that the size of the difference is clinically worthwhile, hypotheses known as the null and alternative hypotheses, respectively. The aim of a trial is to reject one hypothesis in favour of the other; thus if the conclusion is that there is a difference between treatments, the null hypothesis is rejected and the alternative hypothesis accepted.

It is important to minimize the probability of reaching the wrong conclusion when hypothesis testing (see p-value, below); such errors can be minimized by undertaking studies of adequate size.

Kaplan–Meier curves

These curves show the proportion of patients who are event-free throughout follow-up after an initial starting point such as disease diagnosis or treatment. Thus the curve always starts at 100% and typically denotes time to an event such as death and hence can never increase. Patients who do not die contribute to the calculation of these curves and are considered to be at risk up to the time when they were last known to be alive.

Median survival (or time to another event)

The time by which it is estimated that 50% of the individuals will have died or experienced the event under study.

Multivariate analysis

Multivariate analysis is an analysis in which several factors are simultaneously related to outcome, for which an underlying model that defines how the factors interact is required.

Overall survival

Overall survival curves are Kaplan–Meier curves that show how the estimated proportion of patients still alive changes over the period of follow-up.

Parametric and non-parametric

Parametric statistical methods assume that the distribution of data values can be completely described by a few parameters. If the data follow a normal distribution, for example, the average and standard deviation (two parameters) totally specify the range of values and the probability of different values that the data can take. Parametric statistical methods are attractive because of their mathematical tractability.

Non-parametric data cannot be summarized by any simplifying parameters. Statistical methods are typically based on the relative ranks of the data values rather than on the values themselves. Such methods are limited because no assumptions about the distributions that underlie the data can be made.

Positive predictive value and negative predictive value

The positive predictive value is the proportion of cases that are identified as positive by a test and that are actually positive; similarly, the negative predictive value is the proportion of cases that are identified as negative by a test and that are actually negative. (These terms relate to the study of a test's performance in individuals of known status for the disease or condition under examination.)

Power

The power is the probability that the alternative hypothesis is accepted when it is true, and is conventionally set at 90% or more. A power of 90% implies that there is a 10% chance that the alternative hypothesis be rejected when it is true, a probability also known as the type II error.

Progression-free survival

These Kaplan–Meier curves show the proportion of patients who are progression free throughout follow-up. Death may sometimes also be counted as an event.

***p*-value**

The *p*-value is the probability that the null hypothesis (see above)

is wrongly rejected; it is conventionally kept below 5%. The p-value is also known as the type I error.

Relative risk

The relative risk is the relative size of two risk rates. For example, if the mortality rate of insulation workers exposed to asbestos is 58 (per 100,000 person–years) and that of workers who are not exposed is 11, the relative risk of death is 5.3.

Sensitivity

The sensitivity of a test is the proportion of individuals who possess the disease or condition under study who are successfully identified as having the disease or condition by the test. (This terms relates to the study of a test's performance in individuals of known status for the disease or condition under examination.)

Specificity

The specificity of a test is the proportion of individuals who do not have the disease or condition who are correctly identified as not having it. (This terms relates to the study of a test's performance in individuals of known status for the disease or condition under examination.)

Univariate

Univariate analysis is the name given to statistical analyses in which single factors are related to outcome.

Index

T - #0969 - 101024 - C336 - 254/178/18 [20] - CB - 9781901865264 - Gloss Lamination